I0072624

Hepatocellular Carcinoma: Clinical Findings

Hepatocellular Carcinoma: Clinical Findings

Edited by **Jay Amsel**

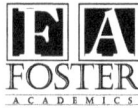

FA
FOSTER
ACADEMICS

New Jersey

Published by Foster Academics,
61 Van Reypen Street,
Jersey City, NJ 07306, USA
www.fosteracademics.com

Hepatocellular Carcinoma: Clinical Findings
Edited by Jay Amsel

© 2015 Foster Academics

International Standard Book Number: 978-1-63242-228-6 (Hardback)

This book contains information obtained from authentic and highly regarded sources. Copyright for all individual chapters remain with the respective authors as indicated. A wide variety of references are listed. Permission and sources are indicated; for detailed attributions, please refer to the permissions page. Reasonable efforts have been made to publish reliable data and information, but the authors, editors and publisher cannot assume any responsibility for the validity of all materials or the consequences of their use.

The publisher's policy is to use permanent paper from mills that operate a sustainable forestry policy. Furthermore, the publisher ensures that the text paper and cover boards used have met acceptable environmental accreditation standards.

Trademark Notice: Registered trademark of products or corporate names are used only for explanation and identification without intent to infringe.

Printed in the United States of America.

Contents

Preface

This book aims to highlight the current researches and provides a platform to further the scope of innovations in this area. This book is a product of the combined efforts of many researchers and scientists, after going through thorough studies and analysis from different parts of the world. The objective of this book is to provide the readers with the latest information of the field.

Hepatocellular carcinoma is the most common type of liver cancer and is also known as malignant hepatoma. This book discusses the clinical features of hepatocellular carcinoma. It is a collective effort of experts from around the globe and showcases the most updated information on the clinical characteristics of hepatocellular carcinoma. This book presents major aspects including Differential Diagnosis, Surgical Treatment, and Non-surgical Treatment. It is a well-researched compilation and discusses various important topics like new diagnostic techniques, molecular targeted therapy, transarterial radioembolization, hepatic lesions imitating hepatocellular carcinoma, laparoscopic liver resection and hepatectomy without allogeneic blood transfusion among others. It will play a vital role in providing a reference for the clinical management of patients with hepatocellular carcinoma. This book will cater to professionals involved in treatment and management of hepatocellular carcinoma, as well as hepatologists, liver surgeons, interventional and diagnostic radiologists and pathologists. Medical trainees, hospital managers and also drug producers will find this book helpful as a reference source.

I would like to express my sincere thanks to the authors for their dedicated efforts in the completion of this book. I acknowledge the efforts of the publisher for providing constant support. Lastly, I would like to thank my family for their support in all academic endeavors.

Editor

Part 1

Diagnosis / Differential Diagnosis

Hepatocellular Carcinoma: Epidemiology and Etiology

Davide Degli Esposti[1,2], Morando Soffritti[3,*], Antoinette Lemoine[1,2],
Eva Tibaldi[3] and Marco Manservigi[3]

*[1]AP-HP, Hôpital Paul Brousse, Service de Biochimie et Biologie
Moléculaire, Inserm; Université Paris-Sud 11;
PRES Universud-Paris; Paul Vaillant Couturier
[2]Laboratoire de Biochimie et Biologie Cellulaire, Faculté de Pharmacie,
Université Paris-Sud 11, Jean Baptiste Clément
[3]Cesare Maltoni Cancer Research Center, Ramazzini Institute,
Castello di Bentivoglio, Via Saliceto, Bentivoglio, Bologna,
[1,2]France
[3]Italy*

1. Introduction

Hepatocellular carcinoma (HCC) is a major public health problem, accounting for about 600,000 deaths in the world in 2004 (WHO, 2008). HCC is the sixth most common cancer worldwide with about 500,000 new cases annually, representing the third largest cause of cancer-related death (Parkin, 2005; Ferlay et al., 2010). A slight decrease in the HCC incidence has been reported in high-rate areas, such as China and Japan (McGlynn et al., 2001). However, a steadily increasing trend has been reported in historically low-rate countries, particularly the United States and some European countries, such as Italy, France, UK and Germany (IARC, 2008a; El-Seragh et al., 2007). In particular, HCC incidence rates doubled in the United States in the period 1985-2002, an earlier age of onset has been observed (with a shift towards 45-60 years old), and HCC has become the fastest growing cause of cancer-related death in men (El-Seragh et al., 2004). Interestingly, it has been reported that in the United States 15-50% of HCC patients had no established risk factors, such as viral hepatitis infections, heavy alcohol consumption or aflatoxin B1 exposure (El-Seragh et al., 2007). Moreover, approximately 10% of all HCC cases in the USA occur in patients with non-cirrhotic livers (Shaw & Shah, 2011). In Europe an analysis of mortality rates from HCC trends in the last 20 years has shown increasing rates for men in 11 countries and for women in 6 countries out of 17 whose data were considered (Bosetti et al., 2008).

The observed increase in the incidence rates of HCC has been concomitant with the obesity epidemic observed in the last 30 years in western countries. Obesity is one of the clinical

---

* Corresponding Author

manifestations of metabolic syndrome and, in the last decade, epidemiological and experimental studies have shown that metabolic syndrome and high fat diets are associated with an increased risk of HCC incidence/mortality (Bugianesi 2007; Starley et al., 2010; Welzel et al., 2011). However, other causes may be involved in the increased incidence of HCC and chemical-induced liver carcinogenesis appears to be a less considered etiology. In this chapter, we will review recent acquisitions in epidemiology and experimental studies on HCC and will focus on chemical risk factors and possible new mechanisms of liver carcinogenesis, in particular those concerning metabolic disruption.

2. Chemical risk agents of hepatocellular carcinoma

Most human HCC occurs following viral hepatitis (mainly HBV or HCV) infections or aflatoxin B1 exposure caused by ingestion of contaminated food (IARC 2008a). However, the epidemiological evidence shows that the human liver is susceptible to chemical-induced carcinogenesis (Blonski et al., 2010; Degli Esposti et al., 2009) and the increased incidence of HCC in patients not having established risk factors (El-Seragh et al., 2007) suggests that some underestimated or new but still not recognized risk factors exist (Blonski et al., 2010). In particular, many natural and artificial agents have been shown by experimental or epidemiological studies to induce HCC (Table 1). In this section we will review the chemical risk factors of HCC as emerging from the epidemiological and experimental data.

2.1 Human hepatocarcinogens

Various classes of chemicals are reported to induce HCC in humans: drugs or hormonal therapies (azathioprine, tamoxifen and estrogen-progesteron oral contraceptives) (IARC, 2011); radioisotopes or heavy metals (Plutonium-239, Radium-224, Thorium-232; arsenic in drinking water) (IARC, 2001; IARC, 2004b); complex mixtures of polyaromatic hydrocarbons (PAH) and combustion products (soots and tobacco smoking)(IARC, 1987; IARC, 2004a); organochlorines such as vinyl chloride monomer (VCM) or 2,3,7,8 tetrachloride-dibenzo-para-dioxin (TCDD) (IARC, 2008b, IARC, 1997); and plant derivatives (betel or *Areca catechu*) (IARC, 2004c). Recently, some psychoactive substances, like cannabinoids, have been reported to worsen liver steatosis and fibrosis, in particular in the presence of HCV infections (Hézode et al., 2008, Parfieniuk & Flisiak, 2008). However, no evidence of carcinogenicity has been shown for delta 9-tetrahydrocannabinol (the principal psychoactive ingredient in marihuana) in rats and mice (Chan et al., 1996). More research is warranted to assess the long-term carcinogenic or co-carcinogenic effects of cannabinoids, particularly in the liver, as assumption of them during cannabis smoking may result in cannabinoid exposure for a large population. Finally, recent reviews have focused on a possible underestimation of non-viral causes of HCC (Blonski et al., 2010; Degli Esposti et al., 2009). In particular, metabolic disorders (Non-Alcoholic Fatty Liver Disease (NAFLD), obesity and diabetes), hormonal drugs (oral contraception, tamoxifen), organochlorine compounds, polycyclic aromatic hydrocarbons, tobacco smoking, betel quid chewing and dietary exposures (in particular arsenic in drinking water and aflatoxin B1, a well known hepatocarcinogen) are indicated as important contributing factors for HCC (Blonski et al., 2010; Degli Esposti et al., 2009).

Agents		Human exposure	Evidence of carcinogenicity		References
Category	Type		Humans	Experimental animals	
Natural	1. Aflatoxins	food contaminant (rice, peanuts, etc.)	+	+	Wogan and Newbern 1967; Wogan et al. 1974; Yeh et al. 1985; Olsen et al. 1988; IARC 1993; Soffritti et al. 1988
	2. Alcohol	lifestyle dependent	+		Hakulinen et al. 1974; Adelstein and White 1976; Hirayama 1981; IARC 1988
	3. Hepatitis B virus	blood transfusion	+	+	Snyder et al. 1982; Buendia 1992
	4. Sterigmatocystin	food contaminant (grain, legumes)		+	Purchase and van der Watt 1970
	5. Luteoschirina	food contaminant rice		+	Uraguchi et al. 1972
	6. Cycloclorotina	food contaminant rice		+	IARC 1976
	7. Pyrazolidinic Alkaloids	plants contaminant		+	Swoboda and Reddy 1972
	8. Cycasin	alimentary exposure		+	Laquer et al. 1963
	9. Safrole	flavouring substance		+	Long et al. 1963; Hagan et al. 1965

+ = strong evidence; (+) = limited evidence

Table 1. Agents inducing Hepatocellular Carcinoma based on experimental/epidemiological evidence (Part I)

Agents		Human exposure	Evidence of carcinogenicity		References
Category	Type		Humans	Experimental animals	
Artificial	1. Thorotrast	iatrogenic	(+)	+	Guimares et al. 1955; Commission of European Communities (CEC) 1984
	2. Radioactive colloidal gold	iatrogenic		+	Upton et al. 1956
	3. Gamma radiation	occupational or accidental		+	Upton et al. 1968
	4. Vinyl Chloride	occupational	(+)	+	Gokel et al. 1976; Koischwitz et al. 1981; Evans et al. 1983; Maltoni et al. 1984; Dietz et al. 1985, Pirastu et al. 1990
	5. Benzidine	occupational		+	IARC 1982
	6. 2-Acetylamino-fluorene	occupational		+	Wilson et al. 1941; Teebor and Becker 1971
	7. 4-Diethylamino-azobenzene	occupational		+	Kinosita 1936 Terayama 1967
	8. Dimethyl-nitrosamina	occupational		+	Magee and Barnes 1956
	9. Diethylnitrosamina	occupational		+	Schmal et al. 1960
	10. Steroidal oral contraceptives	iatrogenic	(+)	(+)	Klatskin 1977; Jick and Hermann 1978; IARC 1979
	11. Androgen steroids	iatrogenic	(+)		Johnson et al. 1972

+ = strong evidence; (+) = limited evidence

Table 1. Agents inducing Hepatocellular Carcinoma based on experimental/epidemiological evidence (Part II)

The diversity of chemical agents that induce liver tumors in humans may be at least partially explained by the multiplicity of molecular pathways that have been found altered both in human and animal hepatic tumors (Degli Esposti et al., 2009; Saffroy et al., 2007).

Hormonal-induced liver tumors, such those observed after estrogen-progesteron oral contraceptives and tamoxifen administration, have been in part explained by promotion of the epithelium proliferation and the generation of reactive oxygen species (ROS) caused by estrogen reactive metabolites (Russo & Russo, 2006) and ER-dependent liver responses, such as hepatocyte mitogenesis (Vickers et al., 1991). Liver carcinogenicity of alpha-particle emitters, in particular Plutonium-239, Radium-224, Thorium-232, and heavy metals such as arsenic may be explained by their ability to induce direct or indirect genotoxic damage (Lehnert et al., 1997; IARC, 2004b). The carcinogenicity of VCM has been linked to the capacity of its two active metabolites (chloroethylene oxide and chloroacetaldehyde) to react with nucleic acid bases to form adducts (IARC, 2008b) and to induce p53 mutations both in humans and in rats (Barbin et al., 1997). It is worth noting that 10-40% of HCC are characterized by global genomic instability as shown by microsatellite analyses and that the exact mechanisms behind this instability still need to be assessed (Salvucci et al., 1999, Chiappini et al., 2004).

Gene polymorphisms and gene-environment interactions may also be risk factors for HCC, particularly concerning gene coding for metabolizing enzymes (glutathione-S-transferase, epoxide hydrolase, cytochrome p4502E1) or DNA repairing enzymes (XRCC1, UDP-glucuronosyltransferase1A7)(Wong et al., 2000, Borentain, 2007). However, until now, these studies have reported contrasting results. Meta-analysis and additional studies with larger samples should be performed in order clarify the role of genetic polymorphisms in the onset of HCC (El-Seragh, 2007; White et al., 2008).

Overall, these data clearly indicate that the human liver is sensitive to chemical-induced carcinogenesis and that xenobiotic exposure could play an underestimated role in inducing hepatocellular carcinomas, alone or associated with already known etiologies.

2.2 Long-term carcinogenicity bioassays as a tool to identify potential hepatocarcinogens

Long-term carcinogenicity bioassays, mainly using rats and mice, have become a consolidated tool for identifying potentially carcinogenic chemical or physical agents (Huff, 2002; Maronpot et al., 2004; Soffritti et al., 2002). The two most extensive bioassay programs in the world are those of the American National Toxicology Program (NTP) and of the Italian Ramazzini Institute (Bucher, 2002; Huff, 2002; Soffritti et al., 2002). Although differences in the etiology exist between rodent and human HCC, there are also significant similarities in the genetic alterations leading to liver cancer in mice, rats and humans (Hoenerhoff et al., 2011; Feo et al., 2009). A recent study performed a global gene profiling of spontaneous (naturally occurring) HCC in B6C3F1 mice used in the NTP two-year bioassay (Hoenerhoff et al., 2011). The authors identified the dysregulation of genes similarly altered in human HCC, namely re-expression of fetal oncogenes, upregulation of protooncogenes, downregulation of tumor suppressor genes, and abnormal expression of cell cycle mediators, growth factors, apoptosis regulators, angiogenesis and extracellular matrix remodeling factors (Hoenerhoff et al., 2011). The use of a pathway-centered approach has lead to the identification of important targets that may be relevant to human HCC and, despite differences in etiology and pathogenesis from human HCC, the molecular readout has proved very similar, thus providing further support for applying this animal model to the study of HCC (Hoenerhoff et al., 2011). Importantly, the results from the two-year carcinogenicity bioassays conducted by the NTP show that 188 out of 577 tested agents induced liver tumors in Fischer 344 rats or B6C3F1 mice (Table 2). Interestingly, 76% of these agents (145 out of 188) induced cancer in other sites than the liver (NTP, 2011). In particular, concerning the use of B6C3F1 mice, it has been suggested that this model might be a very sensitive system to detect chemicals that are likely to cause molecular events leading to cancer (Hoenerhoff et al., 2011). Results from the long term carcinogenicity bioassay program performed by the *Cesare Maltoni* Cancer Research Center of the Ramazzini Institute reveal that, among the studies already concluded and published, 52 agents showed clear evidence of carcinogenicity and 5 of them induced liver tumors in Sprague-Dawley rats or Swiss mice (Table 3). Interestingly, all these agents also induced cancer in other sites than the liver. These results confirm the finding that different strains of rats and mice present a different susceptibility to the development of HCC (Feo et al., 2009; Maronpot 2009). It should be noted that recent studies on genetic susceptibility and epigenetic regulation of the signaling pathways involved in hepatocarcinogenesis in rats have shown that most alterations responsible for a resistant or susceptible phenotype in rats also have a similar contribution to the prognosis of human HCC (Feo et al., 2009). In conclusion, the results of both long-term carcinogenicity studies and of genetic investigation of HCC from rodent models may provide important insights into the mechanisms of hepatocarcinogenesis, helping to identify some critical initiating events that lead to carcinogenesis, as well as progression markers and therapeutic targets (Feo et al., 2009; Hoenerhoff et al., 2011).

	Agents	Route of exposure	Evidence of carcinogenicity[b]				Carcino- genicity in other site	Human exposure
N.	Type		Rats		Mice			
			M	F	M	F		
1	Acetonitrile	Inhalation	E	NE	NE	NE	No	chemical industry
2	Aldrin	Dosed-feed	E	E	CE	NE	Yes	pesticide
3	2-Aminoanthra- quinone	Dosed-feed	CE	IS	CE	CE	Yes	dye industry
4	1-Amino- 2,4-dibromoanthra- quinone	Dosed-feed	CE	CE	CE	CE	Yes	dye industry
5	3-Amino- 9-ethylcarbazole HCl	Dosed-feed	CE	CE	CE	CE	Yes	dye industry
6	11-Aminoundecanoic acid	Dosed-feed	CE	NE	E	NE	Yes	car industry; food packaging
7	Androstenedione	Gavage	E	E	CE	CE	Yes	hormonal treatment
8	Anthraquinone	Dosed-feed	SE	CE	CE	CE	Yes	dye industry
9	Aroclor 1254	Dosed-feed	E	E			Yes	insulator for current transformers
10	Benzofuran	Gavage	NE	SE	CE	CE	Yes	painting industry; food packaging

N.	Type (Agents)	Route of exposure	Evidence of carcinogenicity[b]				Carcinogenicity in other site	Human exposure
			Rats		Mice			
11	Benzophenone	Dosed-feed	SE	E	SE	SE	Yes	printing industry
12	Benzyl acetate	Gavage	E	NE	SE	SE	Yes	cosmetic industry
13	2-Chloro-1-methylethyl ether	Gavage			CE	CE	Yes	dye industry; pharmaceutics
14	Bromodichloromethane	Gavage	CE	CE	CE	CE	Yes	water contaminant
15	1,3 Butadiene	Inhalation			CE	CE	Yes	chemical industry: plastic and rubber
16	2-Butoxyethanol	Inhalation	NE	E	SE	SE	Yes	painting industry
17	Chloral hydrate	Gavage			SE		No	drugs treatment
18	Chloramben	Dosed-feed	NE	NE	E	CE	No	herbicide
19	Chlordane	Dosed-feed	NE	NE	CE	CE	No	pesticide
20	Chlordecone	Dosed-feed	CE	CE	CE	CE	No	insecticide, fungicide
21	Chlorendic acid	Dosed-feed	CE	CE	CE	NE	Yes	plastic industry
22	Chlorinated paraffins: C12 60% chlorine	Gavage	CE	CE	CE	CE	Yes	combustion products; oils
23	Chlorinated paraffins: C23 43% chlorine	Gavage	NE	E	CE	E	Yes	combustion products; oils
24	p-Chloroaniline hydrochloride	Gavage	CE	E	SE	NE	Yes	dye industry
25	Chlorobenzene	Gavage	E	NE	NE	NE	No	chemical industry; solvents
26	Chlorobenzilate	Dosed-feed	E	E	CE	CE	Yes	insecticide
27	Chlorodibromomethane	Gavage	NE	NE	E	SE	No	water contaminant
28	Chloroethane	Inhalation	E	E	IS	CE	Yes	chemical industry; anaesthetic
29	Chloroform	Gavage	CE	NE	CE	CE	Yes	chemical industry; anaesthetic
30	4-Chloro-m phenylenediamide	Dosed-feed	CE	NE	NE	CE	Yes	dye industry

	Agents	Route of exposure	Evidence of carcinogenicity[b]				Carcino-genicity in other site	Human exposure
N.	Type		Rats		Mice			
31	4-Chloro-o phenylenediamide	Dosed-feed	CE	CE	CE	CE	Yes	dye industry
32	Chloroprene	Inhalation	CE	CE	CE	CE	Yes	chemical industry
33	5-Chloro-o-toluidine	Dosed-feed	NE	NE	CE	CE	Yes	dye industry
34	C.I. Acid red 114	Dosed-water	CE	CE			Yes	dye industry
35	C.I. Direct blue 15	Dosed-water	CE	CE			Yes	dye industry
36	C.I. Direct blue 218	Dosed-feed	SE	NE	CE	CE	Yes	dye industry
37	C.I. Disperse blue 1	Dosed-feed	CE	CE	E	NE	Yes	hair colouring
38	C.I. Disperse yellow 3	Dosed-feed	CE	NE	NE	CE	Yes	dye for clothes
39	C.I. Pigment red 3	Dosed-feed	SE	SE	SE	NE	Yes	dye industry
40	C.I. Basic red 9 monohydrochloride	Dosed-feed	CE	CE	CE	CE	Yes	dye industry; clothes, paper, leather
41	Cinnamyl anthranilate	Dosed-feed	CE	NE	CE	CE	Yes	synthetic flavour
42	C.I. solvent yellow 14	Dosed-feed	CE	CE	NE	NE	Yes	dye industry
43	Coconut oil acid diethanolamine	Topical application	NE	E	CE	CE	Yes	cosmetic industry
44	Coumarin	Gavage	SE	E	SE	CE	Yes	pharmaceutical use
45	p-Cresidine	Dosed-feed	CE	CE	CE	CE	Yes	dye industry
46	Cumene	Inhalation	CE	SE	CE	CE	Yes	chemical industry
47	Cupferron	Dosed-feed	CE	CE	CE	CE	Yes	chemical industry
48	Daminozide	Dosed-feed	NE	CE	E	NE	Yes	plants growing regulator
49	D & C red 9	Dosed-feed	CE	E	NE	NE	Yes	cosmetic industry
50	D & C yellow 11	Dosed-feed	SE	SE			Yes	cosmetic industry
51	Decabromodiphenyl oxide	Dosed-feed	Se	SE	E	NE	Yes	plastic industry
52	Decalin	Inhalation	CE	NE	NE	E	Yes	industrial solvent

N.	Type	Route of exposure	Evidence of carcinogenicity[b]			Carcinogenicity in other site		Human exposure
			Rats		Mice			
53	2,4 Diaminotoluene	Dosed-feed	CE	CE	NE	CE	Yes	dye industry
54	1,2 Dibromoethane	Gavage	CE	CE	CE	CE	Yes	gasoline additive; pesticide
55	2,3 Dibromo-1-propanol	Topical application	CE	CE	CE	CE	Yes	pesticide
56	1,4 Dichlorobenzene	Gavage	CE	NE	CE	CE	Yes	moth killer; deodorant
57	2,7 Dichlorodibenzo dioxin-	Dosed-feed	NE	NE	E	NE	Yes	pesticides contaminant
58	p,p'-Dichlorodiphenyl dichloroethylene	Dosed-feed	NE	NE	CE	CE	No	insecticide
59	2,6- Dichloro-p-phenylenediamine	Dosed-feed	NE	NE	CE	CE	No	chemical industry
60	1,2- Dichloropropane	Gavage	NE	E	SE	SE	Yes	chemical industry
61	1,3-Dichloropropene	Gavage	CE	SE	IS	CE	Yes	pesticide
62	Dicofol	Dosed-feed	NE	NE	CE	NE	No	mitecide
63	Dieldrin	Dosed-feed	NE	NE	E	NE	No	insecticide
64	Diethanolamine	Topical application	NE	NE	CE	CE	Yes	chemical industry
65	Di(2-ethylhexyl) adipate	Dosed-feed	NE	NE	CE	CE	No	polivynil plastic
66	Di(2-ethylhexiyl) phthalate	Dosed-feed	CE	CE	CE	CE	No	polivynil plastic
67	Di(p-ethylphenyl) dichloroethane	Dosed-feed	NE	NE	NE	E	No	insecticide
68	Diethyl phthalate	Topical application	NE	NE	E	E	No	plastic industry
69	3,4-Dihydrocoumarin	Gavage	SE	NE	NE	SE	Yes	pharmaceutical use
70	3,3'-Dimetoxybenzidine dihydrochloride	Dosed-water	CE	CE			Yes	dye industry
71	1,4 Dioxane	Dosed-water	CE	CE	CE	CE	Yes	dye, cosmetic and plastic industry

N.	Type	Route of exposure	Evidence of carcinogenicity[b]			Carcinogenicity in other site		Human exposure
	Agents		Rats		Mice			
72	5,5-Diphenylhidantoin	Dosed-feed	E	NE	NE	CE	No	pharmaceutical use
73	2,5-Dithiobiurea	Dosed-feed	NE	NE	NE	E	No	film material
74	Elmiron	Gavage	NE	NE	SE	SE	Yes	pharmaceutical use
75	Ethylbenzene	Inhalation	CE	SE	SE	SE	Yes	chemical industry
76	Ethylene thiourea	Dosed-feed	CE	CE	CE	CE	Yes	rubber industry
77	Eugenol	Dosed-feed	NE	NE	E	E	No	flavouring compound
78	Fluometuron	Dosed-feed	NE	NE	E	NE	No	herbicide
79	Formamide	Gavage	NE	NE	CE	E	No	pharmaceutical use
80	Fumonisin B1	Dosed-feed	CE	NE	NE	CE	Yes	toxin
81	Furan	Gavage	CE	CE	CE	CE	Yes	polymers industry
82	Furfural	Gavage	SE	NE	CE	SE	Yes	food additive
83	Glycidol	Gavage	CE	CE	CE	CE	Yes	plastic industry
84	Goldenseal root powder	Dosed-feed	CE	CE	SE	NE	No	homeopathic use
85	HC blue 1	Dosed-feed	E	SE	CE	CE	Yes	hair colouring
86	HC red 3	Gavage	NE	NE	E	IS	No	hair colouring
87	Heptachlor	Dosed-feed	NE	E	CE	CE	Yes	insecticide
88	1,2,3,6,7,8-Hexachloro dibenzo-p-dioxin	Gavage	E	CE	CE	CE	No	pesticides contaminant
89	Hexachloroethane	Gavage	NE	NE	CE	CE	No	chemical industry; veterinary use
90	Hydrazobenzene	Dosed-feed	CE	CE	NE	CE	Yes	dye industry
91	Hydrochlorothiazide	Dosed-feed	NE	NE	E	NE	No	pharmaceutical use
92	Hydroquinone	Gavage	SE	SE	NE	SE	Yes	rubber and film industry
93	5-(Hydroxymethyl)-2-furfural	Gavage	NE	NE	NE	SE	No	food additive

N.	Type	Route of exposure	Evidence of carcinogenicity[b]		Carcino-genicity in other site		Human exposure
			Rats	Mice			
94	Indium phosphide	Inhalation	CE CE	CE	CE	Yes	electronic industry
95	Isoeugenol	Gavage	E NE	CE	E	Yes	flavouring compound
96	Isophorone	Gavage	SE NE	E	NE	Yes	solvent
97	Lauric acid diethanolamine condensate	Topical application	NE NE	NE	SE	No	pharmaceutical use
98	Leucomalachite green	Dosed-feed	E E		SE	Yes	dye industry
99	Malachite green	Dosed-feed	E		NE	Yes	dye industry
100	2-Mercaptobenzo thiazole	Gavage	SE SE	NE	E	Yes	rubber industry
101	Methyl carbamate	Gavage	CE CE	NE	NE	No	texil industry
102	4,4'-Methylenebis (N,N-dimethyl) benzenamine	Dosed-feed	CE CE	E	CE	Yes	dye industry
103	Methylene chloride	Inhalation	SE CE	CE	CE	Yes	chemical industry
104	4,4' - Methylenedianiline dihydrochloride	Dosed-water	CE CE	CE	CE	Yes	chemical industry
105	Methyleugenol	Gavage	CE CE	CE	CE	Yes	flavouring industry
106	2-Methylimidazole	Dosed-feed	SE CE	SE	SE	Yes	chemical industry
107	Methyl isobutyl ketone	Inhalation	SE E	SE	SE	Yes	solvent
108	2-Methyl-1-nitro anthraquinone	Dosed-feed	CE CE	CE	CE	Yes	dye industry
109	N-Methylolacrylamide	Gavage	NE NE	CE	CE	Yes	adhesive industry
110	Methylphenidate hydrochloride	Dosed-feed	NE NE	SE	SE	No	pharmaceutical use
111	alpha-Methylstyrene	Inhalation	SE NE	E	CE	Yes	plastic industry
112	Michler's Ketone	Dosed-feed	CE CE	CE	CE	Yes	dye industry

N.	Type (Agents)	Route of exposure	Evidence of carcinogenicity[b] Rats		Mice		Carcinogenicity in other site	Human exposure
113	Mirex	Dosed-feed	CE	CE			Yes	insecticide
114	Monuron	Dosed-feed	CE	NE	NE	NE	Yes	herbicide
115	beta-Myrcene	Gavage	CE	E	CE	E	Yes	cosmetic industry
116	1,5-Naphthalene diamine	Dosed-feed	NE	CE	CE	CE	Yes	chemical industry
117	Nithiazide	Dosed-feed	NE	CE	CE	E	Yes	veterinary use
118	5-Nitroacenaphthene	Dosed-feed	CE	CE	NE	CE	Yes	dye industry
119	3-nitro-p-acetophenetide	Dosed-feed	NE	NE	CE	NE	No	pharmaceutical use
120	5-nitro-o-aniside	Dosed-feed	CE	CE	E	CE	Yes	dye industry
121	o-Nitroanisole	Dosed-feed	CE	CE	CE	SE	Yes	chemical industry
122	6-Nitrobenzimidazole	Dosed-feed	NE	NE	CE	CE	No	film industry
123	Nitrofen	Dosed-feed	IS/NE	CE/NE	CE	CE	Yes/No	pesticide
124	Nitromethane	Inhalation	NE	CE	CE	CE	Yes	engine fuel
125	2-Nitro-p-phenyl enediamine	Dosed-feed	NE	NE	NE	CE	No	hair colouring
126	3 Nitropropionic acid	Gavage	E	NE	NE	NE	Yes	chemical industry
127	p-Nitrosodiphenyl-amine	Dosed-feed	CE	NE	CE	NE	No	rubber industry
128	o-Nitrotoluene	Dosed-feed	CE	CE	CE	CE	Yes	dye industry
129	5-Nitro-o-toluidine	Dosed-feed	NE	NE	CE	CE	Yes	dye industry
130	Oxazepam	Dosed-feed			CE	CE	Yes	pharmaceutical use
131	4,4' Oxydianiline	Dosed-feed	CE	CE	CE	CE	Yes	metallurgic industry
132	Oxymetholone	Gavage	E	CE			Yes	pharmaceutical use
133	Petachloroethane	Gavage	E	NE	CE	CE	Yes	chemical industry
134	Pentachlorophenol Dowicide EC-7	Dosed-feed			CE	CE	Yes	insecticide
135	Pentachlorophenol technical	Dosed-feed			CE	SE	Yes	insecticide

	Agents	Route of exposure	Evidence of carcinogenicity[b]			Carcino-genicity in other site		Human exposure
N.	Type		Rats		Mice			
136	Phenazopyridine hydrochloride	Dosed-feed	CE	CE	NE	CE	Yes	pharmaceutical use
137	Phenylbutazone	Gavage	E	SE	SE	NE	Yes	pharmaceutical use
138	Picloram	Dosed-feed	NE	E	NE	NE	No	herbicide
139	Piperonyl sulfoxide	Dosed-feed	NE	NE	CE	NE	No	insecticide
140	Polibrominated biphenyl mixture (Firemaster FF-1)	Dosed-feed and Gavage	CE	CE	CE	CE	No	engine fuel
141	Primidone	Dosed-feed	E	NE	CE	CE	Yes	pharmaceutical use
142	Probenecid	Gavage	NE	NE	NE	SE	No	pharmaceutical use
143	Proflavin hydrochloride	Dosed-feed	E	NE	E	E	Yes	pharmaceutical use
144	Propylene glycol mono-t-butyl ether	Inhalation	E	NE	CE	CE	Yes	solvent
145	Pulegone	Gavage	NE	SE	CE	CE	Yes	cosmetic use
146	Pyridine	Dosed-water	SE	E	CE	CE	Yes	chemical industry
147	Riddelliine	Gavage	CE	CE	CE	CE	Yes	food contaminant
148	Salicylazosulfa-pyridine	Gavage	SE	SE	CE	CE	Yes	pharmaceutical use
149	Selenium sulfide	Gavage	CE	CE	NE	CE	Yes	cosmetic use
150	Stoddard solvent (type 1IC)	Inhalation	SE	NE	NE	E	Yes	solvent
151	Binary mixture PCB 126/153 (TEF evaluation)	Gavage			CE		Yes	chemical industry
152	PECDF (TEF evaluation)	Gavage			SE		Yes	chemical industry
153	PCB 118 (TEF evaluation)	Gavage			CE		Yes	chemical industry

Agents		Route of exposure	Evidence of carcinogenicity[b]				Carcinogenicity in other site	Human exposure
N.	Type		Rats		Mice			
154	PCB mixture PCB 126/118 (TEF evaluation)	Gavage		CE			Yes	chemical industry
155	TCDD (TEF evaluation)	Gavage		CE			Yes	chemical industry
156	3,3',4,4' Tetrachloro azobenzene	Gavage	CE	CE	CE	CE	Yes	pesticide contaminant
157	2,3,7,8 Tetrachloro Dibenzo-p-dioxin	Gavage	CE	CE	CE	CE	Yes	herbicide contaminant
158	1,1,1,2 Tetrachloroethane	Gavage	E	NE	CE	CE	No	solvent
159	1,1,2,2 Tetrachloroethane	Gavage	E	NE	CE	CE	No	solvent
160	Tetrachloroethylene	Gavage	IS	IS	CE	CE	No	stain remover
		Inhalation	CE	SE	CE	CE	Yes	
161	Tetrachlorvinphos	Dosed-feed	NE	CE	CE	CE	Yes	insecticide
162	Tetrafluoroethylene	Inhalation	CE	CE	CE	CE	Yes	chemical industry
163	Tetrahydrofuran	Inhalation	SE	NE	NE	CE	Yes	chemical industry
164	Tetralin	Inhalation	SE	SE	NE	E	Yes	chemical industry
165	4,4'-Thiodianiline	Dosed-feed	CE	CE	CE	CE	Yes	dye industry
166	2,4-& 2,6- Toluene diisocyanate	Gavage	CE	CE	NE	CE	Yes	chemical industry
167	o-Toluidine hydrochloride	Dosed-feed	CE	CE	CE	CE	Yes	dye industry
168	Toxaphene	Dosed-feed	E	E	CE	CE	Yes	insecticide
169	Dioxin mixture (TEF evaluation)	Gavage		CE			Yes	chemical industry
170	PCB 153 (TEF evaluation)	Gavage		E			No	chemical industry
171	PCB 126 (TEF evaluation)	Gavage		CE			Yes	chemical industry

N.	Type	Route of exposure	Rats		Mice		Carcinogenicity in other site	Human exposure
			Rats		Mice			
172	Triamterene	Dosed-feed	E	NE	SE	SE	No	pharmaceutical use
173	1,1,2-Trichloroethane	Gavage	NE	NE	CE	CE	Yes	chemical industry
174	Trichloroethylene	Gavage	NE/IS	NE	CE	CE	No	solvent
175	2,4,6-Trichlorophenol	Dosed-feed	CE	NE	CE	CE	Yes	insecticide
176	1,2,3-Trichloropropane	Gavage	CE	CE	CE	CE	Yes	solvent
177	Triethanolamine	Topical application			E	SE	No	chemical industry
178	Trifluralin	Dosed-feed	NE	NE	NE	CE	Yes	pesticide
179	2,4,5-Trimethylaniline	Dosed-feed	CE	CE	E	CE	Yes	dye industry
180	tris(2,3-Dibromopropyl) phosphate	Dosed-feed	CE	CE	CE	CE	Yes	engine fuel
181	tris(2-Ethylhexyl) phosphate	Gavage	E	NE	NE	SE	Yes	engine fuel
182	Turmeric, oleoresin (curcumin)	Dosed-feed	NE	E	E	E	Yes	pharmaceutical use
183	Urethane	Dosed-water			CE	CE	Yes	chemical industry
184	Bromochloracetic acid	Dosed-water	CE	CE	CE	CE	Yes	water disinfection byproducts
185	Dibromoacetic acid	Dosed-water	SE	SE	CE	CE	Yes	water disinfection byproducts
186	Dibromoacetonitrile	Dosed-water	CE	SE	CE	CE	Yes	water disinfection byproducts
187	2,6 -Xylidine	Dosed-feed	CE	CE			Yes	dye industry
188	Zearalenone	Dosed-feed	NE	NE	CE	CE	Yes	micotoxin

a Data from: http://ntp.niehs.nih.gov/
b CE= clear evidence; SE= some evidence; E= equivocal evidence; NE= no evidence; IS= inadequate experiment

Table 2. Chemicals industrial agents associated with tumor induction in liver based on long term carcinogenicity bioassays performed in Fischer 344 rats and B6C3F1 mice males and females by the *National Toxicology Program (NTP)* USAa

	Agents	Route of exposure	Evidence of carcinogenicity				References
			Rats		Mice		
N.	Type		M	F	M	F	
1	Vynil Chloride	Inhalation	+	+	-	-	Maltoni et al. 1984
2	Trichloroethylene	Ingestion	-	-	NS	NS	Maltoni et al.
		Inhalation	-	-	+	+	1986
3	Benzene	Inhalation	E	(+)	NS	NS	Maltoni et al. 1989
4	Tamoxifen	Ingestion	E	E	-	-	Minardi et al.
		Ingestion	+	+	NS	NS	1994
5	Aspartame	Ingestion	-	-	+	-	Soffritti et al. 2010

Table 3. Agents inducing Hepatocellular Carcinoma identified in the framework of the long term carcinogenicity bioassays program performed by the Cesare Maltoni Cancer Research Center of the Ramazzini Institute

3. New risk factors of hepatocellular carcinoma

The epidemic of obesity has been correlated to an increased risk of various types of cancer (Kaidar-Person et al., 2011). In the last few decades, experimental and epidemiological studies have shown a strong correlation between obesity or its related co-morbidities and HCC incidence or mortality. In this section we will review the data linking metabolic syndrome and HCC risk, as well as some recent results published in the literature suggesting novel paths to be explored in liver cancer etiology.

3.1 Metabolic syndrome and hepatocellular carcinoma: Experimental data

Although no long-term carcinogenic bioassays have been specifically performed to investigate the carcinogenic potential of a high-fat diet, some recent studies provide interesting clues, in particular concerning liver carcinogenesis. A 20-month study on C57BL/6J male mice fed with a high fat western style diet showed that treated animals developed NASH (non-alcoholic steatohepatitis) at 14 months while at 20 months primary liver dysplastic nodules were found (VanSaun et al., 2009). Similar results were found by another group which showed that a high fat diet induced NASH and HCC in C57BL/6J mice but not in A/J mice (Hill-Baskin et al., 2009). Interestingly, the switch from the high-fat to low-fat diet after 100 days of administration until the end of the experiment (400 days of life) in C57BL/6J males prevented the development of obesity by the end of study and reversed the progression of the disease (Hill-Baskin et al., 2009). Again, a study using a diethylnitrosamine-initiated hepatocarcinogenesis model on Sprague-Dawley rats showed that animals fed with high-fat diets had an increased incidence of preneoplastic liver foci after 6 weeks compared to control animals (Wang et al., 2009).

These data may represent an early warning as to a possible liver cancer epidemic in coming decades. While obvious measures to contrast obesity have been undertaken in the last few years in many countries (WHO, 2006; Ministère de la Santé et de la Solidarité, 2006; White House Task Force on Childhood Obesity, 2010) and need to be strengthened, the impact of chemical indoor and outdoor pollution on obesity and HCC risk has been poorly studied and may play an underestimated and synergistic role. In this chapter, we will focus on chemical agents recognized as liver carcinogens and on novel mechanisms of hepatocarcinogenesis, in particular concerning metabolic and endocrine disruption.

3.2 Metabolic syndrome and hepatocellular carcinoma: The dimension

Metabolic syndrome and its characteristic manifestations, such as obesity (or central obesity), insulin resistance/type 2 diabetes, dyslipidemia or hypertension, are the most well-studied emerging risk factors of HCC (Bugianesi 2007; Starley et al., 2010; Welzel et al., 2011). In a recent US study, increase in Body Mass Index (BMI) results in a statistically significant increasing trend for HCC mortality both for women (highest calculated RR 1.68, CI 0.93-3.05, p for trend 0.04) and for men (highest calculated RR 4.52, CI 2.94-6.94, p for trend <0.001) (Calle et al., 2003). Other studies have shown that obesity is a risk factor for developing HCC, increasing the risk from 1.5 to 4 times (Møller et al., 1994; Wolk et al., 2001; Oh et al., 2005). Diabetes has been also shown to be an independent risk factor for HCC, with an increase in the risk ranging from 1.8 to 4 times in Swedish, Danish and Greek cohorts (Adami et al., 1996; Wideroff et al., 1997; Lagiou et al., 2000). Recently, metabolic syndrome has been reported to be more common in persons who developed HCC (37.1%) than in persons who did not (17.1%, p<0.0001) and it was significantly associated with increased risk of HCC after multiple logistic regression analyses (OR=2.13; 95%CI=1.96-2.31, p<0.0001) (Welzel et al., 2011). It is worth noting that a concurrent increase in the incidence and prevalence of NAFLD has been observed with the obesity epidemic (McCullough, 2004; Williams et al., 2011). NAFLD is a spectrum of liver disease ranging from simple steatosis to non-alcoholic steatohepatitis and cirrhosis (Bugianesi, 2007). The prevalence of NAFLD in the general population is estimated to range from 17 to 33% (McCullough, 2004). However, a recent prospective study on 328 persons (average age 54 years) reported that the prevalence of NAFLD was 46%, the global prevalence of NASH was 12.2% (Williams et al., 2011) and 2.7% of patients presented advanced NASH (fibrosis graded more than 2). The results of this study confirmed previous reports, as NAFLD and NASH were more frequently diagnosed in overweight/obese males, with a history of hypertension and diabetes (Williams et al., 2011); it suggests that NAFLD and its complications may be more widespread than previously reported. Importantly, some studies and several case reports have shown a direct relationship between NAFLD and HCC (Page and Harrison, 2009). In a Danish cohort study, the risk for primary liver cancer among NAFLD patients was elevated with a standardized incidence ratio of 4.4 (CI 1.2-11.4) (Sørensen et al., 2003). In a US single center case series, NAFLD accounted for 13% of the cases of HCC (Marrero et al., 2002). Moreover, at least 67 cases of HCC arising in a context of NASH have been reported and in 33% of cases HCC seems to have arisen in the absence of cirrhosis (Page and Harrison, 2009). In this context, it is of major concern that NAFLD is becoming the most common cause of liver disease in children and adolescents (Sundaram et al., 2009). A large pediatric autopsy study found a NAFLD global prevalence of 9.6%, with 38% prevalence in obese children (Schwimmer et al., 2006). The prevalence of fatty liver increased with age from 0.7% in 2-4 year olds to 17.3% in 15-19 year olds (Schwimmer et al., 2006). Of even greater concern is the higher initial incidence of fibrosis or cirrhosis reported in pediatric cases than in adults: a study of obese children with liver steatosis and elevated aminotransferases found NASH in 88% and fibrosis in 71% of patients (Nadeau et al., 2003; Rashid & Roberts 2000).

3.3 Endocrine disruption: Linking metabolic disorder to cancer etiology in the liver?

Endocrine disruption is a term coined in the 1990s which refers to the hormone-like effects of various synthetic chemicals present in the environment (Wingspread consensus statement, 1992; Kavlock et al., 1996). Since then, most laboratory and epidemiological research conducted on endocrine disruptors (ED) has focused on reproductive system pathologies, such as decreased sperm quality, malformations of male genital tract (cryptorchidisme or hypospadia), prostate and breast cancers, and on thyroid dysfunction (Soto & Sonnenschein, 2010). However, in the last decade, several ED, such as derivatives of alkylphenols (i.e. 4-nonylphenol), phthalates, polybrominated diphenyl ethers (PBDEs) or organotin compounds (i.e. tributyltin), have been shown to alter adipose tissue development and to promote fat accumulation in both adipose and liver tissues (Masumo et al., 2002; Grün et al., 2006; Grün & Blumberg 2009). Thus, some ED may also be addressed as "obesogens" and more generally considered as metabolic disruptors, suggesting that the various pathophysiological effects of ED may be due to pleiotropic effects on multiple metabolic pathways and that analyses of toxicological effects should not be limited to the endocrine system, but extended to all organs and tissues, with particular attention to adipose tissue and the liver (Grün & Blumberg, 2009; Casals-Casas & Desvergne, 2011).

Most data on the potential carcinogenic effects of ED derive from studies based on evidence of estrogen carcinogenicity. Estrogen carcinogenicity was experimentally demonstrated on the mouse mammary gland as early as the 1930s by Lacassagne (Lacassagne, 1936). In humans the most notorious case of estrogen carcinogenicity is diethylstilbestrol, a synthetic estrogen prescribed to pregnant women to prevent miscarriage in the 1940s-early 1970s. Diethylstilbestrol has been associated with an increased risk of developing clear-cell carcinoma of the vagina and breast cancer in daughters of exposed women (Herbst et al., 1971; Goodman et al., 2011; Palmer et al., 2006). Other ED, such as bisphenol A, tamoxifen or 2,3,7,8-tetrachlorodibenzodioxin, have been shown to alter mammary development and to induce precancerous and cancerous lesions in rodents (Vandenberg et al., 2008; Fenton et al., 2002; Soto & Sonnenschein, 2010). However, information on the potential carcinogenicity of ED for the liver is still elusive while the marshalling of epidemiological and experimental evidence for a potential carcinogenic effect by ED in the liver remains to be properly addressed. Interaction with nuclear receptors (NR) is one potential mechanism that may be involved in any pathological effects of ED on the liver. Indeed, many NR are signally expressed in the liver and have been reported to play an important role in liver diseases, such as steatosis and HCC (Wagner et al., 2011). Since many ED are small lipophilic compounds, their effects are thought to be mediated mostly by direct interaction with NR, modulating downstream gene expression (Casals-Casas & Desvergne, 2011). However, activation of various receptors, such as G protein-coupled membrane receptors, is also possible, as reported at least in the case of the well-established ED Bisphenol A (Chevalier et al., 2011). The NR superfamily encompasses 48 members and ED are able to alter the signaling pathways mediated by many of them, including estrogen and androgen receptors, thyroid hormone receptor (TR), glucocorticoid receptor (GR), mineralcorticoid receptor (MR), retinoid X receptor (RXR), peroxisome proliferator-activated receptors (PPARs), liver X receptors (LXRs), farnesoid X receptor (FXR), constitutive androstane receptor (CAR), and pregnane X receptor (PXR) (Arrese & Karpen, 2010; Casals-Casas & Desvergne, 2011). The ability of ED to interact with various NR at nanomolar concentrations explains the diversity of induced metabolic perturbation and the increased effects observed particularly when fetal and neonatal exposures occur (Heindel, 2003; Soto & Sonnenschein, 2010; Casals-Casas & Desvergne, 2011). It is worth noting that in addition to sex steroid receptors, this receptor superfamily includes transcription factors playing a central role in integrating metabolic and developmental signaling pathways (Wagner et al.,2011). In particular, data from knockout mice showed that functional PPAR-alpha or FXR are essential in the regulation of hepatic lipid metabolism, as deletion or deficiency of them induces hepatic steatosis in mice. Moreover, PXR and CAR (NRs for which many xenobiotics are ligands) promote hepatic lipid storage by decreasing fatty acid beta-oxidation (Wagner et al., 2011). Importantly, FXR, CAR and PXR are also variously involved in HCC formation. FXR knockout mice suffer from chronic bile acid-induced chronic inflammation and are prone to develop HCC, while CAR and PXR are important in the liver proliferative response, although their exact role in liver tumor promotion is not clear (Yang et al., 2007; Wagner et al., 2011). These data suggest that important interactions exist between NR signaling, lipid metabolism and liver carcinogenesis. This hypothesis is supported by recent findings showing a direct implication of impaired lipid metabolism in the development of hepatocellular carcinoma in animal models. A recent study showed that mice double mutants (due to a growth hormone-activated signal transducer and activator of transcription (STAT5) and GR) developed liver steatosis that progressed to hepatocellular carcinomas (Mueller et al., 2011). Altered STAT5/GR signaling was associated with insulin resistance, high reactive oxygen species levels and increased liver and DNA injuries; that it function correctly was essential for maintenance of lipid homeostasis (Mueller et al., 2011). A second study showed that transgenic CAR -/- mice fed with a NASH-inducing diet are protected from diethylnitrosamine-induced hepatocarcinogenesis (Takizawa et al., 2011). These results suggest that the nuclear receptor CAR might play an important role in promoting hepatocellular carcinomas against a background of NASH. Interestingly, human HCC have been associated with altered lipid metabolism, in particular choline and phospholipid metabolism with an increased synthesis in lysophosphatidic acid, which may provide a mitogenic and proliferative microenvironment through activation of G-protein-coupled receptors (Skill et al., 2011). Moreover, stimulation of lipid biosynthesis and perpetuating chronic hepatic metabolic disease by activation of the transactivator of stress proteins HSF1 promotes HCC development in mice (Jin et al., 2011). Finally, an interesting paper based on a microarray analysis of a hepatitis-induced HCC murine model showed that pro-inflammatory cytokines may promote HCC predominantly in males causing the loss of a gender-identifying hepatic molecular signature (Rogers et al., 2007), suggesting that HCC may be associated with liver-gender disruption in male mice and supporting the idea that endocrine disruption may have broader effects than those reported in reproductive and sexual organs.

Although the scientific data on ED and their effects on liver disease are mostly anecdotal, a few toxicological studies have shown that perinatal exposure to Bisphenol A (BPA) or organotin compounds alters not only adipogenesis in rodents, but also increases both the expression of lipogenic genes and lipid accumulation in the liver of animals exposed (Somm et al., 2009; Grün et al., 2006). Ecotoxicological studies have shown that ED may bioaccumulate and induce altered gene expression in the liver of various animal species (Ter Veld et al., 2008). In particular, BPA, PCBs and PBDE were shown to bioaccumulate in fish livers caught in Italian seas or US lakes (Mita et al., 2011; Pérez-Fuenteaja et al., 2010) and nonylphenol (NP) was reported to induce the expression of female specific proteins in male lizard livers (Verderame et al., 2011). Although the relevance of NR stimulation to human liver cancer is still unclear, this is a well-known non-genotoxic mechanism of rodent liver cancer, in particular concerning PPAR-alpha activation (Ren et al., 2010). Interestingly, it has been shown that rodent carcinogens show higher *in vitro* potency for human NR than do non-carcinogens (Shah et al., 2011). NP was shown to activate human CAR *in vitro* and *in vivo* using transgenic mouse models (Hernandez et al., 2007). Moreover, CAR is involved in hepatic injury and in the development of HCC in a dietary model of NASH, probably by its cell proliferation promoting activity (Takizawa et al., 2011).

Available data on ED-induced hepatic alterations and on their potential action on systemic and hepatic lipid metabolism suggest that ED may have a role in the establishment and progression of some liver diseases, in particular NAFLD and HCC. However, systematic research aiming to investigate interactions between endocrine/metabolic disruption in liver disease/carcinogenesis is still lacking. We will report on some recent advances in the identification of common new subcellular targets in metabolic disease and liver carcinogenesis, with a particular focus on mitochondria and endoplasmic reticulum alterations and their cross-talks with NR signaling perturbation.

4. Molecular aspects of hepatocellular carcinoma

HCC is a cancer caused by a variety of etiologies, including HBV and HCV infection, alcohol over-consumption, aflatoxin B1 exposure and chemical agents. Thus, it is not surprising that a variety of HCC-associated molecular alterations have been detected and no universal molecular signature is definitively associated with all hepatic tumors, either in humans or in experimental animals (Degli Esposti et al., 2009; Pei et al., 2009). In particular, in humans HCC alterations are classically reported in four genetic pathways, namely p53, retinoblastoma (Rb), TGF-beta pathway and Wnt-beta-catenin pathways (Laurent-Puig, 2001; Saffroy et al., 2007). However, the carcinogenic process in the liver looks to be more complex, as a recent review on omics-based studies seems to suggest (Pei et al., 2009). In particular, comparative genomic hybridizations, high-throughput methods used to identify deletion or amplification in genomic DNA, have shown chromosomal aberrations in fourteen human chromosomes, not uniquely associated with viral infections (Pei et al., 2009). Various studies have also reported epigenetic alterations in HCC, in particular hypermethylation and subsequent silencing of some tumor suppressor genes (Pei et al., 2009). Microarray studies have been performed on both mRNA and microRNA (miRNA), but no consistent expression signatures seem to arise, due to alleged differences in technology and experimental design (Pei et al., 2009). All together, these data reinforce the view that the development of HCC, and probably all cancer types, involves multiple factors and interactions at a molecular level. While meta-analysis and integration of –omics data could prove a helpful approach for biomarker identification in cancer (Zender et al., 2006; Ludwig & Weinstein, 2005), it seems urgent we adopt a comprehensive framework including pathophysiological and developmental aspects of the disease with consistent molecular, biochemical and biophysical interactions (Soto & Sonnenschein, 2004).

As we reported in the previous section, the case of endocrine and metabolic perturbation in liver disease and carcinogenesis offers a useful starting point for discussing newly identified or potential carcinogenic pathways and future directions to clarify the complex picture of hepatocellular carcinoma and, maybe more generally, of cancer.

4.1 New aspects of hepatocarcinogenesis: Metabolic disruption and altered cellular homeostasis

Alterations in the metabolism of cancerous tissues have been found since 1930s. Warbug (1930) described that, even in the presence of oxygen, cancer tissues had acquired an irreversible glycolytic metabolism. Increased glycolysis proves to allow the utilization of glycolytic intermediates into the various biosynthetic pathways, including nucleoside and amino acid synthesis, required by highly replicating cells (Potter, 1958, Vander Heiden et al., 2009). This feature is also described in rapidly dividing embryonic tissues, even though they are able to switch to oxidative metabolism as proliferation ceases and cells differentiate, suggesting that cancer development may be understood as altered embryonic development (Barger & Plas, 2010, Cooper, 2009, Soto & Sonnenschein, 2004). As a result of Warburg's observations, defects in mitochondrial function have been suspected as contributing to cancer development and progression (Chatterjee et al., 2011). Recently, not only mitochondria but also endoplasmic reticulum have been found to be implicated in controlling the lipid metabolism, in particular in the liver. Thus, since reprogramming of the energy metabolism has been rediscovered as a hallmark of cancer (Hanahan & Weinberg, 2011) while alteration of the lipid metabolism seems to be associated with HCC development, the role of mitochondria and endoplasmic reticulum in metabolic disruption during liver carcinogenesis forms a testable hypothesis in the context of liver carcinogenesis.

Mitochondria are key organelles both for energy (ATP) production (by oxidative phosphorylation of components of the tricarboxylic acid cycle and lipid beta-oxydation) and for integration of pro-survival/pro-death signaling in cells of every tissue and organ. These functions are essential in determining cellular and tissue homeostasis. In the last decade, a lot of research has focused on the role of mitochondria in liver diseases and mitochondrial dysfunctions have been described both in NAFLD and in HCC (Begriche et al., 2006; Chang et al., 2005; Sato, 2007; Rector et al., 2010). A recent study compared liver histology and function in the obese rodent model Otsuka Long-Evans Tokushima Fatty (OLETF) rat with its lean homolog LETO rat (Rector et al., 2010). The ultrastructure of hepatic mitochondria proved to be impaired and the total mitochondrial content decreased in OLETF rats. Moreover, mitochondrial and total fatty acid oxidation were already reduced as early as the fifth week of age in obese animals, before hepatic steatosis and insulin resistance were observed, suggesting that mitochondrial dysfunction may be a very early event in the natural history of NAFLD (Rector et al., 2010). Various mitochondrial alterations have been reported in patients with NASH. Megamitochondria with ultrastructure abnormalities have been found in NASH patients (Caldwell et al., 1999a; Sanyal et al., 2001). Severe depletion of mitochondrial DNA (mtDNA) has been also reported in patients with NASH or hepatic fibrosis (Caldwell et al., 1999b; Ducluzeau et al., 1999). mtDNA depletion may contribute to impairment of the respiratory chain, a common feature in drug-induced and primary NASH (Begriche et al., 2006). It should be noted that in primary NASH impairment of the respiratory chain is concomitant with an increase in beta-oxidation flux (due to insulin resistance), leading to production of a high level of reactive oxygen species (ROS) (Begriche et al., 2006). Increased ROS generation by mitochondria has also been observed in genetically obese ob/ob mice (Yang et al., 2000) and in rat fed on a choline-deficient diet, a model of steatosis and NASH (Hensley et al., 2000). An increased production of ROS in fatty livers induces lipid peroxidation and subsequently reactive aldehyde formation (Begriche et al., 2006). ROS and aldehydes may further damage mitochondria, generating a vicious circle, and increase the expression of pro-inflammatory cytokines, such as TGF-beta, TNF-alpha, IL-8 or Fas ligand, worsening liver injury (Pessayre & Fromenty, 2005). Mitochondria are also involved in hepatocarcinogenesis. A decrease in mtDNA-dependent cytochromes with disturbed electron transfer has been reported in liver carcinomas, with a subsequent increase in ROS production that can induce nuclear gene mutation in carcinogenesis (Sato, 2007). Moreover, a higher frequency of somatic mutation in regulatory and coding regions of mtDNA has recently been reported in HCC compared to adjacent non-cancerous tissue (Yin et al., 2010). Interestingly, an experimental study showed that long-term administration of L-carnitine, a key molecule in fatty acid transport to mitochondria, decreases the occurrence of hepatic preneoplastic lesions in Long-Evans Cinnamon rats (Chang et al., 2005). These data reinforce the idea that mitochondrial dysfunction, and in particular its role in lipid catabolism, is involved in hepatocarcinogenesis. It is interesting to note that some chemicals with endocrine disruptive properties have been shown to target mitochondrion functionality in various tissues and organs, including the liver (Kovacic, 2010). In particular, five-month exposure to 10-50 ppm diethyl phthalate induced liver impairment, triglyceride accumulation and mitochondrial proliferation in Wistar rats (Pereira et al., 2006). Since phthalates are plasticizers present in plastics used for medical reasons, such as storage bags for blood conservation or instruments for dialysis, it is interesting to note that liver biopsies on dialyzed patients show peroxisome proliferation (Ganning et al., 1984) and that phthalate leakage from blood bags has been proposed as potentially pro-inflammatory (Rael et al., 2009). Furthermore, male mice treated perinatally with 160 or 480 mg/kg of BPA for 14 days showed an increase in cell death mediated by the mitochondrial apoptotic pathway in the testes (Wang et al., 2010). While the hepatic effects on the liver were not evaluated in this study, these results suggest that BPA may directly or indirectly target mitochondria. Other evidence of ED toxicity in mitochondria is provided by results showing that tamoxifen decreased ATP production in a model of isolated perfused rat liver (Marek et al., 2011) and that it impaired mitochondrial respiration, increased cytochrome c release, mitochondrial lipid peroxidation and mitochondrial protein nitration by stimulating mitochondrial nitric oxide synthase (Nazarewicz et al., 2007). Importantly, although epidemiological studies available in humans did not identify any increased risk of liver cancer in women who were administered tamoxifen for breast cancer, several experiments have shown that tamoxifen induces hepatocarcinomas in rats when administered at high doses (Maltoni et al., 1997; IARC, 2011). Another reported ED and human carcinogen, 2,3,7,8 TCDD, has been reported to induce cytotoxicity and mitochondrial dysfunction in isolated rat hepatocytes (Aly & Domènech, 2009) and to mediate tumor progression by activating signaling pathways similar to mtDNA depletion (Biswas et al., 2008). In this context, it would be helpful to consider the interactions between mitochondria, lipid metabolism and nuclear receptors in order to improve our understanding of liver disease and carcinogenesis. In point of fact, several members of the nuclear receptor superfamily are lipid-sensing factors that affect many aspects of lipid metabolism (Alaynick, 2008). PPARs, LXRs, interacting with their transcriptional coactivator PPARgamma Coactivator 1 alpha (PGC-1alpha) have been shown to regulate insulin sensitivity and lipid metabolism (Alaynick, 2008). Interestingly, PGC-1alpha is a known regulator of mitochondrial biogenesis and also able to modulate hepatic steatosis (Puigserver et al., 1998; Sonoda et al., 2007; Wu et al., 1999). Moreover, the mitochondrial protein ANT, a translocase that provides mitochondria with ADP allowing ATP synthesis, has recently been shown to be essential for the functioning of PGC-1 alpha (Kim et al., 2010) while another NR, the estrogen-related receptor alpha (ERR-alpha), important for adaptive energy metabolism (Villena & Kralli, 2008), has been shown to be an effector of PGC-1 alpha, regulating the expression of genes involved in oxidative phosphorylation and mitochondrial biogenesis (Schreiber et al., 2004). Thus, PGC-1 alpha may be a key molecule linking NR signaling to mitochondrial function and activity. Finally, it is important to note that ED and other NR ligands may also act independently on the receptor action and mitochondria can be a direct target of this mechanism, as proposed for PPAR agonists (Scatena et al., 2004). Hence, it has been suggested that characterization of reciprocal influences between mitochondria and PPAR physiology would be fundamental for a better understanding of cancer biology (Scatena et al., 2008).

Endoplasmic reticulum is an organelle responsible for protein synthesis, folding, maturation, quality control and trafficking, as well as for Ca^{2+} homeostasis. Every condition that stresses its folding ability, such as an excess of protein synthesis or alteration of energy availability, causes a physiological response called Unfolded Protein Response (UPR). UPR activation aims to increase the folding capacity of endoplasmic reticulum by inducing transcription of chaperons and by globally decreasing protein synthesis (Schroeder & Kaufman, 2005). In recent years, it has been shown that endoplasmic reticulum plays a central role in the multi-organ coordination of systemic metabolism through the integration of synthetic and catabolic pathways (Kammoun et al., 2009b, Hotamisligil, 2010). Obesity and diabetes have been shown to induce ER stress in both adipose tissue and the liver (Ozcan et al., 2004, Kammoun et al., 2009a). Puri et al., examined the role of endoplasmic reticulum stress in human NAFLD, showing UPR activation in liver biopsies from patients with NAFLD and NASH compared to subjects with the metabolic syndrome and normal liver histology (Puri et al., 2008). Moreover, free fatty acids (FFA) may be important mediators of cell dysfunction (lipotoxicity) not only through death receptors or the mitochondrial-lysosomal pathway, but also via endoplasmic reticulum stress (Alkhouri et al., 2009). Endoplasmic reticulum stress and activation of the UPR are also present in solid cancers, often characterized by hypoxia, nutrient starvation, oxidative stress and other metabolic deregulation, factors that cause endoplasmic reticulum impairment (Li et al., 2011). Depending on the duration and degree of ER stress, the UPR can provide either survival signals by activating adaptive and antiapoptotic pathways, or death signals by inducing cell death programs (Schroeder & Kaufman, 2005; Li et al., 2011). In hepatocellular carcinoma, higher accumulation of the Bip/GRP78 and nuclear localization of ATF6, characteristic of UPR activation, were found in moderately to poorly differentiated human HCC tissue samples (Shuda et al., 2003). Although direct demonstrations at a molecular level are still lacking, the cross-links between endoplasmic reticulum stress, NAFLD and HCC seem to be numerous and future research should address this potential new carcinogenic pathway. However, endoplasmic reticulum seems also to be a target of endocrine disruption. Recently, BPA has been shown, in a murine liver cell line, to increase the gene expression of various actors involved in endoplasmic reticulum stress, such as C/EBP homologous protein, caspase 12 and GRP78 (Asahi et al., 2010). This ties up interestingly with a microarray study in which activation of genetic networks involved in endoplasmic reticulum stress was also detected in mouse testicular Sertoli cells treated with BPA at a concentration of 200 microM (Tabuchi et al., 2006). Furthermore, a number of ED, such as nonylphenol, octylphenol, bisphenol A, and butylated hydroxytoluene, have been shown to inhibit endoplasmic reticulum Ca^{2+} ATPase pumps in a low micromolar concentration (Hughes et al., 2000), suggesting that alterations in endoplasmic reticulum homeostasis may be a common action mechanism by BPA in various different organs. In this connection, some recent papers have highlighted a possible direct interaction between nuclear receptor signaling, lipid metabolism and endoplasmic reticulum stress. A protein deacetylase (SIRT1) has been shown to positively regulate the nuclear receptor PPAR alpha (Purushotham et al., 2009). In particular, hepatic-specific deletion of SIRT1 impairs PPAR alpha signaling and SIRT1 knockout mice develop hepatic steatosis, liver inflammation and endoplasmic reticulum stress (Purushotham et al., 2009). Moreover, the endoplasmic reticulum stress-induced transcription factor ATF6 has been shown to suppress insulin gene expression through the up-regulation of a transcriptional partner of nuclear receptors, SHP, in pancreatic beta-cells and in pancreatic islets of OLETF rats (Seo et al., 2008), suggesting that endoplasmic reticulum stress signaling may also act via NR signaling. As for mitochondria, while no extensive data are available, interactions between endoplasmic reticulum homeostasis and NR physiology have been shown and may play an important yet still under-explored role in the initiation and progression of liver steatosis and HCC. Perturbation of this network by ED is possible, although more research is needed to address the effects of environmental concentrations and to identify the biochemical pathways affected and any long-term pathophysiological consequences, in particular in liver carcinogenesis.

5. Conclusions

In this chapter, we have reviewed some recent acquisitions in HCC epidemiology, in particular regarding the association between obesity and metabolic syndrome and HCC incidence and mortality. We have also reviewed the evidence for liver susceptibility to chemical-induced carcinogenesis, in both rodents and humans, and have shown that long-term carcinogenicity bioassays are a useful tool for identifying potential hepatocarcinogens. In the last part of the chapter, we suggest that endocrine and metabolic disruption, a mechanism involved in the toxic effects of various chemicals, might be a plausible and testable hypothesis in the pathophysiology of NAFLD and its progression toward HCC, in particular concerning the alteration of mitochondria and endoplasmic reticulum in the liver and other tissues. We suggest that long-term carcinogenicity bioassays are a valuable approach to integrating pathological end-points, such as tumor induction, and the analysis of early chronic alteration in tissue and cellular homeostasis, such as mitochondrial and endoplasmic reticulum dysfunctions. This approach could provide important insights into chemical-induced carcinogenic mechanisms, in particular for non-genotoxic carcinogens such as most endocrine disruptors. Moreover, the comparison of experimental results with human biopsies of neoplastic and pre-neoplastic lesions, such as NASH, in well-characterized patients may help to develop specific early markers towards identifying the population at higher risk of HCC.

6. Acknowledgement

The authors thank Ralph Nisbet for his assistance in preparing the manuscript.

7. References

Adami, H.O., Chow W.H., Nyrén, O., et al. (1996). Excess risk of primary liver cancer in patients with diabetes mellitus. *J Natl Cancer Inst*, 88, 1472-1477.

Adelstein, A. & White G. (1976). Alcoholism and mortality. *Popul Trends*, 6, 7-13.

Alaynick, W.A. (2008). Nuclear receptors, mitochondria and lipid metabolism. *Mitochondrion*, 8(4), 329-337.

Alkhouri, N., Dixon, L.,J., Feldstein, A.E. (2009). Lipotoxicity in nonalcoholic fatty liver disease: not all lipids are created equal. *Expert Rev Gastroenterol Hepatol*, 3, 445-451.

Aly, H.A. & Domènech, O. (2009). Cytotoxicity and mitochondrial dysfunction of 2,3,7,8-tetrachlorodibenzo-p-dioxin (TCDD) in isolated rat hepatocytes. *Toxicol Lett*, 191(1), 79-87.

Arrese, M., & Karpen, S.J. (2010). Nuclear receptors, inflammation, and liver disease: insights for cholestatic and fatty liver diseases. *Clin Pharmacol Ther*, 87, 473-478.

Asahi, J., Kamo, H., Baba, R., et al. (2010). Bisphenol A induces endoplasmic reticulum stress-associated apoptosis in mouse non-parenchymal hepatocytes. *Life Sci*, 87(13-14), 431-438.

Barbin, A., Froment, O., Boivin, S. et al. (1997). p53 gene mutation pattern in rat liver tumors induced by vinyl chloride. *Cancer Res*, 57, 1695-1698.

Barger, J.F., & Plas, D.R. (2010). Balancing biosynthesis and bioenergetics: metabolic programs in oncogenesis. *Endocrine-Related Cancer*, 17, R287-R304.

Begriche, K., Igoudjil, A., Pessayre, D., et al. (2006). Mitochondrial dysfunction in NASH: causes, consequences and possible means to prevent it. *Mitochondrion*, 6(1), 1-28.

Biswas, G., Srinivasan, S., Anandatheerthavarada, H.K. et al. (2008). Dioxin-mediated tumor progression through activation of mitochondria-to-nucleus stress signaling. *Proc Natl Acad Sci U S A*, 105(1), 186-191.

Blonski, W., Kotlyar, D.S., Forde, K.A. (2010). Non-viral causes of hepatocellular carcinoma. *World J Gastroenterol*, 16(29), 3603-3615.

Borentain P, Gérolami V, Ananian P, et al. (2007). DNA-repair and carcinogen-metabolising enzymes genetic polymorphisms as an independent risk factor for hepatocellular carcinoma in Caucasian liver-transplanted patients. *Eur J Cancer*, 43(17), 2479-2486.

Bosetti, C., Levi, F., Boffetta, P., et al. (2008). Trends in mortality from hepatocellular carcinoma in Europe, 1980-2004. *Hepatology*, 48, 137-145.

Bucher, JR. (2002). The National Toxicology Program rodent bioassay. Design, interpretations, and scientific contributions. *Ann NY. Acad Sci,* 982, 198-207.

Buendia, M.A. (1992). Hepatitis B viruses and hepatocellular carcinoma. *Adv Cancer Res*, 59, 167-226.

Bugianesi E (2007). Non-alcoholic steatohepatitis and cancer. *Clin Liver Dis*, 11, 191-207.

Caldwell, S.H., Oelsner, D.H., Iezzoni, J.C., et al. (1999a). Cryptogenic cirrhosis: clinical characterization and risk factors for underlying disease. *Hepatology*, 29, 664-669.

Caldwell, S.H., Swerdlow, R.H., Khan, E.M., et al. (1999b). Mitochondrial abnormalities in non-alcoholic steatohepatitis. *J Hepatol*, 31(3), 430-434.

Calle, E.E., Rodriguez C., Walker-Thurmond K., et al. (2003). Overweight, obesity, and mortality from cancer in a prospectively studied cohort of U.S. adults. *N Engl J Med*, 348, 1625-1638.

Casals-Casas, C., & Desvergne, B. (2011). Endocrine disruptors: from endocrine to metabolic disruption. *Annu Rev Physiol*, 73, 135-162.

Chan, P.C., Sills, R.C., Braun, A.G., et al. (1996). Toxicity and carcinogenicity of delta 9-tetrahydrocannabinol in Fischer rats and B6C3F1 mice. *Fundamental Appl Toxicol*, 30, 109-117.

Chang, B., Nishikawa, M., Nishiguchi, S., et al. (2005). L-carnitine inhibits hepatocarcinogenesis via protection of mitochondria. *Int J Cancer*, 113(5), 719-729.

Chatterjee, A., Dasgupta, S., Sidransky, D. (2011). Mitochondrial subversion in cancer. *Cancer Prev Res (Phila)*, 4(5): 638-54.

Chevalier, N., Bouskine, A., Fenichel, P. (2011). Bisphenol A promotes testicular seminoma cell proliferation through GPER/GPR30. *Int J Cancer* In press.

Chiappini, F., Gross-Goupil, M., Saffroy, R., et al. (2004). Microsatellite instability mutator phenotype in hepatocellular carcinoma in non-alcoholic and non-virally infected normal livers. *Carcinogenesis*, 25(4): 541-547.

Commission of the European Communities (CEC). The German thorotrast study. (1984). Directorate general Science, Research and Development, EUR 9504 EN.

Cooper, M. (2009). Regenerative pathologies: stem cells, teratomas and theories of cancer. *Medicine Studies*, 1, 55-66.

Degli Esposti, D., Pham, P., Saffroy, R., et al. (2009). Environmental risk factors in primary liver cancer: a review of the literature and perspectives for primary prevention and early detection. *Eur J Oncol*, 3, 133-150.

Dietz, A., Langbein, G,. & Permatter, W. (1985). Das Vinylchloride induzierte hepatocellulare Karzinom. *Klin Wochenschr*, 63, 325-331.

Ducluzeau, P.H., Lachaux, A., Bouvier, R., et al. (1999). Depletion of mitochondrial DNA associated with infantile cholestasis and progressive liver fibrosis. *J Hepatol*, 30(1), 149-155.

El-Seragh, H.B. (2004). Hepatocellular carcinoma: recent trends in the United States. *Gastroenterology*, 127 Suppl. 5: S27-S34.

El-Seragh, H. & Rudolph, K.L. (2007). Hepatocellular Carcinoma: Epidemiology and Molecular carcinogenesis. *Gastroenterology*, 132: 2557-2576.

Evans, D.M.D., Jones, W.W., & Kung, I.T.M. (1983). Angiosarcoma and hepatocellular carcinoma in vinyl chloride workers. *Histopathology*, 7, 377-388.

Fenton, S.E., Hamm, J.T., Birnbaum, L., et al. (2002). Persistent abnormalities in the rat mammary gland following gestational and lactation exposure to 2,3,7,8-tetrachlorodibenzo-p-dioxin (TCDD). *Toxicol Sci*, 67,63-74.

Feo, F., Frau, M., Tomasi, M.L., et al. (2009). Genetic and epigenetic control of molecular alterations in hepatocellular carcinoma. *Exp Biol Med*, 234, 726-736.

Ferlay, J., Shin, H.R., Bray, F., et al. (2010). GLOBOCAN 2008 v1.2, Cancer Incidence and Mortality Worldwide: IARC CancerBase No. 10. IARC Press, Lyon, France:. Available from: http://globocan.iarc.fr

Ganning, A.E., Brunk, U., Dallner, G. (1984). Phthalate esters and their effect on the liver. *Hepatology*, 4(3), 541-547.

Gokel, J.M., Liebezeit, E. & Eder, M. (1976). Hemangiosarcoma and hepatocellular carcinoma of the liver following vinylchloride exposure: a report of two cases. *Virchows Arch (A)*, 372, 195-203.

Goodman A, Schorge J, Greene MF. (2011). The long-term effects of in utero exposures--the DES story. *N Engl J Med*, 364(22), 2083-2084.

Grün, F., & Blumberg, B. (2009). Endocrine disrupters as obesogens. *Mol Cell Endocrinol*, 304, 19-29.

Grün, F., Watanabe, H., Zamanian, Z., et al. (2006). Endocrine disrupting organotin compounds are potent inducers of adipogenesis in vertebrates. *Mol Endocrinol*, 9, 2141-2155.

Guimaraes, J.P., Lamerton, L.F. & Christensen, W.R. (1955). The late effects of thorotrast administration, a review and an experimental study. *Br J Cancer*, 11, 253-267.

Hagan EC, Jenner PM, Jones WI, Fitzhugh OG, Long EL, Brouwer JG and Webb WK. (1965). Toxic properties of compound related to safrole. *Toxicol Appl Pharmacol*, 7, 18-24.

Hanahan, D., & Weinberg R.A. (2011). Hallmark of cancer: the next generation. *Cell*, 144, 646-674.

Hakulinen, T., Lehtimaki, L., Lehtonen, M. et al. (1974). Cancer morbidity among two male cohorts with increased alcohol consumption in Finland. *J Natl Cancer Inst*, 52, 1711-1714.

Heindel, J.J. (2003). Endocrine disruptors and the obesity epidemic. *Toxicol Sci*, 76(2), 247-249.

Hensley, K., Kotake, Y., Sang, H., et al. (2000). Dietary choline restriction causes complex I dysfunction and increased $H(2)O(2)$ generation in liver mitochondria. *Carcinogenesis*, 21(5), 983-989.

Herbst, A.L., Ulfelder, H., Poskanzer, D.C. (1971). Adenocarcinoma of the vagina. Association of maternal stilbestrol therapy with tumor appearance in young women. *N Engl J Med*, 284(15), 878-881.

Hernandez, J.P., Huang, W., Chapman, L.M., et al. (2007). The environmental estrogen, nonylphenol, activates the constitutive androstane receptor. *Toxicol Sci*, 98(2), 416-426.

Hézode, C., Zafrani, E.S., Roudot-Thoraval, F., et al. (2008). Daily cannabis use: a novel risk factor of steatosis severity in patients with chronic hepatitis C. *Gastroenterology*, 134, 432-439.

Hill-Baskin, A.E., Markiewski, M.M., Buchner, D.A., et al. (2009). Diet-induced hepatocellular carcinoma in genetically predisposed mice. *Hum Mol Genet* 18(16), 2975-2988.

Hirayama T. (1981). A large-scale cohort study on the relationship between diet and selected cancers of digestive organs. In: *Gastrointestinal cancer: endogenous factor*, Bruce, W.R., Correa, P., Lipkin, M., Tannenbaum, S.R., Wilkins, T.D. (Banbury Report 7), 409-429. CSH Press, Cold Spring Harbor, NY.

Hoenerhoff, M.J., Pandiri, A.R., Lahousse, S.A., et al. (2011). Global gene profiling of spontaneous hepatocellular carcinoma in B6CEF1 mice: similarities in the molecular landscape with human liver cancer. *Toxicol Pathol*, 39, 678-699.

Hotamisligil, G.S. (2010). Endoplasmic reticulum stress and the inflammatory basis of metabolic disease. *Cell*, 140, 900-917.

Huff, J. (2002). Chemicals studied and evaluated in long-term carcinogenesis bioassays by both the Ramazzini Foundation and the National Toxicology Program: in tribute to Cesare Maltoni and David Rall. *Ann NY Acad Sci*, 982, 208-230.

Hughes, P.J., McLellan, H., Lowes, D.A., et al. (2000). Estrogenic alkylphenols induce cell death by inhibiting testis endoplasmic reticulum Ca(2+) pumps. *Biochem Biophys Res Commun*, 277(3), 568-574.

International Agency for Research on Cancer (IARC). (1976). Monographs on evaluation of the carcinogenic risk of chemicals to man. Vol. 10. Some naturally occurring substances. IARC Press, Lyon, France.

International Agency for Research on Cancer (IARC). (1979). Monographs on evaluation of the carcinogenic risk of chemicals to humans. Vol. 21. Sex hormones (II). IARC Press, Lyon, France.

International Agency for Research on Cancer (IARC). (1982). Monographs on evaluation of the carcinogenic risk of chemicals to humans. Vol. 29. Some industrial chemicals and dyestuff. IARC Press, Lyon, France.

International Agency for Research on Cancer (IARC). (1987). Monographs on the evaluation of the carcinogenic risk to humans. Suppl. 7. Overall Evaluations of Carcinogenicity: An Updating of IARC Monographs Volumes 1 to 42. IARC Press, Lyon, France.

International Agency for Research on Cancer (IARC). (1988). Monographs on evaluation of the carcinogenic risk of chemicals to man. Vol. 44. Alcohol drinking. IARC Press, Lyon, France.

International Agency for Research on Cancer (IARC). (1993). Evaluation of the carcinogenic risk of chemicals to man. Vol. 56. Some naturally occurring substances. Food items and constituents, heterocyclic aromatic amines and mycotoxins. IARC Press, Lyon, France.

International Agency for Research on Cancer (IARC). (1997). Monographs on the evaluation of the carcinogenic risk of chemical to humans. Vol. 69. Polychlorinated dibenzo-para-dioxins and polychlorinated dibenzofurans. IARC Press, Lyon, France.

International Agency for Research on Cancer (IARC). (2001). Monographs on the evaluation of the carcinogenic risk to humans. Vol. 78. Ionizing radiation part 2: some internally deposited radionucleotides. IARC Press, Lyon, France.

International Agency for Research on Cancer (IARC). (2004a). Monographs on the evaluation of the carcinogenic risk of chemical to humans. Vol. 83. Tobacco smoke and involuntary smoking. IARC Press, Lyon, France.

International Agency for Research on Cancer (IARC). (2004b). Monographs on the evaluation of the carcinogenic risk of chemical to humans. Vol. 84. Some drinking-water disinfectants and contaminants, including arsenic. IARC Press, Lyon, France.

International Agency for Research on Cancer. (2004c). Monographs on the evaluation of the carcinogenic risk of chemical to humans. Vol. 85. Betel quid and areca-nut chewing and some areca-nut-derived nitrosamines. IARC Press, Lyon, France.

International Agency for Research on Cancer. (2008a). World Cancer Report 2008. IARC Press, Lyon, France.

International Agency for Research on Cancer. (2008b). Monographs on the evaluation of the carcinogenic risk of chemical to humans. Vol. 97. 1,3-Butadiene, ethylene oxide, and vinyl halides (vinyl fluoride, vinyl chloride, vinyl bromide). IARC Press, Lyon, France.

International Agency for Research on Cancer (IARC). (2011). Monographs on the evaluation of the carcinogenic risk to humans. Vol. 100A. A review of human carcinogens: pharmaceuticals. IARC Press, Lyon, France.

Jick, H,. & Herman R. (1978). Oral contraceptive-induced benign liver tumors. The magnitude of the problem. *J Am Med Assoc*, 240, 828-829.

Jin, X., Moskophidis, D., Mivechi, N.F. (2011). Heat shock transcription factor 1 is a key determinant of HCC development by regulating hepatic steatosis and metabolic syndrome. *Cell Metab*, 14(1), 91-103.

Johnson, F.L., Lerner, K.G., and Siegal M. (1972). Association of androgenic-anabolic steroid therapy with development of hepatocellular carcinoma. *Lancet*, 2, 1273-1276.

Kaidar-Person, O., Bar-Sela, G., Person B. (2011). The two major epidemics of the twenty-first century: obesity and cancer. *Obes Surg*, in press.

Kammoun, H.L., Chabanon, H., Hainault, I., et al. (2009a). GRP78 expression inhibits insulin and ER stress-induced SREBP-1c activation and reduces hepatic steatosis in mice. *J Clin Invest*, 119(5), 1201-1215.

Kammoun, H.L., Hainault, I., Ferré, P., et al. (2009b). Nutritional related liver disease: targeting the endoplasmic reticulum stress. *Curr Opin Clin Nutr Metab Care*, 12, 575-582.

Kavlock, R.J., Daston, G.P., DeRosa, C., et al. (1996). Research needs for the risk assessment of health and environmental effects of endocrine disruptors: a report of the U.S. EPA-sponsored workshop. *Environ Health Perspect*, 104 Suppl 4, 715-740.

Kim, E.H., Koh, E.H., Park, J.Y., et al. (2010) Adenine nucleotide translocator as a regulator of mitochondrial function: implication in the pathogenesis of metabolic syndrome. *Korean Diabetes J*, 34(3), 146-153.

Kinosita, R. (1936). Researches on the carcinogenesis of the various chemical substances. *Gann*, 30, 423.

Klatskin, G. (1977). Hepatic tumors. Possible relation to use of oral contraceptives. *Gastroenterology*, 73, 386-394.

Koischwitz, V.D., Lelbach, W.K., Lackner, K. et al. (1981). Das vinylchloridinduzierte Leberangiosarkoma und hepatozellulare Karzinom. *Fortschr Rontgenstr*, 134, 283-290.

Kovacic, P. (2010). How dangerous are phthalate plasticizers? Integrated approach to toxicity based on metabolism, electron transfer, reactive oxygen species and cell signaling. *Med Hypotheses*, 74(4), 626-628.

Lacassagne, A. (1936). Hormonal pathogenesis of adenocarcinoma of the breast. *Am J Cancer*, 27: 217–225.

Lagiou, P., Kuper, H., Stuver, S.O., et al. (2000). Role of diabetes mellitus in the etiology of hepatocellular carcinoma. *J Natl Cancer Inst*, 92, 1096-1099.

Laquer, G.L., Mickelsen, O., Whiting, M.G., et al. (1963). Carcinogenic properties of nuts from Cycas circinalis L. indigenous to Guam. *J Natl Cancer Inst*, 31, 919-951.

Laurent-Puig, P., Legoix, P., Bluteau, O., et al. (2001). Genetic alterations associated with hepatocellular carcinomas define distinct pathways of hepatocarcinogenesis. *Gastroenterology*, 120, 1763-1773.

Lehnert, B.E., Goodwin, E.H., Deshpande, A. (1997). Extracellular factor(s) following exposure to alpha particles can cause sister chromatid exchanges in normal human cells. *Cancer Res*, 57, 2164-2171.

Li, X., Zhang, K., Li, Z. (2011). Unfolded protein response in cancer: the physician's perspective. *J Hematol Oncol*, 4 (8) 1-10.

Long, E.L., Nelson, A.A., Fitzhugh, O.G., et al. (1963). Liver tumors produced in rats by feeding safrole. *Arch Pathol*, 75, 595-604.

Ludwig, J.A., & Weinstein, J.N. (2005). Biomarkers in cancer staging, prognosis and treatment selection. *Nat Rev Cancer*, 11, 845-56.

Magee, P.N., & Barnes, J.M. (1956). The production of malignant primary hepatic tumors in the rat by feeding dimethylnitrosamine. *Br J Cancer*, 10, 114-122.

Maltoni, C., Lefemine, G., Ciliberti, A., et al. (1984). *Experimental research on vinyl chloride carcinogenesis. Archives of Research on Industrial Carcinogenesis, vol II*. Princeton Scientific Publishers, Princeton, NJ.

Maltoni, C., Lefemine, G., & Cotti, G. (1986). *Experimental research on trichloroethylene carcinogenesis. Archives of Research on Industrial Carcinogenesis, vol V*. Princeton Scientific Publishers, Princeton, NJ.

Maltoni, C., Ciliberti, A., Cotti, G., et al. (1989). Benzene, an experimental multipotential carcinogen: results of the long-term bioassays performed at the Bologna Institute of Oncology. *Environ Health Perspect*, 82, 109-124.

Maltoni, C., Minardi, F., Pinto C., et al. (1997). Results of three life-span experimental carcinogenicity and anticarcinogenicity studies on tamoxifen in rats. In: Preventive strategies for Living in a chemical World, *Ann NY Acad Sci*, 837, 469-512.

Marek, C.B., Peralta, R.M., Itinose, A.M., et al. (2011). Influence of tamoxifen on gluconeogenesis and glycolysis in the perfused rat liver. *Chem Biol Interact*, 193(1), 22-33.

Maronpot, R.R. (2009). Biological basis of differential susceptibility to hepatocarcinogenesis among mouse strains. *J Toxicol Pathol*, 22, 11-33.

Maronpot, R.R., Flake, G., Huff, J. (2004). Relevance of animal carcinogenesis findings to human cancer predictions and prevention. *Toxicol Pathol* 32(Suppl. 1): 40-48.

Marrero, J.A., Fontana, R.J., Su, G.L., et al. (2002). NAFLD may be a common underlying liver disease in patients with hepatocellular carcinoma in the United States. *Hepatology*, 36, 1349-1354.

Masumo, H., Kidani, T., Sekiya, K., et al. (2002). Bisphenol A in combination with insulin can accelerate the conversion of 3T3L1 fibroblasts to adipocytes. *J Lipid Res*, 43, 676-684.

McCullough, A. (2004). The epidemiology and risk factors of NASH. In: *Fatty liver disease: NASH and related disorders*. Farrel GC, George J, Hall P, McCullough A Eds, 23-37, Blackwell Publishing, Oxford.

McGlynn, K.A., Tsao, L., Hsing A.W., et al. (2001). International trends and pattern of primary liver cancer. *Int J Cancer*, 94, 290-296.

Minardi, F., Belpoggi, F., Soffritti, M., et al. (1994). Studio sperimentale sugli effetti a lungo termine del tamoxifen sul fegato di ratto. In: *I tumori primitivi e secondari del fegato,* Natale, C., Laricchiuta, D. et al. Società Italiana di Prevenzione Diagnosi e Terapia dei Tumori, Monduzzi Editore, Bologna, Italy.

Ministère de la Santé et de la Solidarité. (2006). *Programme National Nutrition Santé*. Retrieved from http://www.sante.gouv.fr/IMG/pdf/synthese_et_sommaire_PNNS_.pdf

Mita, L., Bianco, M., Viggiano, E., et al. (2011). Bisphenol A content in fish caught in two different sites of the Tyrrhenian sea (Italy). *Chemosphere*, 82(3), 405-410.

Møller, H., Mellemgaard, A., Lindvig, K., et al. (1994). Obesity and cancer risk: a Danish record-linkage study. *Eur J Cancer*, 30A, 344-350.

Mueller KM, Kornfeld JW, Friedbichler K, et al. (2011). Impairment of hepatic growth hormone and glucocorticoid receptor signaling causes steatosis and hepatocellular carcinoma in mice. *Hepatology* In press.

Nadeau, K., Klingensmith, G., & Sokol, R.J. (2003). Case report: steatohepatitis in a teenage girl with type 2 diabetes. *Curr Opin Pediatr*, 15(1), 127-131.

National Toxicology Program (NTP). (2011). Chemicals associated with site-specific tumor induction in liver. Available on: http://ntp.niehs.nih.gov/?objectid=E1D17854-123F-7908-7B168177A810AEDC.

Nazarewicz, R.R., Zenebe, W.J., Parihar, A., et al. (2007). Tamoxifen induces oxidative stress and mitochondrial apoptosis via stimulating mitochondrial nitric oxide synthase. *Cancer Res*, 67(3), 1282-1290.

Oh, S.W., Yoon, Y.S., Shin, S.A. (2005). Effects of excess weight on cancer incidences depending on cancer sites and histologic findings among men: Korea National Health Insurance Corporation Study. *J Clin Oncol*, 23, 4742-4754.

Olsen, J.H., Dragsted, L,. & Autrup H. (1988). Cancer risk and occupational exposure to aflatoxins in Denmark. *Br J Cancer*, 58, 392-396.

Ozcan, U., Cao, Q., Yilmaz, E., et al. (2004). Endoplasmic reticulum stress links obesity, insulin action, and type 2 diabetes. *Science*, 306, 457-461.

Page, J.M. & Harrison, S.A. (2009). NASH and HCC. *Clin Liv Dis*, 13, 631-647.

Palmer, J.R., Wise, L.A., Hatch, E.E., et al. (2006). Prenatal diethylstilbestrol exposure and risk of breast cancer. Cancer *Epidemiol Biomarkers Prev* 8, 1509-1514.

Parfieniuk, A. & Flisiak, R. (2008). Role of cannabinoids in chronic liver diseases. World J Gastroenterol, 14, 6109-6114.

Parkin DM, Bray F, Ferlay J et al. (2005). Global cancer statistics 2002. *CA Cancer J Clin*, 55, 74-108.

Pei, Y., Zhang, T., Renault, V.,et al. (2009). An overview of hepatocellular carcinoma study by omics-based methods. *Acta Biochim Biophys Sin (Shanghai)*, 41(1), 1-15.

Pereira, C., Mapuskar, K., Rao, C.V. (2006). Chronic toxicity of diethyl phthalate in male Wistar rats--a dose-response study. *Regul Toxicol Pharmacol*, 45(2), 169-177.

Pérez-Fuenteaja, A., Lupton, S., Clapsadl, M., et al. (2010). PCB and PBDE levels in wild common carp (Cyprinus carpio) from eastern Lake Eire. *Chemosphere*, 81(4): 541-547.

Pessayre, D. & Fromenty, B (2005). NASH: a mitochondrial disease. J Hepatol, 42, 928-940.

Pirastu, R., Comba, P., Reggiani, A., et al. (1990). Mortality from liver disease among Italian vinyl chloride monomer/polyvinyl chloride manufacturers. *Am J Ind Med*, 17,155-161.

Potter, V.R. (1958). The biochemical approach to the cancer problem. *Fed Proc*, 17, 691-697.

Puigserver, P., Wu, Z., Park, C.W., et al. (1998). A cold-inducible coactivator of nuclear receptors linked to adaptive thermogenesis. *Cell*, 92(6), 829-839.

Purchase, I.F.H., & Van der Watt J.J. (1970). Carcinogenicity of sterigmatocystin. *Food Cosmet Toxicol*, 8, 289-295.

Puri, P., Mirshahi, F., Cheung, O., et al. (2008). Activation and dysregulation of the unfolded protein response in nonalcoholic fatty liver disease. *Gastroenterology*, 134, 568-576.

Purushotham, A., Schug, T.T., Xu, Q., et al. (2009). Hepatocyte-specific deletion of SIRT1 alters fatty acid metabolism and results in hepatic steatosis and inflammation. *Cell Metab*, 9(4), 327-338.

Rael, L.T., Bar-Or, R., Ambruso, D.R., et al. (2009). Phthalate esters used as plasticizers in packed red blood cell storage bags may lead to progressive toxin exposure and the release of pro-inflammatory cytokines. *Oxid Med Cell Longev*, 2(3), 166-171.

Rashid, M., Roberts, E.A. (2000). Nonalcoholic steatohepatitis in children. *J Pediatr Gastroenterol Nutr*, 30(1), 48-53.

Rector, R.S., Thyfault, J.P., Uptergrove, G.M., et al. (2010). Mitochondrial dysfunction precedes insulin resistance and hepatic steatosis and contributes to the natural history of non-alcoholic fatty liver disease in an obese rodent model. *J Hepatol*, 52(5), 727-736.

Ren, H., Aleksunes, L.M., Wood, C., et al. (2010). Characterization of peroxisome proliferator-activated receptor alpha--independent effects of PPARalpha activators in the rodent liver: di-(2-ethylhexyl) phthalate also activates the constitutive-activated receptor. *Toxicol Sci*, 113(1), 45-59.

Rogers, A.B., Theve, E.J., Feng, Y., et al. (2007). Hepatocellular carcinoma associated with liver-gender disruption in male mice. *Cancer Res*, 67(24), 11536-11546.

Russo, J. & Russo, I.H. (2006). The role of estrogen in the initiation of breast cancer. *J Steroid Biochem Mol Biol*; 102, 89-96.

Saffroy, R., Pham, P., Reffas, M., et al. (2007). New perspectives and strategy research biomarkers for hepatocellular carcinoma. *Clin Chem Lab Med*, 45, 1169-1179.

Salvucci, M., Lemoine, A., Saffroy, R., et al. (1999). Microsatellite instability in European hepatocellular carcinoma. *Oncogene*, 18(1), 181-187.

Sanyal, A.J., Campbell-Sargent, C., Mirshahi, F., et al. (2001). Nonalcoholic steatohepatitis: association of insulin resistance and mitochondrial abnormalities. *Gastroenterology*, 120, 1183-1192.

Sato N. (2007). Central role of mitochondria in metabolic regulation of liver pathophysiology. *J Gastroenterol Hepatol*, 22 (Suppl1), S1-6.

Scatena, R., Bottoni, P., Giardina, B. (2008). Mitochondria, PPARs, and Cancer: Is Receptor-Independent Action of PPAR Agonists a Key? *PPAR Res*, 2008, 256251.

Scatena, R., Bottoni, P., Martorana, G.E., et al. (2004). Mitochondrial respiratory chain dysfunction, a non-receptor-mediated effect of synthetic PPAR-ligands: biochemical and pharmacological implications. *Biochem Biophys Res Commun*, 319(3), 967-973.

Schmal, D., Preussmann, R., & Hamperl H. (1960). Leberkrebs erzengende Wirkung von Diathylnitrosamin mach oraler Gabe bei Ratten. *Naturwissenschaften*, 47, 89.

Schreiber, S.N., Emter, R., Hock, M.B., et al. (2004). The estrogen-related receptor alpha (ERRalpha) functions in PPARgamma coactivator 1alpha (PGC-1alpha)-induced mitochondrial biogenesis. *Proc Natl Acad Sci U S A*, 101(17), 6472-6477.

Schröder, M. & Kaufman, R.J. (2005). The mammalian unfolded protein response. *Annu Rev Biochem*, 74, 739-789.

Schwimmer, J.B., Deutsch, R., Kahen, T., et al. (2006). Prevalence of fatty liver in children and adolescents. *Pediatrics*, 118(4), 1388-1393.

Seo, H.Y., Kim, Y.D., Lee, K.M., et al. (2008). Endoplasmic reticulum stress-induced activation of activating transcription factor 6 decreases insulin gene expression via up-regulation of orphan nuclear receptor small heterodimer partner. *Endocrinology*, 149(8), 3832-3841.

Shah, I., Houck, K., Judson, R.S., et al. (2011). Using nuclear receptor activity to stratify hepatocarcinogens. *PLoS One*, 6(2), e14584.

Shaw, J.J. & Shah, S.A. 2011. Rising incidence and demographics of hepatocellular carcinoma in the USA: what does it mean? Expert Rev Gastroenterol Hepatol, 5(3), 365-370.

Shuda, M., Kondoh, N., Imazeki, N., et al. (2003). Activation of the ATF6, XBP1 and grp78 genes in human hepatocellular carcinoma: a possible involvement of the ER stress pathway in hepatocarcinogenesis. *J Hepatol*, 38(5), 605-614.

Skill, N.J., Scott, R.E., Wu, J., et al. (2011). Hepatocellular carcinoma associated lipid metabolism reprogramming. *J Surg Res*, 169(1), 51-56.

Snyder, R.L., Tyler, G. & Summers J. (1982). Chronic hepatitis and hepatocellular carcinoma associated with woodchuck hepatitis virus. *Am J Pathol*, 107, 422-425.

Soffritti, M, & McConnell EE. (1988). Liver foci formation during Aflatoxin B1 carcinogenesis in the rat. *Ann NY Acad Sci*, 534, 531-540.

Soffritti, M., Belpoggi, F., Minardi, F., et al. (2002). Ramazzini Foundation cancer program: history and major projects, life-span carcinogenicity bioassays design, chemical studies, and results. *Ann NY Acad Sci*, 982, 26-45.

Soffritti, M., Belpoggi, F., Manservigi, M., et al. (2010). Aspartame administered in feed, beginning prenatally through life span, induces cancers of the liver and lung in male Swiss mice. *Am J Ind Med*, 53, 1197-1206.

Somm, E., Schwitzgebel, V.M., Toulotte, A., et al. (2009). Perinatal exposure to bisphenol a alters early adipogenesis in the rat. *Environ Health Perspect*, 117(10), 1549-1555.

Sonoda, J., Mehl, I.R., Chong, L.W., et al. (2007). PGC-1beta controls mitochondrial metabolism to modulate circadian activity, adaptive thermogenesis, and hepatic steatosis. *Proc Natl Acad Sci U S A*, 104(12), 5223-5228.

Sørensen, H.T., Mellemkjaer, L., Jepsen, P., et al. (2003). Risk of cancer in patients hospitalized with fatty liver: a Danish cohort study. *J Clin Gastroenterol*, 36, 356-359.

Soto, A.M., & Sonnenschein, C. (2004). The somatic mutation theory of cancer: growing problems with the paradigm? *Bioassays*, 26, 1097-1107.

Soto, A.M., & Sonnenschein, C. (2010). Environmental causes of cancer: endocrine disruptors as carcinogens. *Nat Rev Endocrinol* 6(7), 363-370.

Starley, B.Q., Calcagno, C.J., & Harrison, S.A. (2010). Nonalcoholic fatty liver disease and hepatocellular carcinoma: a weighty connection. *Hepatology*, 51, 1820-1832.

Sundaram, S.S., Zeitler, P., & Nadeau, K. (2009). The metabolic syndrome and nonalcoholic fatty liver disease in children. *Curr Opin Pediatr*, 21(4), 529-535.

Swoboda, D.J., and Reddy, J.K. (1972). Malignant tumors in rats given lasiocarpine. *Cancer Res*, 32, 908-912.

Tabuchi, Y., Takasaki, I., Kondo, T. (2006). Identification of genetic networks involved in the cell injury accompanying endoplasmic reticulum stress induced by bisphenol A in testicular Sertoli cells. *Biochem Biophys Res Commun*, 345(3), 1044-1050.

Takizawa, D., Kakizaki, S., Horiguchi, N., et al. (2011). Constitutive active/androstane receptor promotes hepatocarcinogenesis in a mouse model of non-alcoholic steatohepatitis. *Carcinogenesis*, 32(4), 576-583.

Teebor, G.W., & Becker FF. (1971). Regression and persistence of hyperplastic hepatic nodules induced by N-2-Fluorenilacetamide and their relationship to hepatocarcinogenesis. *Cancer Res*, 31, 1-3.

Ter Veld, M.G., Zawadzka, E., van den Berg, J.H., et al. (2008). Food-associated estrogenic compounds induce estrogen receptor-mediated luciferase gene expression in transgenic male mice. *Chem Biol Interact*, 174(2), 126-33.

Terayama, H. (1967). Aminoazo carcinogenesis methods and biochemical problems. *Methods Cancer Res*, 1, 399-449.

Upton AC. Radiation carcinogenesis. (1968). *Methods Cancer Res*, 4, 53-82.

Upton AC., Furth J. and Burnett WT. (1956). Liver damage and hepatomas in mice produced by radioactive colloidal gold. *Cancer Res*, 16, 211-215.

Uraguchi, K., Saito, M., Noguchi, Y., et al. (1972). Chronic toxicity and carcinogenicity in mice of the purified mycotoxins, luteoskyrin and cychloclorotine. *Food Cosmet Toxicol*, 10, 193-207.

Vandenberg, L.N., Maffini, M.V., Schaeberle C.M., et al. (2008). Perinatal exposure to the xenoestrogen bisphenol-A induces mammary intraductal hyperplasias in adult CD-1 mice. *Reprod Toxicol*, 26(3-4), 210-219.

Vander Heiden, M.G., Cantley, L.C., & Thompson, C.B. (2009). Understanding the Warburg effect: the metabolic requirements of cell proliferation. *Science*, 324, 1029-1033.

VanSaun, M.N., Lee, I.K., Washington, M.K., et al. (2009). High fat diet induced hepatic steatosis establishes a permissive microenvironment for colorectal metastases and promotes primary dysplasia in a murine model. *Am J Pathol*, 175(1), 355-364.

Verderame, M., Prisco, M., Andreucci, P., et al. (2011). Experimentally nonylphenol-polluted diet induces the expression of silent genes VTG and Era in the liver of male lizard Podaris sicula. *Environ Pollut*, 159(5), 1101-1107.

Vickers, A.E. & Lucier, G.W. (1991). Estrogen receptor, epidermal growth factor receptor and cellular ploidy in elutriated subpopulations of hepatocytes during liver tumor promotion by 17 alpha-ethinylestradiol in rats. *Carcinogenesis*, 12, 391-399.

Villena, J.A. & Kralli, A. (2008). ERRalpha: a metabolic function for the oldest orphan. *Trends Endocrinol Metab* 19(8), 269-276.

Wagner, M., Zollner, G., Trauner, M. (2011). Nuclear receptors in liver disease. *Hepatology*, 53(3), 1023-1034.

Wang, Q., Zhao, X.F., Ji, Y.L., et al. (2010). Mitochondrial signaling pathway is also involved in bisphenol A induced germ cell apoptosis in testes. *Toxicol Lett*, 199(2), 129-135.

Wang, Y., Ausman, L.M., Greenberg, A.S., et al. (2009). Nonalcoholic steatohepatitis induced by a high-fat diet promotes diethylnitrosamine-initiated early hepatocarcinogenesis in rats. *Int J Cancer*, 124(3), 540-546.

Warburg, O. (1930). The metabolism of tumors: investigation from the Kaiser Wilhelm Institute for Biology, Berlin-Dahlem.

Welzel, T.M., Graubard, B.I., Zeuzem, S., et al. (2011). Metabolic syndome increases the risk of primary liver cancer in the United States: a study in the SEER-medicare database. *Hepatology*, 54(2) 463-471.

White DL, Li D, Nurgalieva Z, El-Serag HB. (2008). Genetic variants of glutathione S-transferase as possible risk factors for hepatocellular carcinoma: a HuGE systematic review and meta-analysis. *Am J Epidemiol*, 167(4), 377-389.

White House Task Force on Childhood Obesity. (2010). *Report to the President*. Retrieved from http://www.letsmove.gov/white-house-task-force-childhood-obesity-report-president

Wideroff, L., Gridley, G., Mellemkjaer, L., et al. (1997). Cancer incidence in a population-based cohort of patients hospitalized with diabetes mellitus in Denmark. *J Natl Cancer Inst*, 89, 1360-1365.

Williams, C.D., Stengel, J., Asike, M.I., et al. (2011). Prevalence of nonalcoholic fatty liver disease and nonalcoholic steatohepatitis among a largely middle-aged population utilizing ultrasound and liver biopsy: a prospective study. *Gastroenterology*, 140, 124-131.

Wingspread consensus statement 1992, as cited in Soto, A.M. & Sonnenschein, C. (2010).

Wilson, R.H., De Eds F., & Cox A.J. (1941). The toxicity and carcinogenic activity of 2-acetaminofluorene. *Cancer Res* 1, 595-608.

Wogan, GN., & Newberne, P.N. (1967). Dose-response characteristics of aflatoxin B1 carcinogenesis in rats. *Cancer Res*, 27, 2370-2376.

Wogan, G.N., Paglialunga, S. & Newberne PN. (1974). Carcinogenic effects of low dietary levels of aflatoxin B1 in rats. *Food Cosmet Toxicol*, 12, 681-685.

Wolk, A., Gridley, G., Svensson, M., et al. (2001). A prospective study of obesity and cancer risk (Sweden). *Cancer Causes Control*, 12, 13-21.

Wong, N., Lai, P., Pang, E., et al. (2000). Genomic aberrations in human hepatocellular carcinomas of differing etiologies. *Clin Cancer Res*, 6, 4000-4009.

World Health Organization. (2006). *European Charter on Counteracting Obesity*. WHO Press, retrieved from
http://www.euro.who.int/__data/assets/pdf_file/0009/87462/E89567.pdf

World Health Organization. (2008). *Global Burden of Disease: 2004 update*. WHO Press , retrieved from
http://www.who.int/healthinfo/global_burden_disease/2004_report_update/en/index.html

Wu, Z., Puigserver, P., Andersson, U., et al. (1999). Mechanisms controlling mitochondrial biogenesis and respiration through the thermogenic coactivator PGC-1. *Cell*, 98(1), 115-124.

Yang, F., Huang, X., Yi, T et al. (2007). Spontaneous development of liver tumors in the absence of the bile acid receptor farnesoid X receptor. *Cancer Res*, 67, 863-867.

Yang, S., Zhu, H., Li, Y., et al. (2000). Mitochondrial adaptations to obesity-related oxidant stress. *Arch Biochem Biophys*, 378(2), 259-268.

Yeh, F.S., Mo, C.C., & Yen RC. (1985). Risk factors for hepatocellular carcinoma in Guangxi, people's Republic of China. *Natl Cancer Inst Monogr*, 69, 47-48.

Yin, P.H., Wu, C.C., Lin, J.C., et al. (2010). Somatic mutations of mitochondrial genome in hepatocellular carcinoma. *Mitochondrion*, 10(2), 174-182.

Zender, L., Spector, M.S., Xue, W., et al. (2006). Identification and validation of oncogenes in liver cancer using an integrative oncogenomic approach. *Cell*, 125(7), 1253-1267.

2

The Relationship Between Nonalcoholic Fatty Liver Disease and Hepatocellular Carcinoma

Misael Uribe, Jesús Román-Sandoval,
Norberto C. Chávez-Tapia and Nahum Méndez-Sánchez
*Medica Sur Clinic and Foundation, Biomedical Research
Department and Liver Research Unit, Mexico City
Mexico*

1. Introduction

Hepatocellular carcinoma (HCC) is the most prevalent type of primary liver cancer, the fifth most common type of solid tumor, and the third highest cause of cancer mortality worldwide (Parkin et al., 2005, Motola-Kuba et al., 2006). On the other hand, nonalcoholic fatty liver disease (NAFLD) is now recognized as one of the most common liver disorders (Lazo and Clark, 2008). The subclinical nature of this disease has prompted research to improve its diagnosis and prevent its progression to nonalcoholic steatohepatitis (NASH), liver cirrhosis, and HCC. An increasing number of reports indicate that NAFLD is the key link between obesity and HCC (Chavez-Tapia et al., 2009, Mendez-Sanchez et al., 2007). It has been suggested that most cases of HCC involve progression of NASH to cirrhosis (Caldwell et al., 2004). In 1980, Ludwig et al. described NASH as an advanced form of fatty liver disease. They defined it as a well-recognized clinical pathological syndrome that occurs primarily in obese women with diabetes mellitus and has histological similarities to alcoholic liver disease in the absence of heavy alcohol consumption (Ludwig et al., 1980). Some reports suggest that 10–24% of the populations of various countries have NAFLD. The prevalence of NAFLD is higher among obese and diabetic patients (70–86%). NASH is estimated to occur in 10% of NAFLD patients. NASH has been posited as a possible cause of cryptogenic cirrhosis (CC) (Bellentani et al., 2000). Patients with CC also develop HCC (Caldwell et al., 1999). In this review, we discuss the associations between obesity and cancer, between metabolic syndrome and NAFLD, and between NAFLD and HCC.

2. Obesity and cancer

The World Health Organization defines obesity as fat accumulation in adipose tissue to the extent that health is impaired. For epidemiological purposes, overweight is defined as a body mass index (BMI) greater than 25 kg/m² and obesity is defined as a BMI greater than 30 kg/m².

Epidemiological studies provide convincing evidence of an association between obesity and cancer of the esophagus (adenocarcinoma), pancreas, colorectum, breast (postmenopausal), endometrium, and kidney (WCR, 2007). The largest meta-analysis to date involved 282,000 patients from prospective observational studies and more than 133 million person-years of follow-up. It showed that a high BMI is associated with a high incidence of cancer. The association is modest and risk estimates range from 1.1 to 1.6 for an increase in BMI of 5 kg/m². For people with an average BMI (23 kg/m²), a 5 kg/m² increase in BMI corresponds to a weight gain of 15 kg (men) or 13 kg (women). The associations between obesity and cancer are sex and site specific but are broadly consistent across geographic populations (Renehan et al., 2008). Emerging evidence suggests that weight loss after bariatric surgery reduces the incidence of cancer (Sjostrom et al., 2009). Furthermore, a prospective study of 900,000 adults in the United States showed that obesity accounts for 14% of all deaths from cancer in men and for 20% of all deaths from cancer in women (Calle et al., 2003) (Fig.1). Men and women with a BMI greater than 40 kg/m² have death rates 52% and 62%, respectively, higher than those of people with normal BMIs. This indicates that obesity also affects the outcome of cancer and this finding is supported by studies showing increased perioperative mortality rates for obese people (Li et al., 2009, Meyerhardt et al., 2003, Haydon et al., 2006, Dignam et al., 2006). There appears to a sex differential with respect to the risk of developing cancer: men have a higher risk than women of developing cancer when their BMI is elevated (Renehan et al., 2008, Moore et al., 2004). This may be due to hormonal differences or it may indicate that BMI is a poor index of central adiposity in females. As females generally only deposit adipose tissue centrally when the total volume of deposited fat is elevated, overweight BMIs do not correspond with visceral fat volume in females to the same extent as in males, which may account for the differences in cancer risk observed when BMI is used to determine obesity status.

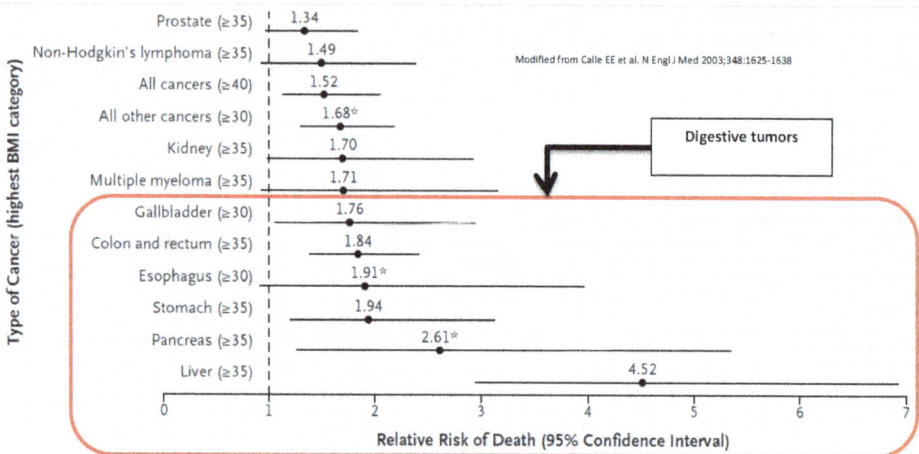

Fig. 1. Mortality from cancer in obese men in the USA.
The highest relative risk was observed in liver cancer. It is also important to note that gastrointestinal tumors are associated with the highest relative risk of death according to BMI and obesity.

In studies in which measures of visceral adiposity such as waist circumference (WC) or visceral fat adiposity (VFA) were used, visceral adiposity was associated with an increased risk of cancer (Moore et al., 2004, Wang et al., 2008, Steffen et al., 2009); it is a stronger predictor of cancer than BMI (Moore et al., 2004), and the cancer risk is similar for males and females (Moore et al., 2004, Wang et al., 2008). Large-scale studies on visceral adiposity across cancer sites are needed to clarify whether there is a clear differential effect of visceral versus subcutaneous obesity. Visceral adiposity (and not subcutaneous adiposity) is associated with development of features of metabolic syndrome (a proxy for a dysmetabolic profile in viscerally obese patients) (Donohoe et al., 2010). Most of the components of the syndrome, alone (Cowey and Hardy, 2006, Giovannucci, 2007) or in combination (Colangelo et al., 2002, Bowers et al., 2006, Trevisan et al., 2001), have been individually linked to cancer at various sites. A prospective international population-based study of 580,000 people (the Me-Can Study) is under way to identify whether metabolic syndrome is independently associated with cancer. Initial findings suggest that a combination of components of metabolic syndrome is associated with colorectal cancer (men RR, 1.25 [95% CI, 1.18–1.32]; women RR, 1.14 [95% CI, 1.02–1.18]) (Stocks et al., 2010), endometrial cancer (RR, 1.37; [95% CI, 1.28–1.46]) (Bjorge et al., 2010), bladder cancer in men (RR, 1.1; [95% CI, 1.01–1.18]) (Stocks et al., 2010), and pancreatic cancer in women (RR, 1.58; [95% CI, 1.34–1.87])(Johansen et al., 2010).

3. Metabolic syndrome and NAFLD

Metabolic syndrome is a condition characterized by a cluster of symptoms, including glucose intolerance/insulin resistance, abdominal obesity, atherogenic dysfunction, dyslipidemia (low concentrations of high-density lipoprotein cholesterol and high concentrations of triglycerides), elevated blood pressure, a proinflammatory state, and a prothrombotic state. It increases morbidity and mortality, especially in respect of cardiovascular disease (Reaven, 2002, Grundy et al., 2004). NAFLD can be considered the hepatic manifestation of metabolic syndrome (Fig. 2) (Rector et al., 2008). NAFLD is strongly associated with metabolic syndrome; 90% of patients with NAFLD have more than one feature of metabolic syndrome and 33% have three or more features (Marchesini et al., 2003). Furthermore, the risk of steatosis increases exponentially as the number of components of metabolic syndrome increases (Marceau et al., 1999). NAFLD has been consistently associated with obesity (60–95%), type 2 diabetes (28–55%), and dyslipidemia (27–92%) (Bugianesi et al., 2005). Metabolic syndrome is associated with liver disease, which may progress and become severe. In addition, the likelihood of developing NASH increases with

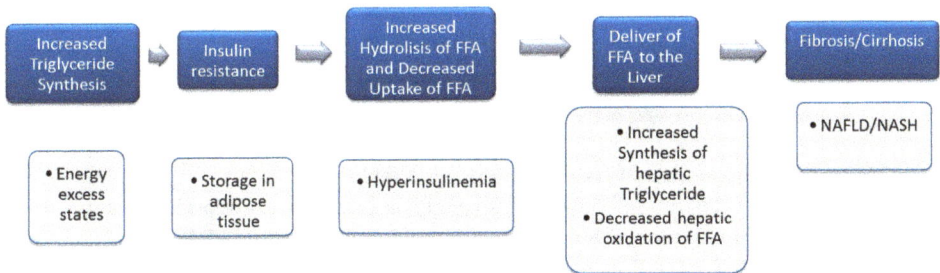

Fig. 2. Triglyceride synthesis and NAFLD.
Triglyceride synthesis increases in states of energy excess. Insulin resistance and hyperinsulinemia increase lipolysis of triglyceride depots in adipose tissue, amplifying the delivery of free fatty acids Free Fatty Acids (FFA) to the liver. Insulin further stimulates liver triglyceride synthesis while inhibiting fatty acid oxidation, inhibiting the production of very-low-density lipoproteins.

the severity of obesity (Bugianesi et al., 2005, Marchesini et al., 2003). There is a universal association between NASH and insulin resistance regardless of BMI, suggesting that insulin resistance is a central factor in the pathogenesis of NASH (Chitturi et al., 2002). The elevated expression of tumor necrosis factor-alpha (TNF-α) in the liver observed in NAFLD may represent a link between insulin resistance and hepatic steatosis. TNF-α has been proposed as an important component of peripheral insulin resistance in obesity and type 2 diabetes. It is linked to increased oxidative stress and cell death in the liver, and potentiates the development of liver fibrosis and progression to NASH (Jiang and Torok, 2008).

4. NAFLD and HCC

It is clear that cirrhosis is linked to the development of HCC regardless of the underlying etiology of liver disease. The exact mechanism responsible for the development of HCC in NASH remains unclear, although the pathophysiological mechanisms responsible for the development of NASH associated with insulin resistance and the subsequent inflammatory cascade likely contribute to the carcinogenic potential of NASH.

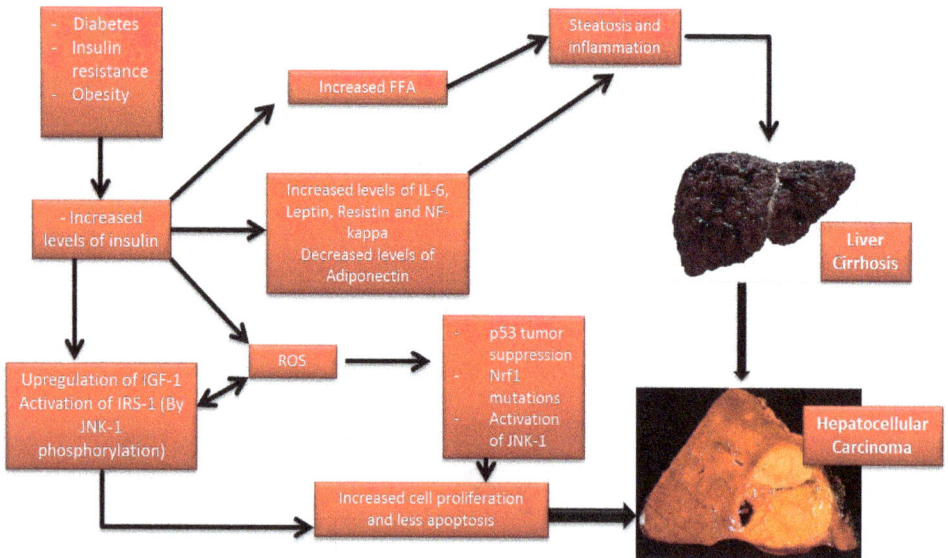

Fig. 3. Proposed pathogeneses of HCC in NAFLD/NASH.
Obesity, diabetes, and insulin resistance are strongly associated with hyperinsulinemia, which can trigger upregulation of IGF-1, activation of IRS-1, increased FFA release, increased secretion of TNF-α, IL-6, leptin, resistin, and NF-κ, and decreased production of adiponectin. Suppression of p53 and activation of JNK-1 result in cell proliferation and decreased apoptosis, which in turn result in HCC. ROS are also important in the pathogenesis of HCC. IGF-1, insulin growth factor-1; IRS-1, insulin receptor substrate-1; FFA, free fatty acid; TNF-α, tumor necrosis factor-alpha; IL-6, interleukin-6; NF-κ, nuclear factor-kappa; JNK-1, Jun amino-terminal kinase-1; HCC, hepatocellular carcinoma; ROS, reactive oxygen species.

Obesity and diabetes are risk factors for NASH and CC and have been implicated in multiple cancers, including HCC (Bugianesi et al., 2007). Insulin resistance associated with obesity, metabolic syndrome, and diabetes results in increased release of FFAs from adipocytes, increased secretion of proinflammatory cytokines such as TNF-α, increased secretion of interleukin-6, leptin, and resistin, and decreased secretion of adiponectin. These processes favor the development of hepatic steatosis and inflammation (Fig. 3) (Bugianesi et al., 2007, Harrison, 2006).

Hyperinsulinemia upregulates the production of insulin-like growth factor-1 (IGF1), a peptide hormone that stimulates growth through cellular proliferation and inhibition of apoptosis (Page and Harrison, 2009, Calle and Kaaks, 2004, Ish-Shalom et al., 1997). Insulin also activates insulin receptor substrate-1 (IRS-1), which is involved in cytokine signaling pathways and has been shown to be upregulated in HCC (Tanaka et al., 1997). The mannose 6-phosphate/IGF2 receptor (M6P/IGF2R) is involved by regulating cell growth and functions as a tumor suppressor. Mutations resulting in loss of heterozygosity for this receptor have been detected in 61% of patients with HCC (Yamada et al., 1997). Adiponectin is an anti-inflammatory polypeptide specific to adipose tissue that is decreased in insulin-resistant states and has been shown to inhibit angiogenesis via modulation of apoptosis in an animal model (Ukkola and Santaniemi, 2002, Brakenhielm et al., 2004). In an insulin-resistant state, these factors promote uninhibited cell growth and appear to play a significant role in the development of HCC in patients with NASH.

NASH is also associated with oxidative stress and the release of reactive oxygen species (ROS), which likely contribute to the development of HCC. An insulin-resistant obese mouse model demonstrated that ROS production is increased in the mitochondria of hepatocytes with fatty infiltration and that oxidative stress may be implicated in hepatic hyperplasia (Bugianesi et al., 2007, Yang et al., 2000). During carcinogenesis, epithelial hyperplasia and dysplasia generally precede cancer by many years (Bugianesi et al., 2007). C-Jun amino-terminal kinase 1 (JNK1) has also recently been linked to obesity, insulin resistance, NASH, and HCC. JNK1 is a ubiquitously expressed mitogen-activated protein kinase. Obesity is associated with abnormally elevated JNK activity (Hirosumi et al., 2002). In hyperinsulinemia, FFA, TNF-α, and ROS are potent activators of JNK, which in turn phosphorylates IRS-1 (Hirosumi et al., 2002, Gomaa et al., 2008). Evidence suggests that statins significantly decrease the risk of HCC in diabetic patients, presumably because of their anti-inflammatory properties (El-Serag and Rudolph, 2007, Huether et al., 2005, Kawata et al., 2001, El-Serag et al., 2009). Interestingly, atorvastatin therapy has been shown to acutely decrease expression of JNK and other inflammatory cells in patients with abdominal aortic aneurysms (Kajimoto et al., 2009). That statin treatment reduces JNK expression may explain, in part, the decreased risk of HCC in diabetic patients who receive statin therapy, although this has yet to be proven. Further studies linking statins and JNK activity with NASH and HCC may enable the development of therapeutic drugs for the prevention and treatment of NASH as well as HCC secondary to NASH. There is a lack of randomized controlled trials on the benefits of bariatric surgery for patients with NASH and obese patients in terms of prevention of HCC (Chavez-Tapia et al., 2010). (Fig. 4)

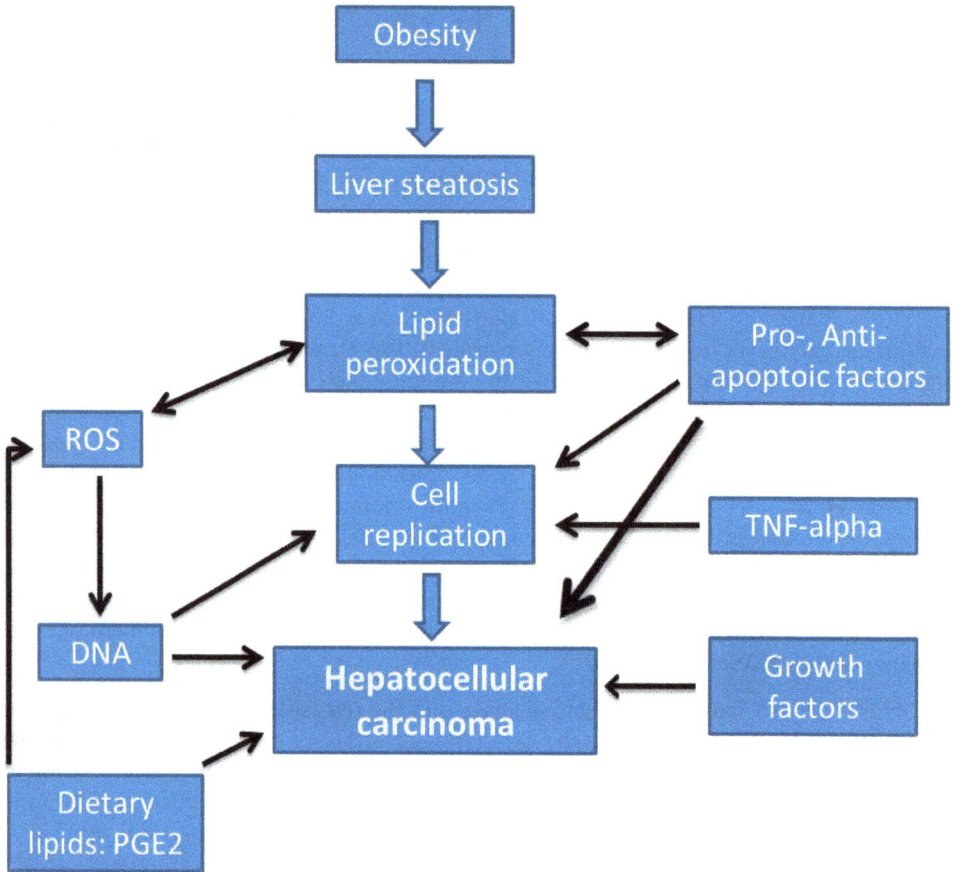

Fig. 4. Proposed progression of and significant factors in the pathogenesis of HCC in NAFLD. ROS, reactive oxygen species; DNA, deoxyribonucleic acid; PGE2, prostaglandin type 2; TNF-α, tumor necrosis factor-alpha

5. Conclusion

The most common cause of liver disease in developed countries is NAFLD, which includes NASH and its associated complications. The prevalence of NAFLD and NASH is likely higher than previously estimated and is associated with the growing epidemics of obesity and diabetes. There is increasing evidence showing that NASH may progress to HCC. The overall prevalence of HCC in patients with NAFLD remains low, although the incidence of HCC in developed countries is rising. HCC secondary to NASH typically develops when cirrhosis is present, although rare cases of HCC arising in cases of NASH without cirrhosis raise the possibility that carcinogenesis secondary to NAFLD can occur in the absence of advanced liver disease. The connection between NAFLD and progression to HCC is becoming clearer, and the increasing burden of NASH, diabetes mellitus, and obesity is becoming heavier. Community awareness of the potential for this disease to progress to

HCC is critical. Complications of NASH are expected to increase with the continuing epidemics of obesity and diabetes. Once a diagnosis of cirrhosis is made, screening for HCC should be pursued. Given recent epidemiological data on diabetes, thought should be given to the use of statins for NASH patients, particularly those with diabetes and hyperlipidemia. Further research is urgently needed to better elucidate the signaling pathways that result in HCC when insulin resistance is present. Studies evaluating potential targets for the treatment of NASH and HCC, including those targeting JNK activation, should be actively pursued.

6. References

Bellentani, S., Saccoccio, G., Masutti, F., Croce, L. S., Brandi, G., Sasso, F., Cristanini, G. & Tiribelli, C. 2000. Prevalence of and risk factors for hepatic steatosis in Northern Italy. *Annals of internal medicine*, 132, 112-7.

Bjorge, T., Stocks, T., Lukanova, A., Tretli, S., Selmer, R., Manjer, J., Rapp, K., Ulmer, H., Almquist, M., Concin, H., Hallmans, G., Jonsson, H., Stattin, P. & Engeland, A. 2010. Metabolic syndrome and endometrial carcinoma. *American journal of epidemiology*, 171, 892-902.

Bowers, K., Albanes, D., Limburg, P., Pietinen, P., Taylor, P. R., Virtamo, J. & Stolzenberg-Solomon, R. 2006. A prospective study of anthropometric and clinical measurements associated with insulin resistance syndrome and colorectal cancer in male smokers. *American journal of epidemiology*, 164, 652-64.

Brakenhielm, E., Veitonmaki, N., Cao, R., Kihara, S., Matsuzawa, Y., Zhivotovsky, B., Funahashi, T. & Cao, Y. 2004. Adiponectin-induced antiangiogenesis and antitumor activity involve caspase-mediated endothelial cell apoptosis. *Proceedings of the National Academy of Sciences of the United States of America*, 101, 2476-81.

Bugianesi, E., Mccullough, A. J. & Marchesini, G. 2005. Insulin resistance: a metabolic pathway to chronic liver disease. *Hepatology*, 42, 987-1000.

Bugianesi, E., Vanni, E. & Marchesini, G. 2007. NASH and the risk of cirrhosis and hepatocellular carcinoma in type 2 diabetes. *Current diabetes reports*, 7, 175-80.

Caldwell, S. H., Crespo, D. M., Kang, H. S. & Al-Osaimi, A. M. 2004. Obesity and hepatocellular carcinoma. *Gastroenterology*, 127, S97-103.

Caldwell, S. H., Oelsner, D. H., Iezzoni, J. C., Hespenheide, E. E., Battle, E. H. & Driscoll, C. J. 1999. Cryptogenic cirrhosis: clinical characterization and risk factors for underlying disease. *Hepatology*, 29, 664-9.

Calle, E. E. & Kaaks, R. 2004. Overweight, obesity and cancer: epidemiological evidence and proposed mechanisms. *Nature reviews. Cancer*, 4, 579-91.

Calle, E. E., Rodriguez, C., Walker-Thurmond, K. & Thun, M. J. 2003. Overweight, obesity, and mortality from cancer in a prospectively studied cohort of U.S. adults. *The New England journal of medicine*, 348, 1625-38.

Colangelo, L. A., Gapstur, S. M., Gann, P. H., Dyer, A. R. & Liu, K. 2002. Colorectal cancer mortality and factors related to the insulin resistance syndrome. *Cancer epidemiology, biomarkers & prevention : a publication of the American Association for Cancer Research, cosponsored by the American Society of Preventive Oncology*, 11, 385-91.

Cowey, S. & Hardy, R. W. 2006. The metabolic syndrome: A high-risk state for cancer? *The American journal of pathology*, 169, 1505-22.

Chavez-Tapia, N. C., Mendez-Sanchez, N. & Uribe, M. 2009. Role of nonalcoholic fatty liver disease in hepatocellular carcinoma. *Annals of hepatology : official journal of the Mexican Association of Hepatology,* 8 Suppl 1, S34-9.

Chavez-Tapia, N. C., Tellez-Avila, F. I., Barrientos-Gutierrez, T., Mendez-Sanchez, N., Lizardi-Cervera, J. & Uribe, M. 2010. Bariatric surgery for non-alcoholic steatohepatitis in obese patients. *Cochrane database of systematic reviews,* CD007340.

Chitturi, S., Abeygunasekera, S., Farrell, G. C., Holmes-Walker, J., Hui, J. M., Fung, C., Karim, R., Lin, R., Samarasinghe, D., Liddle, C., Weltman, M. & George, J. 2002. NASH and insulin resistance: Insulin hypersecretion and specific association with the insulin resistance syndrome. *Hepatology,* 35, 373-9.

Dignam, J. J., Polite, B. N., Yothers, G., Raich, P., Colangelo, L., O'connell, M. J. & Wolmark, N. 2006. Body mass index and outcomes in patients who receive adjuvant chemotherapy for colon cancer. *Journal of the National Cancer Institute,* 98, 1647-54.

Donohoe, C. L., Pidgeon, G. P., Lysaght, J. & Reynolds, J. V. 2010. Obesity and gastrointestinal cancer. *The British journal of surgery,* 97, 628-42.

El-Serag, H. B., Johnson, M. L., Hachem, C. & Morgana, R. O. 2009. Statins are associated with a reduced risk of hepatocellular carcinoma in a large cohort of patients with diabetes. *Gastroenterology,* 136, 1601-8.

El-Serag, H. B. & Rudolph, K. L. 2007. Hepatocellular carcinoma: epidemiology and molecular carcinogenesis. *Gastroenterology,* 132, 2557-76.

Giovannucci, E. 2007. Metabolic syndrome, hyperinsulinemia, and colon cancer: a review. *The American journal of clinical nutrition,* 86, s836-42.

Gomaa, A. I., Khan, S. A., Toledano, M. B., Waked, I. & Taylor-Robinson, S. D. 2008. Hepatocellular carcinoma: epidemiology, risk factors and pathogenesis. *World journal of gastroenterology : WJG,* 14, 4300-8.

Grundy, S. M., Brewer, H. B., Jr., Cleeman, J. I., Smith, S. C., Jr. & Lenfant, C. 2004. Definition of metabolic syndrome: Report of the National Heart, Lung, and Blood Institute/American Heart Association conference on scientific issues related to definition. *Circulation,* 109, 433-8.

Harrison, S. A. 2006. Liver disease in patients with diabetes mellitus. *Journal of clinical gastroenterology,* 40, 68-76.

Haydon, A. M., Macinnis, R. J., English, D. R. & Giles, G. G. 2006. Effect of physical activity and body size on survival after diagnosis with colorectal cancer. *Gut,* 55, 62-7.

Hirosumi, J., Tuncman, G., Chang, L., Gorgun, C. Z., Uysal, K. T., Maeda, K., Karin, M. & Hotamisligil, G. S. 2002. A central role for JNK in obesity and insulin resistance. *Nature,* 420, 333-6.

Huether, A., Hopfner, M., Baradari, V., Schuppan, D. & Scherubl, H. 2005. EGFR blockade by cetuximab alone or as combination therapy for growth control of hepatocellular cancer. *Biochemical pharmacology,* 70, 1568-78.

Ish-Shalom, D., Christoffersen, C. T., Vorwerk, P., Sacerdoti-Sierra, N., Shymko, R. M., Naor, D. & De Meyts, P. 1997. Mitogenic properties of insulin and insulin analogues mediated by the insulin receptor. *Diabetologia,* 40 Suppl 2, S25-31.

Jiang, J. & Torok, N. 2008. Nonalcoholic steatohepatitis and the metabolic syndrome. *Metabolic syndrome and related disorders,* 6, 1-7.

Johansen, D., Stocks, T., Jonsson, H., Lindkvist, B., Bjorge, T., Concin, H., Almquist, M., Haggstrom, C., Engeland, A., Ulmer, H., Hallmans, G., Selmer, R., Nagel, G., Tretli,

S., Stattin, P. & Manjer, J. 2010. Metabolic factors and the risk of pancreatic cancer: a prospective analysis of almost 580,000 men and women in the Metabolic Syndrome and Cancer Project. *Cancer epidemiology, biomarkers & prevention : a publication of the American Association for Cancer Research, cosponsored by the American Society of Preventive Oncology,* 19, 2307-17.

Kajimoto, K., Miyauchi, K., Kasai, T., Shimada, K., Kojima, Y., Shimada, A., Niinami, H., Amano, A. & Daida, H. 2009. Short-term 20-mg atorvastatin therapy reduces key inflammatory factors including c-Jun N-terminal kinase and dendritic cells and matrix metalloproteinase expression in human abdominal aortic aneurysmal wall. *Atherosclerosis,* 206, 505-11.

Kawata, S., Yamasaki, E., Nagase, T., Inui, Y., Ito, N., Matsuda, Y., Inada, M., Tamura, S., Noda, S., Imai, Y. & Matsuzawa, Y. 2001. Effect of pravastatin on survival in patients with advanced hepatocellular carcinoma. A randomized controlled trial. *British journal of cancer,* 84, 886-91.

Lazo, M. & Clark, J. M. 2008. The epidemiology of nonalcoholic fatty liver disease: a global perspective. *Seminars in liver disease,* 28, 339-50.

Li, D., Morris, J. S., Liu, J., Hassan, M. M., Day, R. S., Bondy, M. L. & Abbruzzese, J. L. 2009. Body mass index and risk, age of onset, and survival in patients with pancreatic cancer. *JAMA : the journal of the American Medical Association,* 301, 2553-62.

Ludwig, J., Viggiano, T. R., Mcgill, D. B. & Oh, B. J. 1980. Nonalcoholic steatohepatitis: Mayo Clinic experiences with a hitherto unnamed disease. *Mayo Clinic proceedings. Mayo Clinic,* 55, 434-8.

Marceau, P., Biron, S., Hould, F. S., Marceau, S., Simard, S., Thung, S. N. & Kral, J. G. 1999. Liver pathology and the metabolic syndrome X in severe obesity. *The Journal of clinical endocrinology and metabolism,* 84, 1513-7.

Marchesini, G., Bugianesi, E., Forlani, G., Cerrelli, F., Lenzi, M., Manini, R., Natale, S., Vanni, E., Villanova, N., Melchionda, N. & Rizzetto, M. 2003. Nonalcoholic fatty liver, steatohepatitis, and the metabolic syndrome. *Hepatology,* 37, 917-23.

Mendez-Sanchez, N., Arrese, M., Zamora-Valdes, D. & Uribe, M. 2007. Current concepts in the pathogenesis of nonalcoholic fatty liver disease. *Liver international : official journal of the International Association for the Study of the Liver,* 27, 423-33.

Meyerhardt, J. A., Catalano, P. J., Haller, D. G., Mayer, R. J., Benson, A. B., 3rd, Macdonald, J. S. & Fuchs, C. S. 2003. Influence of body mass index on outcomes and treatment-related toxicity in patients with colon carcinoma. *Cancer,* 98, 484-95.

Moore, L. L., Bradlee, M. L., Singer, M. R., Splansky, G. L., Proctor, M. H., Ellison, R. C. & Kreger, B. E. 2004. BMI and waist circumference as predictors of lifetime colon cancer risk in Framingham Study adults. *International journal of obesity and related metabolic disorders : journal of the International Association for the Study of Obesity,* 28, 559-67.

Motola-Kuba, D., Zamora-Valdes, D., Uribe, M. & Mendez-Sanchez, N. 2006. Hepatocellular carcinoma. An overview. *Annals of hepatology : official journal of the Mexican Association of Hepatology,* 5, 16-24.

Page, J. M. & Harrison, S. A. 2009. Nash and HCC. *Clinics in liver disease,* 13, 631-47.

Parkin, D. M., Bray, F., Ferlay, J. & Pisani, P. 2005. Global cancer statistics, 2002. *CA: a cancer journal for clinicians,* 55, 74-108.

Reaven, G. 2002. Metabolic syndrome: pathophysiology and implications for management of cardiovascular disease. *Circulation,* 106, 286-8.

Rector, R. S., Thyfault, J. P., Wei, Y. & Ibdah, J. A. 2008. Non-alcoholic fatty liver disease and the metabolic syndrome: an update. *World journal of gastroenterology : WJG*, 14, 185-92.

Renehan, A. G., Tyson, M., Egger, M., Heller, R. F. & Zwahlen, M. 2008. Body-mass index and incidence of cancer: a systematic review and meta-analysis of prospective observational studies. *Lancet*, 371, 569-78.

Sjostrom, L., Gummesson, A., Sjostrom, C. D., Narbro, K., Peltonen, M., Wedel, H., Bengtsson, C., Bouchard, C., Carlsson, B., Dahlgren, S., Jacobson, P., Karason, K., Karlsson, J., Larsson, B., Lindroos, A. K., Lonroth, H., Naslund, I., Olbers, T., Stenlof, K., Torgerson, J. & Carlsson, L. M. 2009. Effects of bariatric surgery on cancer incidence in obese patients in Sweden (Swedish Obese Subjects Study): a prospective, controlled intervention trial. *The lancet oncology*, 10, 653-62.

Steffen, A., Schulze, M. B., Pischon, T., Dietrich, T., Molina, E., Chirlaque, M. D., Barricarte, A., Amiano, P., Quiros, J. R., Tumino, R., Mattiello, A., Palli, D., Vineis, P., Agnoli, C., Misirli, G., Boffetta, P., Kaaks, R., Rohrmann, S., Bueno-De-Mesquita, H. B., Peeters, P. H., May, A. M., Spencer, E. A., Allen, N. E., Bingham, S., Tjonneland, A., Halkjaer, J., Overvad, K., Stegger, J., Manjer, J., Lindkvist, B., Hallmanns, G., Stenling, R., Lund, E., Riboli, E., Gonzalez, C. A. & Boeing, H. 2009. Anthropometry and esophageal cancer risk in the European prospective investigation into cancer and nutrition. *Cancer epidemiology, biomarkers & prevention : a publication of the American Association for Cancer Research, cosponsored by the American Society of Preventive Oncology*, 18, 2079-89.

Stocks, T., Borena, W., Strohmaier, S., Bjorge, T., Manjer, J., Engeland, A., Johansen, D., Selmer, R., Hallmans, G., Rapp, K., Concin, H., Jonsson, H., Ulmer, H. & Stattin, P. 2010. Cohort Profile: The Metabolic syndrome and Cancer project (Me-Can). *International journal of epidemiology*, 39, 660-7.

Tanaka, S., Mohr, L., Schmidt, E. V., Sugimachi, K. & Wands, J. R. 1997. Biological effects of human insulin receptor substrate-1 overexpression in hepatocytes. *Hepatology*, 26, 598-604.

Trevisan, M., Liu, J., Muti, P., Misciagna, G., Menotti, A. & Fucci, F. 2001. Markers of insulin resistance and colorectal cancer mortality. *Cancer epidemiology, biomarkers & prevention : a publication of the American Association for Cancer Research, cosponsored by the American Society of Preventive Oncology*, 10, 937-41.

Ukkola, O. & Santaniemi, M. 2002. Adiponectin: a link between excess adiposity and associated comorbidities? *Journal of molecular medicine*, 80, 696-702.

Wang, Y., Jacobs, E. J., Patel, A. V., Rodriguez, C., Mccullough, M. L., Thun, M. J. & Calle, E. E. 2008. A prospective study of waist circumference and body mass index in relation to colorectal cancer incidence. *Cancer causes & control : CCC*, 19, 783-92.

WCR, F. 2007. Food, nutrition, physical activity and the prevention of cancer: a global perspective. *American Institute for Cancer Research*, 2nd edition.

Yamada, T., De Souza, A. T., Finkelstein, S. & Jirtle, R. L. 1997. Loss of the gene encoding mannose 6-phosphate/insulin-like growth factor II receptor is an early event in liver carcinogenesis. *Proceedings of the National Academy of Sciences of the United States of America*, 94, 10351-5.

Yang, S., Zhu, H., Li, Y., Lin, H., Gabrielson, K., Trush, M. A. & Diehl, A. M. 2000. Mitochondrial adaptations to obesity-related oxidant stress. *Archives of biochemistry and biophysics*, 378, 259-68.

3

The Histomorphological and Immunohistochemical Diagnosis of Hepatocellular Carcinoma

Daniela Fanni, Clara Gerosa and Gavino Faa
University of Cagliari
Italy

1. Introduction

Hepatocellular carcinoma is one of the most common malignancies worldwide, and its incidence is growing in association with viral and nonviral chronic liver diseases (Sherman M, 2010). Hepatocellular carcinoma is a lethal cancer, and improved survival relies on the detection of early tumors smaller then 2 cm, which are less likely to have dissemination (Di Tommaso, 2011). The diagnosis of hepatocellular carcinoma is based on a multidisciplinary approach, including imaging modalities and serum markers, such as alphafetoprotein (Zhou L 2006). However, such diagnosis still rests on the incontrovertible histological evidence obtained by CT scan or echo-guided needle biopsy. Radiology is the main technique used to detect hepatocellular carcinoma in the setting of cirrhosis; the typical imaging shows hepatocellular carcinoma bigger then 2 cm in more than 90% of cases. When the radiological features of hepatic liver nodules in cirrhosis are not typical, the American Association for the Study of Liver Diseases (AASLD) guidelines recommend the use of liver biopsy. The potential risks of bleeding and seeding due to liver biopsy can be minimized with very thin, 20- to 21-gauge needles, so this invasive technique is recommended now and will be recommended in the future for approximately 50% of dubious hepatic nodules between 1 and 2 cm in size. Indeed, the cumulative experience of several internationally recognized hepatology centers (Bolondi L, 2005)(Forner A, 2008)(Sangiovanni A, 2010)(Leoni S, 2010) has shown that 30% of 1 to 2 cm nodules are not malignant. Recently, Leoni et al. have reported that the application of international guidelines, even with three imaging techniques, leads to a false-negative rate of 20% for nodules ultimately shown to be hepatocellular carcinoma (Leoni S, 2010), whereas Sangiovanni et al. (Sangiovanni A, 2010) have documented in a single-technique scenario that 55% of patients will need to undergo biopsy for a final diagnosis. Thus, biopsy has a very crucial role when radiology fails and pathologists are asked to document malignancies in lesions that are also the most difficult to ascertain (Sherman M, 2010). Regarding the application of needle biopsy for small liver nodules, the American Association for the Study of Liver Diseases recommends that biopsy should be performed for nodules less than 2 cm if their radiologic findings are not characteristic of hepatocellular arcinoma, whereas biopsy is not needed for lesions showing characteristic radiologic findings (Bruix J, 2005). This recommendation has been supported by prospective validation (Forner A, 2008) (Bruix J, 2011). Core liver biopsy is definitely superior to fine needle aspiration, because the specimen obtained is suitable for the assessment of both architectural and cytologic features. Furthermore, the tissue block obtained provides materials for marker studies. Fine needle aspiration is usually adequate for the evaluation of large lesions that are likely to be moderately to poorly differentiated, where diagnostic criteria are easier to evaluate (ICGHN, 2009). An International Working Party of the World Congresses of Gastroenterology proposed a consensus nomenclature and diagnostic criteria for hepatocellular nodular lesions (International Working Party, 1995). The International Working Party classified nodular lesions found in chronic liver disease into large regenerative nodule, low-grade dysplastic nodule, high-grade dysplastic nodule, and hepatocellular carcinoma; this nomenclature has been widely adopted. In addition, the International Working Party introduced the concept of dysplastic focus as a cluster of hepatocytes with features of early neoplasia (in particular small cell change or iron-free foci in a siderotic background) measuring less than 0.1 cm, and defined small hepatocellular carcinoma as a tumor measuring less than 2 cm (International Working Party, 1995). More recent studies support the division of small hepatocellular carcinoma into two clinico-pathological groups that have been termed early hepatocellular carcinoma and progressed hepatocellular carcinoma. Early hepatocellular carcinoma has a longer time to recurrence and a higher 5-year survival rate compared with progressed hepatocellular carcinoma (ICGHN, 2009).

2. Morphological features

The histological appearance of hepatocellular carcinoma has been described in detail over the years and criteria for diagnosis and nomenclature have been clarified (Lopez JB 2005). Distinct morphological features have been reported and, in the majority of cases, hepatocellular can be identified by routine haematoxylin-eosin stained sections, that show a malignant lesion with evidence of hepatocellular differentiation (ICGHN, 2009). The hepatocellular carcinoma's cells are variably similar to the normal liver cells, depending on the degree of differentiation (Ishak KG, 2001). The nuclei are usually hyperchromic and irregular with prominent nucleoli and a high nuclear/cytoplasmic ratio. The tumor cells usually have distinct cell membranes and a moderate amount of eosinophilic, finely granular cytoplasm and may contain a variety of cellular products, mimicking normal and pathologic liver cell function (Goodman ZD, 2007). The cytoplasm could give a clear cell appearance due to the presence of cytoplasmic fat and/or glycogen. Cytoplasmic Mallory bodies and hyaline globules, representing alpha-1-antitrypsin storage, lightly eosinophilic ground-glass-like cytoplasmic inclusions, due to fibrinogen and other plasma proteins can be found. Bile pigment may be present in tumor cells or in dilated canaliculi, that can be easily observed even in hematoxylin eosin stained sections (Goodman ZD, 2007). The cells of hepatocellular carcinoma generally try to grow in ways that mimic the cell plates of normal liver, producing well-recognized growth trabecular pattern (Ishak KG, 2001). The histological picture could remember the early architecture of embryonic and foetal liver (fig. 1), suggesting the hypothesis that carcinogenesis follows liver developing ontogenesis. The architectural feature show different growth patterns. Most often the tumor grows in a **trabecular pattern** with thickened cords of cells separated by vascular sinusoids, mimicking the cell plates and sinusoids of normal liver; a rapid growth of the tumor cells causes the plates to become thickened and contorted, producing trabeculae that are surrounded by endothelial cells. The trabeculae may contain very dilated canaliculi, producing a

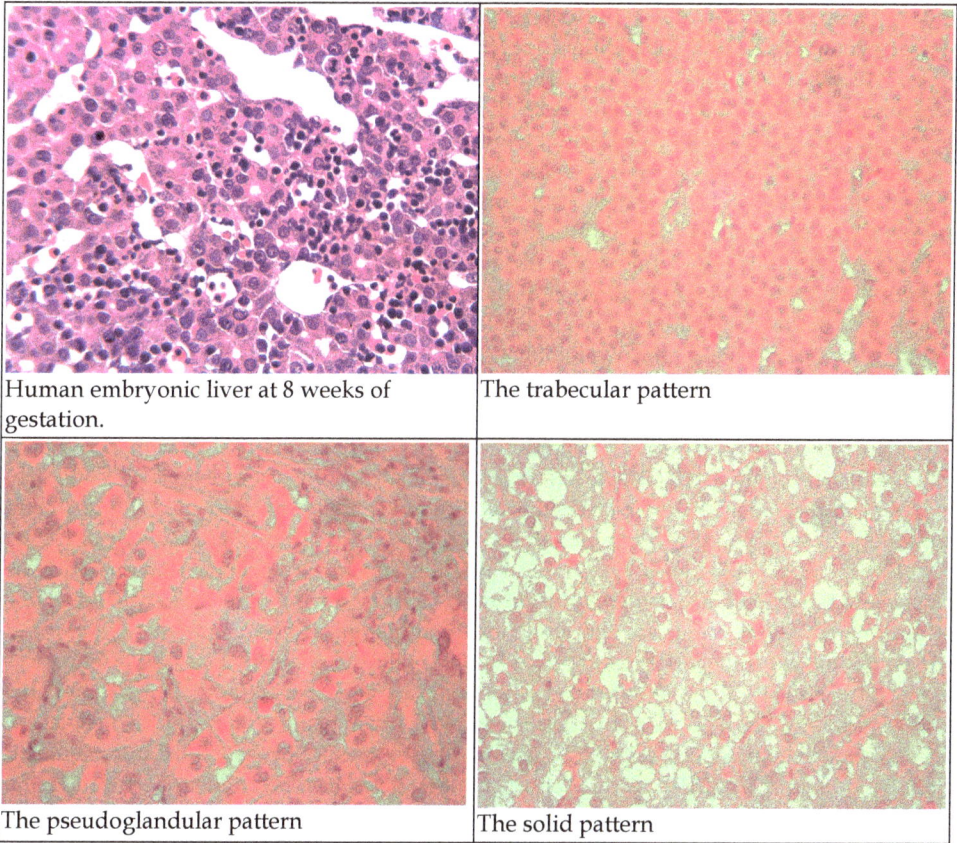

| Human embryonic liver at 8 weeks of gestation. | The trabecular pattern |
| The pseudoglandular pattern | The solid pattern |

Fig. 1. The architecture of a human embryonic liver at 8 weeks of gestation compared with the growth patterns of hepatocellular carcinoma.

pseudoglandular pattern, in other fields, trabeculae may grow together, compressing the sinusoids and forming sheets of tumor cells, producing a **solid or compact pattern** (Goodman ZD, 2007). Early hepatocellular carcinoma has a vaguely nodular appearance and is well differentiated. Progressed hepatocellular carcinoma has a distinctly nodular pattern and is mostly moderately differentiated, often with evidence of microvascular invasion (ICGHN, 2009). Small lesions with malignant potential show only subtle differences from the surrounding parenchyma, making them difficult to assess reproducibly. The International Working Party criteria of 1995 have led to remarkable progress in global standardization of nomenclature of liver nodules (International Working Party, 1995). However, although these criteria have been widely adopted, their application is challenging in equivocal lesions. Perhaps the most significant problem is that most histologic criteria are arrayed on a gradual spectrum and cannot be easily summarized as "present or absent". Additionally, the number of criteria suggested in the literature are too numerous to achieve interobserver consensus, and the diagnostic weight carried by each of these criteria is uncertain. Frequently, criteria used for malignancy in other tissues, such as mitotic activity and cellular atypia, are not represented to a significant degree in well differentiated hepatocellular carcinoma. In addition, the liver lacks a layered structure as seen in the gastrointestinal tract, it is difficult to determine the presence of destructive growth in early hepatocellular carcinomas. Despite these difficulties, current histologic criteria for these nodules clearly yield reliable diagnoses at both ends of the spectrum; most pathologists will correctly identify nodules up to low grade dysplastic nodule as benign, whereas even small well differentiated hepatocellular carcioma with distinct nodular pattern or small moderately differentiated hepatocellular carcinomas will be correctly identified as malignant. The remaining gray zone includes high grade dysplastic nodule and early hepatocellular carcinoma. In evaluation of these lesions, the presence of stromal invasion is a useful criterion of malignancy. Accordingly, pathologists can decide whether the equivocal tumor is hepatocellular carcinoma or high grade dysplastic nodule by recognizing the presence or absence of tumor cell invasion into the intratumoral portal tracts. When obvious stromal invasion is not found in an equivocal tumor, the lesion may be diagnosed as either high grade dysplastic nodules or early hepatocellular carcinomas without detectable invasion (ICGHN, 2009). The diagnosis of stromal invasion is subjective and may require the assistance of histochemical (Victoria Blue or reticulin stains) and immunohistochemical stains (keratin 7 or 19) for differentiation from pseudoinvasion (Park YN, 1998). Biopsy diagnosis of equivocal nodules remains a challenge, because minute biopsy specimens may not contain intratumoral portal tracts, thus precluding the detection of stromal invasion. Similarly, the detection of unpaired arteries, mitoses, and various immunohistochemical markers are prone to sampling error (Senes G, 2007). Connective tissue stroma is typically sparse, and reticulin fibers are absent or reduced, being found only at the periphery of trabeculae. In contrast to most other malignant epithelial neoplasms, hepatocellular carcinoma is soft and the lack of a desmoplastic stroma is a helpful diagnostic clue (Goodman ZD, 2007). A subset of tumors, that has been named **fibrolamellar epatocellular carcinoma**, differs from other types of hepatocellular carcinoma in clinical features and prognosis (Craig JR, 1980)(Soreide O, 1986). Fibrolamellar carcinoma is a unique type of liver carcinoma that arises in non-cirrhotic livers of young individuals (Torbenson M, 2007). Its etiology is unknown. Histologically, the tumor is made up of large polygonal cells characterized by abundant granular eosinophilic cytoplasm, large vesiculated nuclei, prominent nucleoli and abundant stroma composed of lamellae of collagen. Lamellar bands of fibrosis are present within the tumor and can be seen in both primary and metastatic tumors (Ross HM, 2011). Rarely, hepatocellular carcinoma will produce abundant stroma, producing the scirrhous pattern of hepatocellular carcinoma (Goodman ZD, 2007).

3. Immunohistochemistry

Immunostains can be used to study hepatocellular carcinoma and to distinguish hepatocellular carcinoma from other focal lesion or other malignancies, especially intrahepatic cholangiocarcinoma and metastatic adenocarcinoma (Ishak KG, 2001)(Varma V, 2004). As the cells of hepatocellular cacinoma attempt to mimic normal liver cells, they may produce any of the cellular products that can be found in hepatocytes both in health and in disease, and, if present, these are readily demonstrated by immunostaining. Unfortunately, they are not specific and many of these can also be found in tumors other than hepatocellular carcinoma (Goodman ZD, 2007). There are no stains that can absolutely distinguish well-differentiated hepatocellular carcinoma from hepatic benign lesions, such as hepatocellular adenoma or dysplastic nodules, and similarly, no single stain can always distinguish poorly differentiated hepatocellular carcinoma from poorly differentiated cholangiocarcinoma or metastatic adenocarcinoma. However, selected immunostains, taken in the context of other morphologic features, can be very helpful in establishing the diagnosis of hepatocellular carcinoma in difficult cases.

The **polyclonal antiserum to carcinoembryonic antigen (pCEA)** is useful in demonstrating bile canaliculi (fig. 2), both in normal liver and in hepatocellular carcinoma, due to the presence of a CEA-like cross-reactive substance called biliary glycoprotein I (Saad RS, 2004)(Goodman ZD, 2007) (Onofre AS, 2007) (Lau SK, 2002).

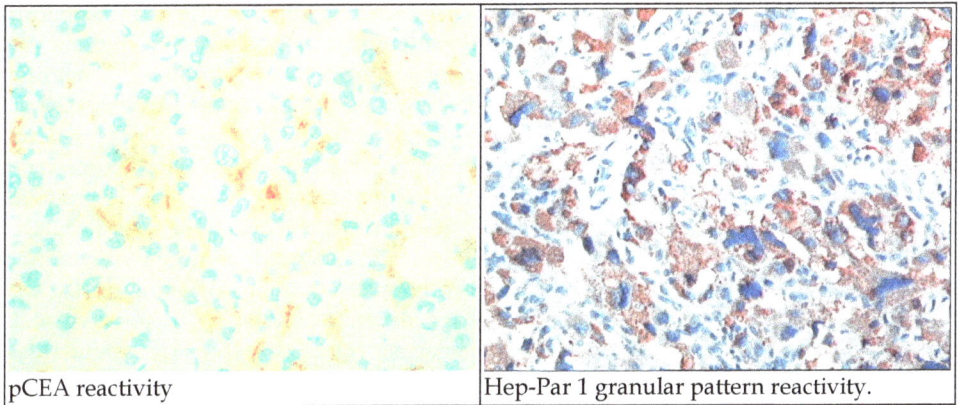

| pCEA reactivity | Hep-Par 1 granular pattern reactivity. |

Fig. 2. Immunohistochemistry for pCEA and Hep-Par 1.

HepPar-1 (Hepatocyte Paraffin 1) is a monoclonal antibody that reacts with an epitope of liver mitochondria, with a typical granular pattern (fig. 2) in most liver specimens (Lugli A, 2004)(Minervini MI, 1997) (Leong AS , 1998) (Zimmerman , 2001). It also sometimes reacts with other normal or pathological structure, such as renal tubules and intestinal epithelium as well as with intestinal metaplasia in the stomach and esophagus (Goodman ZD, 2007). It produces positive staining in the vast majority of cases of hepatocellularr carcinoma (Saad RS, 2004)(Siddiqui MT, 2002) and only a small percentage of other tumors, including some cholangiocarcinomas and metastatic adenocarcinomas from the stomach and other sites (Terracciano LM, 2003), but when used in the context of morphology, clinical setting and other stains, HepPar-1 is very useful in distinguishing hepatocelluar carcinoma from other malignancies (Wang L, 2006). The scientific literature reported cases of hepatocellular carcinoma negative for HepPar-1 (Sugiki T, 2004), probably due to the uneven distribution of HepPar-1 in hepatocellular carcinoma, as reported by our group (Senes G, 2007). What's more the degree of positive staining could varies from case to case (Goodman ZD, 2007): some tumors have a very patchy distribution of positive cells, which can be easily missed in a small biopsy.

Glypican 3 (GPC3), a cell-surface heparan sulfate proteoglycans that is secreted into the plasma, is a member of the glypican family of heparinsulfate proteoglycan linked to the cell surface through a glycosylphosphatidylinositol anchor (Filmus J, 2001). Glypican 3 has been suggested to play a negative role in cell proliferation and an apoptosis-inducing role in specific tissues (Cano-Gauci DF, 1999). The gene is frequently methylated in various tumors and cell lines, suggesting a tumor-suppressive role in tumorigenesis (Di Tommaso, 2007). It is also overexpressed in hepatocellular carcinoma (Zhu ZW, 2001). Glypican-3 has recently become established as a serum and tissue marker for hepatocellular carcinoma, both at messenger and protein level (Capurro, 2003)(Libbrecht L 2006) (ICGHN, 2009). At the beginning, by using a home-made antibody, glypican 3 weak and focal staining was observed in hepatocellular carcinoma precursor lesions and a diffuse staining in the vast majority of hepatocellular carcinomas (Yamauchi N, 2005). Glypican-3 immunoreactivity has a reported sensitivity of 77% and specificity of 96% in the diagnosis of small hepatocellular carcinoma; therefore, glypican-3 positivity is a strong argument for malignancy but the absence of immunoreactivity does not help in the differential diagnosis (Libbrecht L 2006)(ICGHN, 2009). The staining pattern is usually cytoplasmic but may be membranous or canalicular. The monoclonal antibody from Biomosaics (IG12 clone) at a dilution of 1:50 to 1:100 as amplified with the new short polymer systems (Advance [Dako], Novolink [Novocastra], and Super-picture + [Zymed]) yields reliable results. Since glypican-3 staining may be only focal, additional markers or a panel of markers may be necessary. Glypican-3 staining must be interpreted in context, because it may also be seen in regenerating hepatocytes in a setting of hepatitis and in melanocytic lesions (ICGHN, 2009). A recent work from our group (Sollai M, 2011) sowed immunoreactivity for glypican-3 in the fetal human liver, caracterized by a strong immunostaning during the first month of gestation and by a progressive decrease, ending with a very weak expression at birth. This work may add new data to the theory of strict similarities between cell programs utilized during development, silenced at birth, and re-activated by tumor cells during liver cancerogenesis.

HSP70 (heat shock protein 70) belongs to a class of genes (heat shock proteins) implicated in tumorigenesis, in the regulation of cell-cycle progression and apoptosis (Garrido C, 2001)(Helmbrecht K, 2000)(ICGHN, 2009). Most hepatocellular carcinomas are associated with chronic inflammation and fibrosis, acting as stressful conditions that lead to heat shock protein synthesis. HSP70 is, in particular, a potent antiapoptotic survival factor (ICGHN, 2009); it was reported as the most abundantly up-regulated gene among a set of 12,600 genes in early hepatocellular carcinoma (Chuma et al, 2003). Furthermore, it was significantly overexpressed in progressed hepatocellular carcinoma as compared with early hepatocellular carcinoma, and in the latter as compared with precancerous lesions. HSP70 immunoreactivity was recently reported in the majority of hepatocellular carcinomas, including early and well-differentiated forms, but not in non-malignant nodules (Di Tommaso L, 2007), thus suggesting its use as a marker of malignancy. HSP70 immunoreactivity (SC-24 clone, dilution 1:250 to 1:500 amplified with short polymer systems; Santa Cruz Biotechnology, Santa Cruz, CA) is nucleocytoplasmic and mostly focal with 70% sensitivity for hepatocellular carcinoma detection in surgically resected specimens (Haussinger D, 1985).

GS (glutamine synteatse) catalyzes the synthesis of glutamine from glutamate and ammonia in the mammalian liver (Haussinger D, 1985) where it has been shown to be restricted to hepatocytes surrounding the terminal hepatic venules in the murine and human liver

(Moorman AF, 1988, 1989). It is known that glutamine, the end product of glutamine synteatse activity, is the major energy source of tumor cells (Reitzer LJ, 1979). Based on findings on experimental hepatocarcinogenesis, GS positive tumor cells are believed to be derived from GS positive hepatocytes that have been affected by carcinogens. Thus, GS was suggested as a specific marker for tracing cell lineage relationships during hepatocarcinogenesis (Gebhardt R, 1999). Most importantly, GS is a target gene of β-catenin so that its overexpression is associated with mutations of β -catenin or with activation of this pathway (Christa et al, 1994)(ICGHN, 2009). Then up-regulation of GS mRNA, protein, and activity has been demonstrated in human hepatocellular carcinoma (Christa et al, 1994). Interestingly, a stepwise increase in GS immunoreactivity from precancerous lesions to early and to advanced hepatocellular carcinoma was also reported, proposing for GS a role in the promotion of the metastatic potential of hepatocellular carcinogenesis (Osada et al, 1999). The monoclonal antibody from Chemicon International (clone MB302) at a dilution of 1:500 to 1:1000 and amplified with a new short polymer system yields reliable results. In order to increase its specificity as a marker of malignancy, GS immunostaining should be diffuse and strong, a pattern that can be seen in 50% of hepatocellular carcinomas, including early forms (Haussinger D, 1985).

CHC (clathrin heavy chain) is an endothelial marker overexpressed in hepatocellular carcinoma (Seimiya M, 2008). CHC was chosen because it is an endothelial marker, it works well as an internal standard for non parenchymal liver cells and, as already suggested in a surgical series, is overexpressed in the cytoplasm of malignant hepatocytes (Seimiya M, 2008). In contrast, most non malignant hepatocytes were reported to be negative or to have weak to moderate staining intensity (Seimiya M, 2008).

Alpha-fetoprotein is frequently elevated in the serum of patients with hepatocellular carcinoma, even when the tumor is negative at immunostaining (Zhou L, 2006)(Wang L 2006). In most published series, it has been found in less than an half of hepatocellular carcinomas: for that reason, it is less useful for diagnostic purposes (Goodman ZD, 2007) (Chu PG, 2002) (Onofre AS , 2007) (Lau SK , 2002).

Cytokeratins are sometimes suggested as a means of tumor classification, especially **cytokeratin 7** (Maeda , 1996)(Chu , 2000)(Durnez A et al 2006) and **cytokeratin 20** (Chu P, 2000) (Faa G , 1998), but in rare cases the tumor cells display aberrant keratin expression, suggesting that the staining pattern should be interpreted with caution (Fanni D, 2009). Cytokeratin 7 can be present in some hepatocelluar carcinomas, as well as cytokeratin 20, the latter in a minority of case. For that reason, cytokeratin 7 and 20 profiles are not very useful in the diagnosis of hepatocellular carcinoma (Goodman ZD, 2007). **Cytokeratin 8-18** (Porcell , 2000) (Van Eyken P, 1988), **cytokeratin 19** (Maeda T, 1996)(Van Eyken P, 1988) as well as the staining with a **pancytokeratin cocktail (AE1/AE3)**, that usually produces negative or weak staining, are less frequently used (Goodman ZD, 2007).

CD34 is present and demonstrable in endothelial cells of large blood vessels and most capillary beds throughout the body, with the exception of normal hepatic sinusoidal endothelium. The trabeculae of hepatocellular carcinoma are surrounded by endothelial cells which phenotypically resemble capillary endothelium and are usually positive for CD34. On the contrary, normal hepatic sinusoidal endothelium and benign hepatocellular lesions typically have CD34 positive sinusoids only in areas that receive increased arterial blood: cirrhotic nodules tend to be positive only around the periphery of regenerative nodules and focal nodular hyperplasia may show immunoreactivity for CD34 restricted to the sinusoids bordering fibrous septa (Goodman ZD, 2007). A diffuse, regular CD34 positivity of sinusoids can be helpful in distinguishing a cirrhotic nodule from a well-differentiated hepatocellular carcinoma. The staining for CD34 in hepatocellular adenomas is variable: this means that caution should be taken in the interpretation of CD34 reactivity in well differentiated tumor lesions, because a positive stain does not necessarily indicate malignancy (Varma V 2004)(Gouysse G, 2004).

CD68 is a transmembrane glycoprotein located within lysosomes and endosomes. Thus, macrophages as well as other cell types rich in lysosomes/endosomes are CD68-positive (Ross HM, 2011). The staining pattern of CD68 was explored in the epithelial cells of both fibrolamellar and typical hepatocellular carcinomas In the romer, CD68 reactivity was found in the majority of cases, whereas it was absent in classical hepatocellular carcinoma (Ross HM, 2011).

4. Differential diagnosis

The diagnosis of hepatocellular carcinoma is sometimes very straightforward, not requiring anything other than hematoxylin eosin stained sections, whereas in most cases it requires the proper evaluation of several fine histological features, the reticulin framework, and the type of neo-vascularization. Two types of benign lesions enter into the differential diagnosis of hepatocellular carcinoma: hepatocellular adenoma in a noncirrhotic liver, and dysplastic nodules in the setting of cirrhosis (Ishak KG, 2001)(International Working Party, 1995)(Theise ND, 2002). The most frequent problem is distinguishing poorly differentiated hepatocellular carcinoma from other malignancies, especially metastases but also from poorly differentiated cholangiocarcinoma. A large cell carcinoma with eosinophilic cytoplasm, prominent nuclei and nucleoli may well be hepatocellular but that diagnosis should not be made without definite evidence of hepatocellular differentiation. Bile, recognizable canaliculi on haematoxylin-eosin or CEA stain, a positive stain for alphafetoprotein, a granular staining pattern with HepPar-1, or a trabecular growth pattern allow a diagnosis of hepatocellular origin of tumor cells with more or less certainty. However, the very rare cases of liver metastasis from a gastrointestinal adenocarcinoma with hepatoid features should be excluded, particularly when no other evidence of hepatocellular differentiation is found (Porcell , 2000). The tumor could be metastatic than primary in the liver, especially in the absence of cirrhosis. Cholangiocarcinomas and metastatic adenocarcinomas typically have a desmoplastic stroma, in contrast to hepatocellular carcinoma. A tumor with abundant stroma is almost always an adenocarcinoma, with the exception of the rare fibrolamellar type and even rarer scirrhous type of hepatocellular carcinoma (Craig JR, 1980)(Soreide O, 1986). Other metastatic malignant tumors may also be confused with hepatocellular carcinoma, in particular those characterized by large tumor cells with abundant cytoplasm, including melanomas (especially amelanotic) carcinoids, some poorly differentiated neuroendocrine tumors and renal cell carcinomas.

4.1 Hepatocellular carcinoma versus hepatocellular adenoma

Hepatocellular adenoma typically develops in women in the reproductive age group, and is often associated with oral contraceptive steroid use. Microscopically, they are composed of benign-looking hepatocytes arranged in sheets and cords without acinar architecture.

Adenoma cells are usually larger and paler than nontumor hepatocytes of the surrounding liver, due to increased cytoplasmic glycogen and/or fat. The nuclei of the tumor cells are typically uniform and regular, the nuclear/cytoplasmic ratio is low, and mitoses are almost never seen (Tab. 1). A well-developed reticulin framework is usually present in the tumor (Goodman ZD, 2007). The sinusoids, with flattened endothelial lining cells, are usually compressed, thus contributing to the sheet-like appearance. Sometimes the sinusoids are dilated, a finding which can be mistaken for peliosis hepatis. Bile ducts are not found in hepatocellular adenoma, but ductules and progenitor cells may be present. The presence of dilated sinusoids and ductules has caused some tumors to be classified as a telangiectatic variant of focal nodular hyperplasia, but molecular studies have shown these to be a variant of hepatocellular adenoma (Paradis V, 2004).

4.2 Hepatocellular carcinoma versus dysplastic nodule

Dysplastic nodule is the term used for a benign lesion that can be confused with hepatocellular carcinoma (International Working Party, 1995)(Theise ND, 2002)(Hytiroglou P, 2004). These are nodules in a cirrhotic liver that are macroscopically distinct from the surrounding cirrhotic nodules. They are usually larger than surrounding nodules and may be detected by imaging studies. They may also differ in colour or texture and may bulge from the surface of the liver (Goodman ZD, 2007). Distinguishing a well-differentiated hepatocellular carcinoma from a regenerative nodule or from a dysplastic nodule may be very difficult, particularly in small needle aspiration or core biopsies (Libbrecht L 2006). Histological examination is required to distinguish a dysplastic nodule from a small hepatocellular carcinoma (Tab. 2), and they are further classified as low-grade or high-grade, based on morphologic features (Goodman ZD, 2007).

Low-grade dysplastic nodules

Low-grade dysplastic nodules are sometimes vaguely nodular but are often distinct from the surrounding cirrhotic liver because of the presence of peripheral fibrous scar. This is not a true capsule, but rather condensation of scarring as is seen around all cirrhotic nodules (ICGHN, 2009). Architectural changes beyond clearly regenerative features are not present; these lesions do not contain pseudoglands or markedly thickened trabeculae. Unpaired arteries and portal areas are sometimes present in small numbers (Park YN, 1998). Nodule-in-nodule lesions are not present. Low-grade dysplastic nodules are composed of liver cells that are minimally abnormal, showing mild increase in cell density with a monotonous pattern, and they have no cytologic atypia, though they may have large cell change, formerly referred to as large cell dysplasia and or atipia (Anthony PP, 1973). The nuclear/cytoplasmic ratio is normal or slightly increased and there are no mitoses. The large cell atipia is charcterized by slightly nuclear pleomorfism (aneuploidia), multinucleation, abundant cytoplasm, mixed with normal hepatocyte. Steatosis may be present and there may be Mallory bodies (Goodman ZD, 2007). Low-grade dysplastic nodules may have diffuse siderosis or diffusely increased copper retention (ICGHN, 2009). Iron may be increased or decreased compared to the surrounding cirrhotic liver (Goodman ZD, 2007). Among members of the consensus panels ICGHN, 2009 there was no serious difficulty in differentiating Low-grade dysplastic nodules from early hepatocellular carcinoma. At the opposite end of the spectrum, distinction between Low-grade dysplastic nodules and large regenerative nodules was often found to be difficult or impossible. Therefore, there is currently consensus that distinction between these two diagnostic categories cannot be made confidently by morphology alone and remains a task for the future. Fortunately, this distinction does not appear to have significant practical consequences at present (ICGHN, 2009).

High-grade dysplastic nodules

High-grade dysplastic nodules may be distinctly or vaguely nodular in the background of cirrhosis, although they also lack a true capsule, similar to low-grade dysplastic nodules; however, they are more likely to show a vaguely nodular pattern than low-grade dysplastic nodules. An high-grade dysplastic nodules is defined as having architectural and/or cytologic atypia, but the atypia is insufficient for a diagnosis of hepatocellular carcinoma. These lesions most often show increased cell density, sometimes more than 2 times higher than the surrounding nontumoral liver, often with an irregular trabecular pattern (ICGHN, 2009). Small cell change, also known as small cell dysplasia or atipia is the most frequently seen form of cytologic atypia in high-grade dysplastic nodules (Watanabe S, 1983). Small cell atipia refers to clusters of cells with features that suggest increased cellular proliferation. Hepatocytes show small or regular size, with hypercromic irregular nuclei, nuclear groove, anphophilic cytoplasm, nodular pattern, decreased reticolin small cell change. Plates more than two cells thick, pseudogland formation, cytoplasmic basophilia, higher nuclear/cytoplasmic ratio, nuclear hyperchromasia or an irregular nuclear contour are the most suggestive diagnostic elements (Goodman ZD, 2007). These features often confined to one or more foci within the nodule, giving the appearance 'nodule-in-nodule' formation (Goodman ZD 2007). This form of atypia may also occur in small hepatocellular foci outside of high-grade dysplastic nodules; the term dysplastic focus (International Working Party, 1995) may be appropriately used for such lesions. Large cell change may or may not be present in high-grade dysplastic nodules. Unpaired arteries are found in most lesions, but usually not in great numbers. A nodule-in-nodule appearance is occasionally found in high-grade dysplastic nodules, and subnodules often have a higher labeling index of proliferating cell nuclear antigen or Ki-67 than that of high-grade dysplastic nodules parenchyma. When a nodule with largely high-grade dysplastic features contains a subnodule of hepatocellular carcinoma, the subnodule of hepatocellular carcinoma is usually well-differentiated with a well-defined margin. The diagnostic discrepancy between high-grade dysplastic nodules and early hepatocellular carcinoma was frequent at the first consensus meeting, but it remarkably improved at the second meeting, due to the recognition of stromal invasion as a diagnostic criterion for the differentiation of high-grade dysplastic nodules from early hepatocellular carcinoma (ICGHN, 2009). If areas of questionable invasion are present, immunostaining for keratins 7 or 19 may be useful; if such stainings demonstrate a ductular reaction, the focus is considered a pseudoinvasion and does not warrant a diagnosis of hepatocellular carcinoma (Park YN, 2007). It is generally accepted that high-grade dysplastic nodule are precursors of hepatocellular carcinoma based on several lines of evidence, including morphologic features intermediate between low grade nodules and hepatocellular carcinoma, the presence of foci of hepatocellular carcinoma in otherwise high-grade dysplastic nodules, and follow-up showing progression to malignancy in a few cases. In some cases in clinical practice, it may be impossible to distinguish a high-grade dysplastic nodule from a well differentiated hepatocellular carcinoma, especially in needle biopsies. The current ability to increase the survival of patients with hepatocellular carcinoma relies upon the surveillance of cirrhotic patients. Surveillance allows hepatocellular carcinoma precursors (dysplastic nodules) and malignant tumors to be recognized at an earlier stage making cure possible. Radiology plays a major role in hepatocellular carcinoma diagnosis because hepatocellular carcinoma is characterized by neoarterial vascularisation with a typical imaging pattern. Current international guidelines have restricted the use of the liver biopsy to the characterization of hepatocellular nodules which remain diagnostically equivocal after imaging. Thus pathologists are today facing very challenging and often well differentiated lesions, leading to difficulties in distinguishing high grade dysplasia and well differentiated hepatocellular carcinoma. In this scenario novel concepts obtained through international consensus have been proposed with emphasis on hepatocellular carcinoma of small size (up to 2 cm) which includes 2 distinct types, the early and progressed hepatocellular carcinoma (Roncalli M, 2011). High nuclear/cytoplasmic ratio of tumor cells is the most reliable sign of malignancy, even when the nuclei are not atypical, and this feathures, in combination with trabecular or pseudoglandular growth patterns distinguishes well-differentiated hepatocellular carcinoma from benign hepatocellular lesions (Goodman ZD, 2007). One of the main features used in this distinction is stromal invasion, which is usually not present in needle biopsy material (Park YN, 2007). Sampling errors in the biopsies may significantly influence the final diagnosis. It is indeed these small and limited tissue samples that pathologists rely upon, to make real diagnoses. The differential diagnosis of small, well-differentiated hepatocellular nodules mainly rests on fine histological criteria which can be difficult to adequately evaluate on tiny samples (Goodman ZD, 2007).

Early or small well-differentiated hepatocellular carcinoma

Early hepatocellular are vaguely nodular and are characterized by various combinations of the following major histologic features (Hytiroglou P, 2004)(Kojiro M, 2006)(Hytiroglou P, 2007):

1. increased cell density more than 2 times that of the surrounding tissue, with an increased nuclear/cytoplasm ratio and irregular thin-trabecular pattern;
2. varying numbers of portal tracts within the nodule (intratumoral portal tracts);
3. pseudoglandular pattern;
4. diffuse fatty change; and
5. varying numbers of unpaired arteries.

Among these features, diffuse fatty change is observed in approximately 40% of cases (Kutami R, 2000). The characteristic features of early hepatocellular carcinoma are sometimes seen in larger tumors. Including well-differentiated tumors that measure over 2 cm and thus do not qualify for the designation of small hepatocellular carcinoma set forth by the IWP. The prevalence of fatty change decreases along with increasing tumor size; therefore, fatty change is uncommon in tumors larger than 3 cm. Fatty change is also uncommon in moderately differentiated hepatocellular carcinomas. Any of the features listed above may be diffuse throughout the lesion or may be restricted to an expansile subnodule (nodule-in-nodule). Most importantly, because all of these features may also be found in high dysplastic nodules, it is important to note that stromal invasion remains most helpful in differentiating early hepatocellular carcinoma from high dysplastic nodules (ICGHN, 2009).

Pathologists today are asked to provide timely and conclusive diagnostic reports for the management and therapy of radiologically equivocal hepatocellular nodules found in small biopsy samples. Although the traditional hematoxylin-eosin-based morphology remains the milestone, integration with biological information is required to make biopsy interpretation more objective and reproducible. To support the morphological criteria, additional and more objective criteria of malignancy, such as stromal invasion and the composite expression of a number of tissue biomarkers (translated to clinical practice from expression studies of human hepatocarcinogenesis (Chuma M, 2007)(Paradis V, 2003)(Nam SW, 2005)(Llovet JM, 2006)(Wurmbach E, 2007)(Di Tommaso L, 2007), have been proposed. Some have already been validated, as recently emphasized by Roskams and Kojiro (Roskams T, 2010), and their use in clinical practice has been suggested in the recent update of the AASLD practice guidelines (Bruix J, 2011). Indeed, the use of these tools can make pathologists, even those not specialized in liver pathology and in the diagnosis of liver tumor, more confident in the fine diagnostics of this challenging field. This is particularly true for small hepatocellular carcinoma, which is the most curable form and is particularly difficult to recognize with imaging. Non invasive imaging techniques were successful in 1- to 2 cm hepatocellular carcinoma detection in patients with cirrhosis in only 33% of cases (Forner A, 2008). In these cases the application of a panel of putative markers, such as glypican3, HSP70 and GS was thought to help to address the diagnostic challenge (Di Tommasi 2007). Hepatocelluar carcinoma is supported by the immunoreactivity of at least 2 markers while lack of immunoreactivity does not conclusively rule out malignancy. When morphological features suggest a non-malignant nodule an immunonegative profile is expected. In these cases, the staining of 2 markers should prompt reconsideration of the diagnosis. The panel may also be useful in clinically obvious but tangentially or minimally sampled tumors. It should be noted that in this setting the sparse peripheral neoplastic cells that might have been insufficient for a conclusive diagnosis of malignancy on hematoxylin eosin can easily be highlighted by the panel (Di Tommasi, 2009). The endothelial marker clathrin heavy chain (CHC) has been recently suggested to be diagnostically useful as well, particularly in combination with GPC3 (Seimiya M, 2008); its value was initially tested in surgical specimens (Seimiya M, 2008), and really also in liver biopsy samples (Di Tommasi 2011). A homogeneous series of small hepatocellular carcinoma no more then 2 cm in diameter and, for comparison, non small hepatocellular carcinomas sampled by a fine-needle approach (20-21 gauge) were immunostained for CHC with the aim of determining whether the addition of a novel marker (CHC) to the previously validated panel could increase the panel's diagnostic accuracy in the detection of small hepatocellular carcinoma (Di Tommasi 2011). The performance of the 4 markers' panel was superior to the performance of the same panel without CHC (the 3 markers' panel). With staining at least two markers, the accuracy was 97% and 84.3% in non small and small hepatocellular carcinomas, respectively, superior to the accuracy of the panel without the addition of CHC (86% and 76.9%, respectively). For small hepatocellular carcinomas, the addition of CHC to the panel consistently increased the sensitivity from 46.8% to 63.8%. Interestingly enough, for non small hepatocellular carcinomas, in cases in which the liver nodule was sampled with a 20 to 21 gauge needle, the accuracy of the novel panel (97%) was higher than the the previously reported (78.4%) with a 3M panel in an analogous hepatocellular carcinoma series sampled with 16- to 18-gauge needles. This means that the addition of CHC not only counterbalances the putative loss of sensitivity of thinner core materials but also increases the diagnostic accuracy. Although the use of a 4 markers' panel is more elaborate and time-consuming for pathologists, the unitary cost of an additional immunoreaction to the panel is much less expensive than confirmatory additional imaging (Sangiovanni A, 2010) or repeat liver biopsies. When hepatocellular carcinoma series were dissected into subpopulations according not only to size but also to grading (G1 versus G2/G3), the panel accuracy remained excellent and greater than 90% for G2/G3 hepatocellular carcinomas, regardless of the size. This datum confirms that the performance of the 4 markers' panel is optimal when tumor differentiation is compromised; in other words, the individual markers of the panel cooperatively stain hepatocellular carcinomas that have progressed. Unfortunately, these are cases for which the pathological diagnosis can be rendered on morphological grounds without the use of staining beyond hematoxylin eosin. Interestingly, although the tumor size was not an issue in G2/G3 hepatocellular carcinomas, it was a major issue in well-differentiated (G1) hepatocellular carcinomas. Indeed, in this hepatocellular carcinoma group, which is the most difficult to evaluate in routine clinical practice, the accuracy of the panel was still excellent in non small G1 hepatocellular carcinomas (93.9%) but dropped to 67.4% in small G1 hepatocellular carcinomas. In the latter, the sensitivity for hepatocellular carcinoma detection was 50%, with 100% specificity, and the performance of the 4 markers' panel was much better than that of the 3 markers' panel. In addition, we noticed that a consistent fraction of these tumors showed negative staining (6/30, 20%) or one marker only (9/30, 30%). The most likely (though speculative) explanation for these conflicting results is that G1 hepatocellular carcinomas greater than 2 cm and G1 hepatocellular carcinomas smaller than 2 cm are not the same disease. An international agreement between Eastern and Western pathologists has recently been obtained for a new hepatocellular carcinoma entity: very well-differentiated, no more then 2 cm, hepatocellular carcinoma (which is also called very early hepatocellular carcinoma) (International Consensus Group for Hepatocellular Neoplasia, 2009). This is the earliest described and well-differentiated form of hepatocellular carcinoma and is likely the morphological link between high grade dysplastic nodule and hepatocellular carcinoma that has progressed. Very early hepatocellular carcinoma type is very difficult to recognize on imaging because of the immature vascular supply. A consistent fraction of the small G1 hepatocellular carcinoma cases likely belong to this very early type. The phenotypic profile of these cases is clearly distinct from that of other hepatocellular carcinomas of the present series, and this provides indirect proof of an earlier disease. Indeed, the small G1 hepatocellular carcinomas were less likely to be stained with the combination of the panel markers, their profile being intermediate between dysplasia (usually not staining) and hepatocellular carcinoma that has progressed (mostly staining). It is, therefore, reasonable to assume that when an hepatocellular carcinoma is just born, its phenotypic profile is not yet settled (e.g., the vascular support), and these markers are individually and progressively acquired and detectable. The most represented marker in small G1 hepatocellular carcinomas seemed to be CHC (58.8%), followed by GS (41.2%), HSP70 (17.6%), and GPC3 (11.8%). This means that in small G1 hepatocellular carcinomas, CHC is the most overexpressed marker. Thus, its evaluation, particularly in tumor core biopsy samples, is important, needs attention, and requires preliminary individual training. In particular, as for all the other markers under study, its staining should decorate putative malignant hepatocytes, and should appear as antigen overexpression in comparison with surrounding, adjacent nonneoplastic parenchymal cells. The prospective evaluation of nodules that remain diagnostically uncertain after biopsy could be very valuable for assessing the diagnostic strength of the present panel. Clearly, the search for additional and early markers has just started and is far less than completed. In conclusion, in core biopsy specimens of hepatocellular carcinomas sampled with a 20-to 21-gauge needle, the addition of CHC to a panel composed of GPC3,

HSP70, and GS increases the overall diagnostic accuracy in both small hepatocellular carcinomas (from 76.9% to 84.3%) and nonsmall hepatocellular carcinomas (from 86% to 97%), and there is an important gain in sensitivity in the detection of small hepatocellular carcinomas (from 46.8% to 63.8%). Absolute specificity was obtained only when two of the four markers were positive (regardless of which ones). Accuracy for hepatocellular carcinoma detection was not affected by the tumor size in G2/G3 hepatocellular carcinomas (>90%). In G1 hepatocellular carcinomas, tumor size played a major role in discriminating cases, with higher accuracy for nonsmall hepatocellular carcinomas (93.9%) and lower accuracy for small hepatocellular carcinomas (67.4%); likewise, the sensitivity was 88.2% for nonsmall hepatocellular carcinomas and 50% for small hepatocellular carcinomas. This results suggest that small G1 hepatocellular carcinomas include early tumors characterized by a relatively silent phenotype and the progressive acquisition of the markers is under study. The use of the present panel of markers supports the recognition of both small and nonsmall HCCs in the diagnostic pathology of challenging cases sampled by core biopsy (Di Tommasi 2011).

The combination of more than one putative marker of malignancy raises the overall accuracy. Glypican 3, HSP70 and GS have been found to be valuable in the differential diagnosis of hepatocellular carcinoma. A 3 markers' panel composed by HSP70, GPC3, and GS was demonstrated to be very useful in distinguishing between dysplastic and early malignant hepatocellular nodules arising in cirrhosis (Di Tommaso, 2007, 2009). When applying a panel of these three markers (GPC3, HSP70, and GS) to resected small lesions, the finding of any two positive markers had a sensitivity of 72% and a specificity of 100% to detect malignancy (Di Tommaso 2007, 2009). The diagnostic accuracy of this 3 markers' panel in liver biopsies of hepatocellular nodules has not been yet tested (ICGHN, 2009).

Immunohistochemistry should not be use as a diagnostic tool without consideration for morphology; on the contrary, it should always be carefully considered and dictated by morphology, and should serve as an ancillary tool to support a diagnostic conclusion. Hepatocellular carcinoma is often characterized by marked morphological and phonotypical intratumoral variability. Senes et al (2006) observed a striking variability in the degree of differentiation of the tumor cells among the 17 different sub-nodules detected in a case of hepatocellular carcinoma. Moreover, even the expression of the immunohistochemical markers utilized in this study varied greatly among different tumor regions (Senes et al 2006). As a consequence, in the case that, before the surgical resection, a needle biopsy had been performed, it was hypothesized that the interpretation of the bioptic core could have lead to different diagnoses, depending on the different tumor region sampled. This case underlines a previously unreported major role for sampling variability in the interpretation of needle biopsies and the possibility that, in clinical practice, when a very small fragment of the liver tumor is obtained by an ultrasound guided biopsy, immunoreactivity of the observed tumor cells could not sorely represent the distribution of tumor markers in the whole neoplasm, leading to sampling variability related diagnostic mistakes, not only for defining tumor grading but even in the differential diagnosis between primary and secondary liver tumor.

4.3 Hepatocarcinoma versus other malignant neoplasia

The differential diagnosis between hepatocellular carcinoma, cholangiocarcinoma and metastatic colorectal adenocarcinoma may be difficult when only based on morphology

(Terracciano , 2003). In fact, a subset of extrahepatic adenocarcinomas of different origin may show a solid "hepatoid" pattern virtually indistinguishable from hepatocellular carcinoma (Porcell , 2000). Similarly, metastases to the liver from various hepatoid variants of extra-hepatic neoplasms and other primary hepatic tumors, such as cholangiocarcinoma, may be mistaken for hepatocellular carcinoma (Varma V and Cohen C 2004). On the other hand, undifferentiated hepatocellular carcinoma may mimic poorly differentiated tumors of different origin, while its tubular and adenoid variants may be indistinguishable from cholangiocarcinoma or from metastatic colorectal adenocarcinoma. Furthermore, some of the unusual morphologic variants, including clear-cell, pleomorphic, and sarcomatoid variants, may be mistaken for metastases. The current literature shows that difficulties in histological typing of liver tumors, particularly in the differential diagnosis between hepatocellular carcinoma and cholangiocarcioma and metastases can be minimized by using immunohistochemistry (Varma V and Cohen C 2004)(Ma CK et al 1993). For that reason, in these cases, immunohistochemical analyses are often required (Stroescu , 2006). The panel of antibodies utilized to solve this differential diagnosis includes (tab. 2): cytokeratin 8-18 (Porcell , 2000)(Van Eyken P, 1988) Hep-Par1 (Leong AS , 1998) (Zimmerman , 2001) (Lugli A, 2004)(Minervini MI, 1997), glypican 3 (Yamauchi , 2005) (Libbrecht L 2006) (Zhu ZW et al 2001) (Capurro M et al 2003), cytokeratin 7 (Maeda , 1996) (Chu , 2000) (Durnez A et al 2006), cytokeratin 20 (Chu P, 2000)(Faa G , 1998), cytokeratin 19 (Maeda T, 1996)(Van Eyken P, 1988), CEA (Saad RS, 2004)(Goodman ZD, 2007) (Onofre AS , 2007) (Lau SK , 2002) and Alpha-fetoprotein (Onofre AS , 2007) (Lau SK , 2002) (Zhou L, 2006)(Wang L 2006). Among the numerous diagnostic immunohistochemical markers studied, alphafetoprotein (Wang L 2006), cytokeratin 7 (Durnez A et al 2006), cytokeratin 20 (Chu P et al 2000), cytokeratin 19 (Van Eyken P et al 1988), Hep-Par-1 (Zimmerman RL et al 2001)(Siddiqui MT et al 2002) and glypican 3 (Libbrecht L 2006) (Zhu ZW et al 2001) (Capurro M et al 2003) have been found to be the most valuable in the differential diagnosis between hepatocellular carcinoma and metastatic tumors. Immunoreactivity of tumour cells for cytokeratin 8-18, Hep-Par 1 and glypican 3 is considered suggestive of hepatocellular carcinoma; a diffuse immunoreactivity for cytokeratin 7 and cytokeratin 19 favours the diagnosis of cholangiocarcinoma; diffuse positivity for cytokeratin 20 and negativity for cytokeratin 7 are normally associated with metastatic colorectal adenocarcinoma. The sensitivity and specificity of the monoclonal antibody Hep-Par-1 for hepatocellular carcinoma are considered very high; as a consequence, the usefulness of this marker in the differential diagnosis of hepatic tumors is widely accepted (Chu PG et al 2002)(Saad RS et al 2004), although it stains normal hepatocytes as well. Moreover, expression profiling of primary hepatic tumors has demonstrated that glypican 3, a membrane-anchored heparan sulphate proteoglycan, is markedly expressed in hepatocellular carcinoma, particularly in well differentiated cases (Yamauchi N et al 2005). In spite of the availability of such armamentarium, daily experience shows that diagnostic mistakes can occur more frequently than generally expected. Indeed, some cases of hepatocellular carcinoma have been reported do not show immunoreactivity for Hep Par1 (Sugiki T et al 2004), nor for glypican 3 (Zhu ZW et al 2001). We reported a case of hepatocellular carcinoma with a peculiar immunohistochemical profile, characterized by the association of the typical immunoreactivity of hepatocellular carcinoma with a diffuse and strong positivity for cytokeratin 20 (Fanni D, 2009), generally considered typical of metastatic colorectal adenocarcinoma. The reason for this heterogeneity in immunoreactivity of hepatocellular carcinomas could be related to multiple factors: different etiology, variable degree of differentiation, size of the bioptic core and sampling variability (Maharaj B et al 1998). The differential diagnosis of these lesions is often difficult, especially because of the scant material obtained by needle biopsy (Zhu ZW et al 2001).

5. Fibrolamellar carcinoma

Despite the distinctive clinical and histological features of fibrolamellar carcinoma, this entity can be a diagnostic challenge, because of lack of consistency of the diagnosis of fibrolamellar carcinomas due by pathologists (Ross HM, 2011). Even among experts, weak reproducibility was seen in the histological diagnosis of primary liver tumors with fibrous stroma in non-cirrhotic patients and a consensus diagnosis was achieved in only 32% of the cases (Malouf G, 2009). A large difference is seen in the average age of diagnosis for cases of fibrolamellar carcinoma published in the peer reviewed literature versus cases diagnosed in the SEER database, a difference most likely explained by inconsistencies in making the diagnosis of fibrolamellar carcinoma (El-Serag HB, 2004). Histologically, a common diagnostic pitfall is the overinterpretation of intratumoral fibrosis as being diagnostic of fibrolamellar carcinoma. In addition, another common reason for misdiagnosis is a misperception that most cases of primary liver carcinoma in children and young adults are fibrolamellar carcinomas, leading to overdiagnosis of fibrolamellar carcinoma in this age group, especially with tumors arising in livers without underlying disease (Ross HM, 2011). To improve the reproducibility of the histological diagnosis, over the past several years immunohistochemical stains that may be of assistance have been searched. The role for immunohistochemical markers as an aide in the diagnosis of fibrolamellar carcinomas has been previously explored but sought for additional markers among the currently used panel of antibodies available in most hospital laboratories (Vivekanandan P, 2004)(Klein WM, 2005). Fibrolamellar carcinomas show routinely strong immunoreactivity for CK7, while only about one third of typical hepatocellular carcinomas are CK7-positive (Klein WM, 2005)(Abdul-Al HM, 2010)(Ward SC, 2010). Further analysis of previously reported gene expression studies showed a modest increase in the expression of CD68 (Kannangai R, 2007). The immunohistochemical profile of fibrolamellar carcinomas was further extended to include CD68 staining, because of the routine availability of CD68 in most hospital laboratories: this approach can be helpful in routine surgical practice. CD68 staining among cases from four different institutions have been shown that metastatic tumors do not lose their CD68 positivity (Ross HM, 2011). A distinctive pattern of immunostaining for CD68 in fibrolamellar carcinomas was demonstrated. Nearly all cases showed a granular, stippled pattern, or a dot-like pattern of positivity. This staining pattern is highly sensitive for fibrolamellar carcinoma, but is not specific. In terms of its possible role in routine clinical use, given its high negative predictive value, a diagnosis of fibrolamellar carcinoma in a primary liver carcinoma that is CD68 negative should be strongly re-considered to ensure that fibrolamellar carcinoma is the appropriate diagnosis (Ross HM, 2011). In addition to the fibrolamellar carcinomas, this distinctive pattern was also seen in a minority of conventional hepatocellular carcinoma in both of hepatocellular carcinomas arising in cirrhotic and non-cirrhotic livers. Although not statistically significant, a larger percentage of conventional hepatocellular carcinomas that arose in non-cirrhotic livers showed CD68 staining. Whether this represents dysregulation of similar biological pathways is unclear. Also of note, CD68 positivity was seen adjacent to necrosis and CD68 staining in this context should be interpreted cautiously. Another point that bears emphasis is that none of the cases in the control groups that were CD68 positive had the typical histological features of fibrolamellar carcinoma. Thus, combining the histological findings with CD68 would likely increase the specificity of CD68 staining for fibrolamellar carcinoma. The reproducibility of the histological diagnosis of fibrolamellar carcinoma can be substantially improved by careful attention to the full pattern of histological features, including large polygonal tumor cells with abundant eosinophilic cytoplasm, large vesiculated nuclei, large nucleoli, and lamellar fibrosis (Torbenson M, 2007). Moreover, most cases should be CK7 positive (Klein WM, 2005)(Abdul-Al HM, 2010)(Ward SC, 2010) as well as CD68 positive (Ross HM, 2011). In the absence of CK7 and/or CD68 positivity, a diagnosis of fibrolamellar carcinoma should be carefully re-considered. These findings also extend our understanding of the biology of

Morphological feature	Hepatocellular carcinoma	Hepatocellular adenoma	Low grade dysplastic nodule	High grade dysplastic nodule
Cirrhosis background	80%	Absent	100%	100%
Portal space	Variable	Absent	Present	Present
Bile duct	Variable	Absent	Present	Present
Isolated thick wall arteries	Present	Present	Rare	Rare
Architecture	Tick trabecular, pseudo-glandular or solid pattern	Sheet-like	Regenerative feature	Irregular trabecular pattern
Nodularity	Present	Not specific	Absent	Nodule in nodule
Reticolin	Absent	Present	Present	Increased and irregular
Cytological atipia	Present	Focal	Absent	Present
N/C, nuclear pleomorphism	Variable	Focal	Large cell dysplasia	Small cell dysplasia
Nucleoli	Present	Absent	Absent	Absent or small
Steatosis	Present	Present	Absent	Absent
Mitoses	Rare	Absent	Absent	Absent
Stromal and vascular invasion	Present	Absent	Absent	Absent
Ductular reaction (Ck7 e Ck19)	Variable	Absent	Present	Present
CD34	Diffuse	Variable	Variable	Variable
Ki67	High	Low	Low	Variable

Table 1. The morphological features that differentiate the hepatocellular carcinoma from hepatocellular adenoma and from dysplastic nodules.

fibrolamellar carcinomas. Their oncocytic appearance has typically been attributed to cytoplasmic swelling by numerous packed mitochondria, as seen in electron microscopy studies. The CD68 positivity indicates that fibrolamellar carcinomas also have increased lysosomal or endosomal accumulations in their cytoplasm, which may suggest that abnormalities in endosomal/lysosomal trafficking are characteristic of fibrolamellar carcinomas. Overexpression of CD68 protein occurs at the level of both mRNA and protein (Ross HM, 2010). Of note, one previous study examined a case of fibrolamellar carcinoma and found it to be CD68-positive when using clone KP1 but not clone PG-M1 (Kaiserling E, 1995). They also reported that fibrolamellar carcinoma was weakly positive for Ki-M1P and 3A5, and negative for an anti-lysozyme antibody (Kaiserling E, 1995). These authors also reported that the non-neoplastic liver in a case of biliary atresia was CD68 positive (using clone KP1) and that, based on electron microscopy, immunoreactivity correlated with lysosome-like granules as well as electron dense structures representing probably bile components. Thus, some caution is likely warranted when staining a tumor rich in cytoplasmic bilirubin for CD68, as the bilirubin may be stored in lysosomes within tumor cells. In sum, CD68 immunostaining is a sensitive marker for fibrolamellar carcinoma that may be of use in routine diagnostic surgical pathology. In addition, it may be of use in research studies by helping properly classify cases of fibrolamellar carcinoma. This is of importance because it can help ensure a uniform biological entity, being investigated by different groups, as the incorporation of non-fibrolamellar carcinoma cases in such studies is unlikely to improve our understanding of the biology of this disease.

Immunohistochemical markers	Hepatocellular carcinoma	Cholangiocarcinoma	Metastatic colorectal adenocarcinoma
Alpha-fetoprotein	+	-	-
pCEA	+	-	-
Hep-Par1	+	-	-
Glypican 3	+	-	-
Cytokeratin 8-18	+	-	-
Cytokeratin 7	-	+	-
Cytokeratin 19	-	+	-
Cytokeratin 20	-	-/+	+

Table 2. The panel of immunohistochemistry that helps to solve the differential diagnosis between the hepatocellular carcinoma from other malignant neoplasms

6. References

Abdul-Al HM, Wang G, Makhlouf HR, et al. Fibrolamellar hepatocellular carcinoma: an immunohistochemical comparison with conventional hepatocellular carcinoma. Int J Surg Pathol 2010;18:313–318.

Anthony PP, Vogel CL, Barker LE. Liver cell dysplasia: a premalignant condition. J Clin Pathol 1973;26:217-223.

Bolondi L, Gaiani S, Celli N, Golfieri R, Grigioni WF, Leoni S, et al. Characterization of small nodules in cirrhosis by assessment of vascularity: the problem of hypovascular hepatocellular carcinoma. HEPATOLOGY 2005;42:27-34.

Bruix J, Sherman M. Management of hepatocellular carcinoma.HEPATOLOGY 2005;42:1208-1236.

Bruix J, Sherman M. Management of hepatocellular carcinoma: an update. HEPATOLOGY 2011;53:1020-1022.

Cano-Gauci DF, Song HH, Yang H, Mckerlie C, Choo B, Shi W, et al. Glypican-3-deficient mice exhibit developmental overgrowth and some of the abnormalities typical of Simpson-Golabi-Behmel syndrome. J Cell Biol 1999;146:255-264.

Capurro M, Wanless IR, Sherman M, Deboer G, Shi W, Miyoshi E, Filmus J. Glypican-3: a novel serum and histochemical marker for hepatocellular carcinoma. Gastroenterology 2003; 125:89-97

Chu P, Wu E, Weiss LM. Cytokeratin 7 and cytokeratin 20 expression in epithelial neoplasms: a survey of 435 cases. Mod Pathol 2000; 13: 962-972

Chu PG, Ishizawa S, Wu E, Weiss LM. Hepatocyte antigen as a marker of hepatocellular carcinoma: an immunohistochemical comparison to carcinoembryonic antigen, CD10, and alphafetoprotein. Am J Surg Pathol 2002; 26: 978-988

Chuma M, Sakamoto M, Yamazaki K, Ohta T, Ohiki M, Asaka M, et al. Expression profiling in multistage hepatocarcinogenesis: identification of HSP70 as a molecular marker of early hepatocellular carcinoma.HEPATOLOGY 2003;37:198-207.

Craig JR, Peters RL, Edmondson HA, et al. Fibrolamellar carcinoma of the liver. Cancer 1980;46:372–379.

Christa L, Simon MT, Flinois JP, Gebhardt R, Brechot C, Lasserre C. Overexpression of glutamine synthetase in human primary liver cancer. Gastroenterology 1994;106:1312-1320.

Di Tommaso L, Franchi G, Park YN, Fiamengo B, Destro A, Morenghi E, Montorsi M, Torzilli G, Tommasini M, Terracciano L, Tornillo L, Vecchione R, Roncalli M. Diagnostic value of HSP70, glypican 3, and glutamine synthetase in hepatocellular nodules in cirrhosis. Hepatology. 2007 Mar;45(3):725-34.

Di Tommaso L, Destro A, Seok JY, Balladore E, Terracciano L, Sangiovanni A, Iavarone M, Colombo M, Jang JJ, Yu E, Jin SY, Morenghi E, Park YN, Roncalli M. The application of markers (HSP70 GPC3 and GS) in liver biopsies is useful for detection of hepatocellular carcinoma. J Hepatol. 2009 Apr;50(4):746-54. Epub 2008 Dec 25.

Durnez A, Verslype C, Nevens F, Fevery J, Aerts R, Pirenne J, Lesaffre E, Libbrecht L, Desmet V, Roskams T. The clinicopathological and prognostic relevance of cytokeratin 7 and 19 expression in hepatocellular carcinoma. A possible progenitor cell origin. Histopathology 2006; 49: 138-151

El-Serag HB, Davila JA. Is fibrolamellar carcinoma different from hepatocellular carcinoma? A US population-based study. Hepatology 2004;39:798–803.

Faa G, Van Eyken P, Roskams T, Miyazaki H, Serreli S, Ambu R, Desmet VJ. Expression of cytokeratin 20 in developing rat liver and experimental models of ductular and oval cell proliferation. J Hepatol 1998; 29:628-633

Fanni D, Nemolato S, Ganga R, Senes G, Gerosa C, Van Eyken P, Geboes K, Faa G. Cytokeratin 20-positive hepatocellular carcinoma. Eur J Histochem. 2009 Dec 1;53(4):269-73.

Filmus J. Glypicans in growth control and cancer. Glycobiology 2001;11: 19R–23R.

Forner A, Vilana R, Ayuso C, Bianchi L, Sole´ M, Ayuso JR, et al. Diagnosis of hepatic nodules 20 mm or smaller in cirrhosis: prospective validation of the noninvasive diagnostic criteria for hepatocellular carcinoma. HEPATOLOGY 2008;47:97-104.

Garrido C, Gurbuxani S, Ravagnan L, Kroemer G. Heat shock proteins: endogenous modulators of apoptotic cell death. Biochem Biophys Res Commun 2001;286:433-442.

Gebhardt R, Tanaka T, Williams GM. Glutamine synthetase heterogeneous expression as a marker for the cellular lineage of preneoplastic and neoplastic liver populations. Carcinogenesis 1989;10:1917-1923.

Gouysse G, Frachon S, Hervieu V, et al. Endothelial cell differentiation in hepatocellular adenomas: implications for histopathological diagnosis. J Hepatol 2004;41:259–266.

Goodman ZD. Neoplasms of the liver. Modern Pathology (2007) 20, S49–S60

Haussinger D, Sies H, Gerok W. Functional hepatocyte heterogeneity in ammonia metabolism. The intercellular glutamine cycle. J Hepatol 1985;1:3-14.

Helmbrecht K, Zeise E, Rensing L. Chaperones in cell cycle regulation and mitogenic signal transduction: a review. Cell Prolif 2000;33:341-365.

Hytiroglou P, Theise ND. Differential diagnosis of hepatocellular nodular lesions. Semin Diagn Pathol 1998; 15: 285-299

Hytiroglou P. Morphological changes of early human hepatocarcinogenesis. Semin Liver Dis 2004;24:65–75.

Hytiroglou P, Park YN, Krinsky G, Theise ND. Hepatic precancerous lesions and small hepatocellular carcinoma. Gasteroenterol Clin N Am 2007;36:867-887.

International Working Party. Terminology of nodular hepatocellular lesions. Hepatology 1995;22:983–993.

International Consensus Group for Hepatocellular Neoplasia. Pathologic diagnosis of early hepatocellular carcinoma: a report of the international consensus group for hepatocellular neoplasia. HEPATOLOGY 2009;49:658-664.

Ishak KG, Goodman ZD, Stocker JT. Tumors of the Liver and Intrahepatic Bile Ducts. Atlas of Tumor Pathology, Third Series, Fascicle 31. Armed Forces Institute of Pathology: Washington DC, 2001.

Jolly C, Morimoto RI. Role of the heat shock response and molecular chaperones in oncogenesis and cell death. J Natl Cancer Inst 2000;92: 1564-1572.

Kaiserling E, Ruck P, Xiao JC. Immunoreactivity of neoplastic and non-neoplastic hepatocytes for CD68 and with 3A5, Ki-M1P, and MAC387 light and electron microscopic findings. Int Hepatol Commun 1995;3:322–329.

Kannangai R, Vivekanandan P, Martinez-Murillo F, et al. Fibrolamellar carcinomas show overexpression of genes in the RAS, MAPK, PIK3, and xenobiotic degradation pathways. Hum Pathol 2007;38:639-644.

Kojiro M. Pathology of Hepatocellular Carcinoma. Oxford: Blackwell Publishing, 2006.

Klein WM, Molmenti EP, Colombani PM, et al. Primary liver carcinoma arising in people younger than 30 years. Am J Clin Pathol 2005;124:512–518.

Kutami R, Nakashima Y, Nakashima O, Shiota K, Kojiro M. Pathomorphologic study on the mechanism of fatty change in small hepatocellular carcinoma of humans. J Hepatol 2000;33:282-289.

Lau SK, Prakash S, Geller SA, Alsabeth R. Comparative immunohistochemical profile of hepatocellular carcinoma, cholangiocarcinoma, and metastatic adenocarcinoma. Hum Pathol 2002; 33:1175-1181

Leong AS, Sormunen RT, Tsui WM, Liew CT. Hep-Par1 and selected antibodies in the immunohistological distinction of hepatocellular carcinoma from cholangiocarcinoma, combined tumours and metastatic carcinoma. Histopathology 1998; 33:318-324

Leoni S, Piscaglia F, Golfieri R, Camaggi V, Vidili G, Pini P, et al. The impact of vascular and nonvascular findings on the non invasive diagnosis of small hepatocellular carcinoma based on EASL and AASLD criteria. Am J Gastroenterol 2010;105:599-609.

Libbrecht L, Severi T, Cassiman D, Vander Borght S, Pirenne J, Nevens F, Verslype C, van Pelt J, Roskams T. Glypican-3 expression distinguishes small hepatocellular carcinomas from cirrhosis, dysplastic nodules, and focal nodular hyperplasia like nodules. Am J Surg Pathol 2006; 30: 1405-1411

Lopez JB. Recent developments in the first detection of hepatocellular carcinoma. Clin Biochem Rev 2005; 26: 65-79

Llovet JM, Chen Y, Wurmbach E, Roayaie S, Fiel MI, Schwartz M, et al. A molecular signature to discriminate dysplastic nodules from early hepatocellular carcinoma in HCV cirrhosis. Gastroenterology 2006;131:1758-1767.

Lugli A, Tornillo L, Mirlacher M, et al. Hepatocyte paraffin 1 expression in human normal and neoplastic tissues: tissue microarray analysis on 3,940 tissue samples. Am J Clin Pathol 2004;122:721-727.

Ma CK, Zarbo RJ, Frierson HF Jr, Lee MW. Comparative immunohistochemical study of primary and metastatic carcinomas of the liver. Am J Clin Pathol 1993; 99: 551-557

Maeda T, Kajiyama K, Adachi E, Takenaka K, Sugimachi K, Tsuneyoshi M. The expression of cytokeratins 7, 19, and 20 in primary and metastatic carcinomas of the liver. Mod Pathol 1996; 9:901-909

Maharaj B, Maharaj RJ, Leary WP, Cooppan RM, Naran AD, Pirie D, Pudifi n DJ. Sampling variability and its influence on the diagnostic yield of percutaneous needle biopsy of the liver. Lancet 1986; 1: 523-525

Malouf G, Falissard B, Azoulay D, et al. Is histological diagnosis of primary liver carcinomas with fibrous stroma reproducible among experts? J Clin Pathol 2009;62:519-524.

Minervini MI, Demetris AJ, Lee RG, et al. Utilization of hepatocyte-specific antibody in the immunocytochemical evaluation of liver tumors. Mod Pathol 1997;10:686-692.

Moorman AF, de Boer PA, Geerts WJ, van de Zande L, Lamers WH, Charles R. Complementary distribution of carbamoylphosphate synthetase (ammonia) and glutamine synthetase in rat liver acinus is regulated at a pretranslational level. J Histochem Cytochem 1988;36:751-755.

Moorman AF, Vermeulen JL, Charles R, Lamers WH. Localization of ammonia-metabolizing enzymes in human liver: ontogenesis of eterogeneity. HEPATOLOGY 1989;9:367-372.

Nam SW, Park JY, Ramasamy A, Shevade S, Islam A, Long PM, et al. Molecular changes from dysplastic nodule to hepatocellular carcinoma through gene expression profiling. HEPATOLOGY 2005;42:809-818.

Onofre AS, Pomjanski N, Buckstegge B, Bocking A. Immunocytochemical diagnosis of hepatocellular carcinoma and identification of carcinomas of unknow primary metastatic to the liver on fine-needle aspiration cytologies. Cancer 2007; 111:259-268

Osada T, Sakamoto M, Nagawa H, Yamamoto J, Matsuno Y, Iwamatsu A, et al. Acquisition of glutamine synthetase expression in human hepatocarcinogenesis: relation to disease recurrence and possible regulation by ubiquitin-dependent proteolysis. Cancer 1999;85:819-831.

Paradis V, Bie`che I, Darge`re D, Laurendeau I, Laurent C, Bioulac Sage P, et al. Molecular profiling of hepatocellular carcinomas (HCC) using a large-scale real-time RT-PCR approach: determination of a molecular diagnostic index. Am J Pathol 2003;163:733-741.

Paradis V, Benzekri A, Dargere D, et al. Telangiectatic focal nodular hyperplasia: a variant of hepatocellular adenoma. Gastroenterol 2004;126:1323–1329.

Park YN, Yang C-P, Fernandez GJ, Cubukcu O, Thung SN, Theise ND. Neoangiogenesis and sinusoidal "capillarization" in dysplastic nodules of the liver. Am J Surg Path 1998;22:656-662.

Park YN, Kojiro M, Di Tommaso L, Dhillon AP, Kondo F, Nakano M, et al. Ductular reaction is helpful in defining early stromal invasion, small hepatocellular carcinomas, and dysplastic nodules. Cancer 2007;109:915–923.

Porcell AI, De Young BR, Proca DM, Frankel WL Immunohistochemical analysis of hepatocellular and adenocarcinoma in the liver: MOC31 compares favorably with other putative markers. Mod Pathol 2000 13:773-778

Reitzer LJ, Wice BM, Kennell D. Evidence that glutamine, not sugar, is the major energy source for cultured HeLa cells. J Biol Chem 1979;254:2669-2676.

Roncalli M, Terracciano L, Di Tommaso L, David E, Colombo M. Liver precancerous lesions and hepatocellular carcinoma: the histology report. Dig Liver Dis. 2011 Mar;43 Suppl 4:S361-72.

Roskams T, Kojiro M. Pathology of early hepatocellular carcinoma: conventional and molecular diagnosis. Semin Liver Dis 2010;30:17-25.

Ross HM, Daniel HD, Vivekanandan P, Kannangai R, Yeh MM, Wu TT, Makhlouf HR, Torbenson M. Fibrolamellar carcinomas are positive for CD68. Mod Pathol. 2011 Mar;24(3):390-5.

Saad RS, Luckasevic TM, Noga CM, Johnson DR, Silverman JF, Liu YL. Diagnostic value of HepPar1, pCEA, CD10, and CD34 expression in separating hepatocellular carcinoma from metastatic carcinoma in fine-needle aspiration cytology. Diagn Cytopathol 2004; 30: 1-6

Sangiovanni A, Manini MA, Iavarone M, Romeo R, Forzenigo LV, Fraquelli M, et al. The diagnostic and economic impact of contrast imaging technique in the diagnosis of small hepatocellular carcinoma in cirrhosis. Gut 2010;59:638-644.

Seimiya M, Tomonaga T, Matsushita K, Sunaga M, Ohishi M, Kodera M, et al. Identification of novel immunohistochemical tumor markers for primary hepatocellular carcinoma; clathrin heavy chain and formiminotransferase cyclodeaminase. HEPATOLOGY 2008;48:519-530.

Senes G, Fanni D, Cois A, Uccheddu A, Faa G. Intratumoral sampling variability in hepatocellular carcinoma: a case report. World J Gastroenterol. 2007 Aug 7;13(29):4019-21.

Sherman M. Hepatocellular carcinoma: epidemiology, surveillance, and diagnosis. Semin Liver Dis 2010;30:3-16.

Siddiqui MT, Saboorian MH, Gokaslan ST, Ashfaq R. Diagnostic utility of the HepPar1 antibody to differentiate hepatocellular carcinoma from metastatic carcinoma in fine needle aspiration samples. Cancer 2002; 96: 49-52

Sollai M, Fanos V, Fanni D, Gerosa C, Senes G, Dessì A, Locci A, Van Eyken P, Faa G. GLYPICAN 3 IMMUNOREACTIVITY IN THE HUMAN FETAL LIVER DURING GESTATION. J Matern Fetal Neonatal Med (in press).

Soreide O, Czemiak A, Bradpiece H, et al. Characteristics of fibrolamellar hepatocellular carcinoma: a study of nine cases and a review of the literature. Am J Surg 1986;151:518–523.

Stroescu C, Herlea V, Dragnea A, Popescu I. The diagnostic value of cytokeratins and carcinoembryonic antigen immunostaining in differentiating hepatocellular carcinomas from intrahepatic cholangiocarcinomas. J Gastrointestin Liver Dis 2006; 15:9-14

Sugiki T, Yamamoto M, Aruga A, Takasaki K, Nakano M. Immunohistological evaluation of single small hepatocellular carcinoma with negative staining of monoclonal antibody Hepatocyte Paraffin 1. J Surg Oncol 2004; 88: 104-107

Terracciano LM, Glatz K, Mhawech P, Vasei M, Lehmann FS, Vecchione R, Tornillo L. Hepatoid adenocarcinoma with liver metastasis mimicking hepatocellular carcinoma: an immunohistochemicaland molecular study of eight cases. AM J Surg Pathol 2003; 27:1302-1312

Theise ND, Park YN, Kojiro M. Dysplastic nodules and hepatocarcinogenesis. Clin Liver Dis 2002;6:497–512.

Torbenson M. Review of the clinicopathologic features of fibrolamellar carcinoma. Adv Anat Pathol 2007;14:217–223.

Van Eyken P, Sciot R, Paterson A, Callea F, Kew MC, Desmet VJ. Cytokeratin expression in hepatocellular carcinoma: an immunohistochemical study. Hum Pathol 1988; 19: 562-568

Varma V, Cohen C. Immunohistochemical and molecular markers in the diagnosis of hepatocellular carcinoma. Adv Anat Pathol 2004; 11: 239-249

Vivekanandan P, Micchelli ST, Torbenson M. Anterior gradient-2 is overexpressed by fibrolamellar carcinomas. Hum Pathol 2009;40:293–299.

Wang L, Vuolo M, Suhrland MJ, Schlesinger K. HepPar1, MOC-31, pCEA, mCEA and CD10 for distinguishing hepatocellular carcinoma vs. metastatic adenocarcinoma in liver fine needle aspirates. Acta Cytol 2006; 50: 257-262

Watanabe S, Watanabe S, Okita K, Harada T, Kodama T, Numa Y, et al. Morphologic studies of the liver cell dysplasia. Cancer 1983;51:2197-2205

Ward SC, Huang J, Tickoo SK, et al. Fibrolamellar carcinoma of the liver exhibits immunohistochemical evidence of both hepatocyte and bile duct differentiation. Mod Pathol 2010;23:1180–1190.

Watanabe S, Watanabe S, Okita K, Harada T, Kodama T, Numa Y, et al. Morphologic studies of the liver cell dysplasia. Cancer 1983;51:2197-2205

Wurmbach E, Chen YB, Khitrov G, Zhang W, Roayaie S, Schwartz M, et al. Genome-wide molecular profiles of HCV-induced dysplasia and hepatocellular carcinoma. HEPATOLOGY 2007;45:938-947.

Yamauchi N, Watanabe A, Hishinuma M, Ohashi K, Midorikawa Y, Morishita Y, Niki T, Shibahara J, Mori M, Makuuchi M, Hippo Y, Kodama T, Iwanari H, Aburatani H, Fukayama M. The glypican 3 oncofetal protein is a promising diagnostic marker for hepatocellular carcinoma. Mod Pathol 2005; 18: 1591-1598

Zhou L, Liu J, Luo F. Serum tumor markers for detection of hepatocellular carcinoma. World J Gastroenterol 2006; 12:1175-1181

Zhu ZW, Friess H, Wang L, Abou-Shady M, Zimmermann A, Lander AD, Korc M, Kleeff J, Buchler MW. Enhanced glypican-3 expression differentiates the majority of hepatocellular carcinomas from benign hepatic disorders. Gut 2001; 48: 558-564

Zimmerman RL, Burke MA, Young NA, Solomides CC, Bibbo M. Diagnostic value of hepatocyte paraffin 1 antibody to discriminate hepatocellular carcinoma from metastatic carcinoma in fine-needle aspiration biopsies of the liver. Cancer 2001; 93: 288-291

4

Recent Advances in the Immunohistochemistry-Aided Differential Diagnosis of Benign Versus Malignant Hepatocellular Lesions

Péter Tátrai, Ilona Kovalszky and András Kiss
Semmelweis University
Hungary

1. Introduction

Rather than obliterating the need for histopathologic examination, the availability of modern imaging modalities and efficient antitumor therapies heighten the importance of timely and accurate histologic diagnosis of hepatocellular carcinoma (HCC). More than ever before, there is now real hope of curative intervention for HCC discovered in an early stage. Thus, a key diagnostic role is assigned to histopathology whenever radiologic findings are inconclusive. While classical micromorphologic (cytologic and architectural) features are still at the heart of histopathologic evaluation, there is ongoing effort to complement histologic findings with the analysis of characteristic immunohistochemical (IHC) markers. In all modern pathology centers, IHC has become a cornerstone of the diagnostic process. The aid provided by immunomarkers is particularly resorted to when ambiguous cases are encountered. This review focuses on the role of IHC in one of the major differential diagnostic dilemmas related to HCC: the benign versus malignant problem. The question of malignant character may arise either when evaluating biopsies of suspicious nodules obtained from high-risk patients, or when analyzing tissue from hepatocellular tumors discovered in a non-cirrhotic background. Accordingly, the review will separately discuss the problem of small nodular lesions in cirrhosis, and the issue of large tumors arising in the normal liver. In our attempt to summarize state-of-the-art expert opinion, we have largely built on two outstanding reviews (Park, 2011; Roncalli et al., 2011), and tried to provide an update on recent progress made in the field.

Since it is very challenging to propose a logical and non-overlapping classification of all IHC markers, molecules will be presented in an alphabetical order. Brief introduction of each marker at its first mentioning will be followed by evaluation of its diagnostic utility, with regard to both benefits and potential pitfalls.

2. Differentiation of HCC from small precursor lesions

2.1 Dysplastic nodules and small HCC: Definitions and the role of biopsy

It is now commonly accepted that, at least in the setting of chronic hepatitis, HCC evolves through several stages of premalignant lesions. In the current view, HCC may either evolve directly from microscopic (< 1 mm) clusters of atypical hepatocytes called dysplastic foci, or arise within macroscopic lesions termed dysplastic nodules (DNs). The following definitions conform to the latest recommendations by the International Consensus Group for Hepatocellular Neoplasia (2009). DNs with no or minimal cytologic/architectural atypia are referred to as low-grade (LG) and are unlikely to be immediately precancerous, while those with marked atypia (that is nevertheless insufficient for the diagnosis of HCC) are termed high-grade (HG), and often harbor overtly malignant subnodules. The term large regenerative nodule (LRN) has also been in use; however, LRN cannot be confidently discriminated on a purely morphologic basis from LGDN, and due to its supposed polyclonal origin it is not considered as a distinct step in the hepatocarcinogenic process (Libbrecht et al., 2005). Finally, small HCC (sHCC) is a histologically malignant tumor below the size of 2 cm, and may present as a vaguely or distinctly demarcated nodular mass, denoted as early and progressed sHCC, respectively.

Unlike dysplastic foci that are too small to be detected by any radiological technique, DNs and sHCC may often be clearly distinguished from the surrounding parenchyma by ultrasound. Hence, ultrasound screening has become an integral part of surveillance for the high-risk populations, i.e. for hepatitis B carriers and cirrhotics with various etiologies. According to the international guidelines (Bruix & Sherman, 2005) based on the Barcelona Clinic Liver Cancer Group recommendations, nodules discovered by ultrasound, if smaller than 1 cm, are followed up strictly and monitored for enlargement; nodules between 1-2 cm are subjected to examination by two contrast-enhanced dynamic imaging modalities; and nodules greater than 2 cm are examined by one dynamic imaging technique. Being a hypervascular tumor with dominantly arterial blood supply, typical HCCs show enhancement in the arterial phase followed by washout in the portal venous phase. Nodules between 1-2 cm with characteristic imaging findings by two methods, and nodules greater than 2 cm showing typical vascular pattern by one method, are treated as HCC. On the other hand, nodules with atypical vascular pattern or inconsistent radiologic findings require confirmation of benign versus malignant character by biopsy.

2.2 Individual markers for the discrimination of dysplastic nodules vs. small HCC

alpha-Smooth muscle actin (a-SMA) is a cytoskeletal component specific to cells with smooth muscle differentiation, including vascular smooth muscle cells and activated hepatic stellate cells. Hence, α-SMA immunostaining can be used to highlight both arteries and capillarized sinusoids. Although α-SMA IHC alone is not informative enough to solve the problem in question, it may help recognize unpaired arteries (i.e., arteries not accompanied by other portal structures) characteristic of DNs and sHCC (Park et al., 1998; Roncalli et al., 1999), and reveal pericytes around capillarized blood vessels.

Agrin is a large heparan sulfate proteoglycan deposited in biliary and vascular basement membranes of the liver (Tátrai et al., 2006). Since it is missing from the sinusoids of the normal liver and cirrhotic regenerative nodules, but appears in the wall of HCC microvessels very early during malignant transformation, the presence of agrin associated to microvascular structures is suggestive of HCC. Applying semi-quantitative evaluation criteria, agrin IHC discriminated sHCC from DNs with a sensitivity of 87% and a specificity of 97% (Tátrai et al. 2009). The chief practical difficulty with the use of agrin IHC is positive

Recent Advances in the Immunohistochemistry-Aided Differential Diagnosis of Benign Versus
Malignant Hepatocellular Lesions

75

labeling of ductular reaction and, although with lesser intensity, transitional cells differentiating from ductular cells into hepatocytes. Agrin-positive basement membranes on the periphery, or occasionally in the interior, of regenerative nodules due to the presence of reactive ductules and active parenchymal regeneration may confound the untrained observer. Thus, evaluation of agrin IHC requires some caution and expertise, and agrin immunopositivity is indicative of HCC only when it colocalizes with vascular markers such as CD31 or CD34. On the other hand, positive labeling of reactive ductules may be seen as an advantage, since the presence or absence of ductular reaction in and around a nodule is a diagnostic factor *per se* (see *Cytokeratin-7 and -19* below). Agrin IHC has been tested on resected specimens but not on core biopsies; hence, its performance with small samples is as yet unknown.

Annexin A2 (ANXA2). Annexins, calcium-dependent phospholipid-binding proteins with multiple functions in the regulation of vesicular trafficking, cell division, and apoptosis, are known to be differentially expressed in many forms of human neoplasia (Mussunoor & Murray, 2008). ANXA2 is upregulated in several cancer types but silenced in others; in HCC, it is overexpressed by tumor hepatocytes, as well as by endothelial cells of tumor neovessels (Yu et al., 2007). Increased ANXA2 expression was observed in proliferating benign hepatocytes, but not in sinusoidal endothelial cells, during liver regeneration (Masaki et al., 1994). Accordingly, diffuse vascular endothelial staining of ANXA2 was seen in 28/34 (84%) of HCCs but 0/7 DNs, whereas diffuse sinusoidal CD31 staining was observed in 43% of the same lesions (Longerich et al., 2011). Thus, diffuse vascular ANXA2 staining was proposed to be specific to HCC, and was successfully applied to improve the diagnostic accuracy of the GPC3 + GS + HSP70 panel (see below).

CD31/CD34. CD31, also known as platelet endothelial cell adhesion molecule-1 or PECAM-1, is a member of the immunoglobulin superfamily, and acts as a cell adhesion and signaling receptor on hematopoietic and endothelial cells (Newman, 1997). Pathologists routinely use CD31 for the immunostaining of vascular endothelia (e.g., the vasculature of tumors), or tumors with endothelial differentiation. CD34, a glycoprotein with poorly defined functions (proposed roles include regulation of adhesion and proliferation), is expressed on endothelial cells, as well as on hematopoietic and tissue stem/progenitor cells (Nielsen & McNagny, 2008). Although in clinical practice CD34 is used as a stem cell marker for the separation of hematopoietic progenitors, and as an immunomarker it has broad applications in pathology elsewhere (e.g. in the differential diagnosis of mesenchymal neoplasms, see Ponsaing et al., 2007), in the present context it is merely regarded as a vascular endothelial marker alternative to CD31. Normal sinusoidal endothelium is nearly devoid of these markers, in contrast with capillarized sinusoids, unpaired arteries, and HCC microvessels that all exhibit CD31/CD34 immunopositivity (Couvelard et al., 1993; Park et al., 1998). Normal liver is at one end of the spectrum, with virtually no CD31/CD34 immunostaining except for portal blood vessels, and typical HCC is at the other extreme with complete and ubiquitous CD31/CD34-positive vascular pattern. Thus, CD31/CD34 IHC may in theory facilitate distinction between regenerative and dysplastic nodules, as well as between DNs and HCC. However, an abrupt jump in the number of CD31/CD34-positive capillaries was observed between LGDN and HGDN, while the transition from regenerative nodules to LGDN and from HGDN to HCC was rather smooth. CD31-positive capillary units were significantly more abundant in HGDN relative to both cirrhotic regenerative nodules and

LGDN; however, HGDN did not differ significantly from HCC in this respect (Roncalli et al., 1999). Similarly, CD34 immunostaining was shown to increase gradually from normal sinusoids through capillarized sinusoids to neovessels, but failed to discriminate between HGDN and HCC (Park et al., 1998; Tátrai et al., 2009). In conclusion, endothelial markers may confirm suspicion of malignant character, but without exact cutoff values determined for each lesion type they are hardly diagnostic on their own (Park, 2011). In addition, similar to α-SMA, endothelial markers may be suitable for the detection of unpaired arteries (see above).

Cyclase-associated protein 2 (CAP2) is the human homologue of CAP, a protein originally isolated from budding yeast and only poorly characterized in mammals; in the yeast, CAP is known to associate with both the adenylyl cyclase complex and actin cytoskeleton. CAP2 levels were found to increase gradually during the process of hepatocarcinogenesis. CAP2 was overexpressed in early HCC relative to noncancerous and precancerous lesions, and further upregulated in progressed HCC (Shibata et al., 2006). In the normal and cirrhotic liver, smooth muscle cells strongly expressed CAP2, but normal hepatocytes were negative, and only weak staining was occasionally seen on the periphery of regenerative nodules. Precancerous lesions were either negative or only focally positive (5-10% of total area immunostained), whereas all early HCCs exhibited some CAP2 positivity, and 40% of them showed rather diffuse (70-100%) CAP2 immunostaining (Sakamoto, 2009). When examining nodule-in-nodule type early HCC lesions, the more advanced component exhibited stronger CAP2 reaction. While these results are encouraging, neither sensitivity and specificity values nor data on biopsy specimens have been reported.

Cytokeratin-7 and -19 (CK7/19). In the context of liver histology, CK-7 and -19 are cholangiocytic cytokeratins that highlight bile ducts and reactive ductules. Stromal invasion, i.e., invasion of (pre)malignant hepatocytes into the portal tract or septal stroma, is one of the earliest signs of hepatocellular transformation, and the scarceness or lack of outer and inner ductular reaction (DR) due to invasive growth has been reported to sensitively reflect malignant character of hepatic nodules in both resected and biopsied specimens (Park et al., 2007). The recognition of stromal invasion may be especially challenging in biopsy specimens and in well-differentiated, vaguely nodular sHCC where invasive growth is focal and obscure. The authors propose that visualization of CK7-positive DR may help resolve this diagnostic dilemma. By scoring the intensity of DR semiquantitatively on a scale between 0 and 4+, most non-invasive lesions (diagnosed as such by trained experts) scored 3+ or 4+, while overtly invasive HCCs typically scored 0 or 1+. In our own calculation, considering 0 to +2 as "missing or scant DR" and 3+ to 4+ as "present or florid DR", the lack of strong CK7-positive DR identified histologically invasive lesions with sensitivity and specificity parameters as follows: 83% and 97% (inner DR in resected nodules); 67% and 98% (outer DR in resected nodules); 95% and 90% (biopsied nodules). As expected, well-differentiated, vaguely nodular type HCCs proved to be the most problematic because they often had significant amount of (probably residual) DR both within and around.

Enhancer of zeste homologue 2 (EZH2). As the catalytically active subunit of the polycomb repressive complex 2, EZH2 is responsible for histone methylation-mediated gene silencing, and has been reported to be upregulated in a variety of human cancers (Xiao, 2011). Overexpression of EZH2 was detected in both HCC cell lines and tissue samples, and siRNA-mediated knockdown of EZH2 decreased tumorigenicity of human HCC cells

Recent Advances in the Immunohistochemistry-Aided Differential Diagnosis of Benign Versus
Malignant Hepatocellular Lesions

77

xenografted into nude mice (Chen et al., 2007). In a testing cohort containing 121 HCCs and 121 nontumorous liver tissues, nuclear EZH2 immunoreaction was observed in 66% of tumor cells but only 2.4% of nonneoplastic hepatocytes, and by selecting an appropriate cut-off value, discrimination with 96% sensitivity and 98% specificity could be obtained (Cai et al., 2011). Subsequently, in a validation series consisting of core biopsies, EZH2 alone was able to discriminate between nonmalignant nodules and HCC with a sensitivity of 78% and a specificity of 93%. In fact, EZH2 as an individual marker outperformed both GPC3 and HSP70 in this study, and additional refinement of diagnostic accuracy could be achieved by combining EZH2 with the latter two markers (see below).

Glutamine synthetase (GS) is a metabolic enzyme that converts glutamate and ammonia into glutamine, a main fuel for tumor cells. In contrast with the normal liver where GS expression is restricted to pericentral and periportal hepatocytes, most HCCs exhibit upregulation of GS (Christa et al., 1994) and diffuse, intense cytoplasmic GS immunostaining (Di Tommaso et al., 2007). This is thought to be due to overactivation of the β-catenin pathway, since GS is among the target genes of β-catenin (Zucman-Rossi et al., 2007). Expression levels of GS were found to increase in parallel with HCC progression (Osada et al., 1999). GS as an individual marker yielded 70% sensitivity and 94% specificity in discriminating resected benign vs. malignant nodules in cirrhosis (Di Tommaso et al., 2007). Over 50% of tumor cells were strongly GS-positive in the majority of HCCs, including early tumors; however, to gain more sensitivity, GS immunostaining was already considered homogeneous and positive with little more than 10% of immunoreactive cells. Similar diagnostic efficacy was obtained with biopsy specimens (GS as an individual marker, sensitivity: 59%, specificity: 98%) (Di Tommaso et al., 2009).

Glypican-3 (GPC3), a glycosyl-phosphatidylinositol anchored cell surface heparan sulfate proteoglycan, is overexpressed in the majority of HCCs (Zhu et al., 2001), and is currently accepted as the best-performing individual IHC and serum marker of HCC (Capurro et al., 2003; International Consensus Group, 2009). GPC3 regulates multiple growth factor signaling pathways including those of Wnts, Hhs, IGF, FGF2, and BMPs, and is therefore thought to be directly involved in HCC pathogenesis (reviewed by Akutsu et al., 2010). Being an oncofetal antigen, it is absent from the healthy adult liver and becomes re-expressed upon hepatocytic transformation only. GPC3 immunostaining in malignant hepatocytes may present as granular or strong diffuse cytoplasmic pattern, and may also appear on the cell membrane. With the detection threshold set very low (lesions with a single GPC3-immunoreactive cell were treated as positive), a sensitivity of 77% and a specificity of 96% could be achieved when discriminating sHCC from benign hepatic nodules in resected specimens (Libbrecht et al., 2006). The same values were 83% and 100% for needle biopsies. Of course, like with any other method, some lesions were in the 'grey zone': occasionally, foci of hepatocytes with marked atypia and GPC3 positivity were discovered in HGDNs; and a proportion of HCCs, especially the well-differentiated and less aggressive ones, remained negative in spite of maximum possible sensitivity. Di Tommaso et al. (2007, 2009) applied somewhat stricter criteria for positivity (threshold was set at 5% immunoreactive cells), and could nevertheless nicely reproduce previous results, achieving 74% sensitivity and 96% specificity on resected specimens, and 71% / 94% on core biopsies. Wang et al. (2010) found 83% of HCC needle biopsies to be GPC3-positive. Impressive as these values are, GPC3 IHC also has its potential pitfalls and, not coincidentally, GPC3 is currently recommended for use in combination with one or more additional markers (see below). As much as 40% of early HCCs arising in cirrhosis may be GPC3-negative (Wang et al., 2006). On the other hand, Abdul-Al et al. (2008) and Shafizadeh et al. (2008) pointed out that focal positive staining for GPC3 in active chronic hepatitis C is not an infrequent finding, and may correlate with the acquisition of a fetal-like phenotype during hepatocytic regeneration. Intriguingly, other authors claimed that cirrhotic nodules were invariably negative in core needle biopsies (Anatelli et al., 2008). In a high case number tissue microarray-based study, 9% of non-neoplastic and 16% of preneoplastic liver samples were GPC3-positive (Baumhoer et al., 2008). Thus, while the utility of GPC3 is undisputed, awareness of its limitations in terms of both sensitivity and specificity is advisable.

Heat shock protein 70 (HSP70). The 70-kDa member of the heat shock protein family was identified as the most abundantly upregulated gene during HCC progression by a gene expression array comparing early vs. progressed components of nodule-in-nodule type lesions (Chuma et al., 2003). Overexpression of HSP70, observed in other cancer types as well, enhances proliferation, and confers resistance to attacks of the immune system and apoptosis (Khalil et al., 2011). In IHC studies, HSP70 was strongly expressed by cholangiocytes that hence served as internal positive control, but not by normal hepatocytes, and only faintly and focally in cirrhotic nodules. The intensity of HSP70 immunostaining seemed to increase in parallel with the transition from DN through early HCC to progressed HCC (Chuma et al., 2003). Sensitivity and specificity of HSP70 alone in discriminating HGDN from early HCC was 78% and 95% in resected specimens (Di Tommaso et al., 2007). The criterion for positivity was nucleocytoplasmic staining in at least 5% of lesional hepatocytes. In needle biopsies, however, HSP70 recognized malignant nodules with a sensitivity as low as 48% (Di Tommaso et al., 2009). The fall in sensitivity was probably due to scattered focal positivity in highly differentiated lesions which made them especially prone to sampling error.

2.3 Marker panels for the discrimination of dysplastic nodules vs. small HCC

Agrin + CD34. The discriminative power of agrin IHC could be slightly improved by taking into account the CD34 immunostaining pattern of small nodular lesions. By handling only those nodules as malignant that exhibited complete immunostaining with both agrin and CD34, sHCC could be identified in 87% of the cases, and 100% specificity was attained (Tátrai et al., 2009).

Clathrin heavy chain (CHC) + formiminotransferase cyclodeaminase (FTCD). These two potential markers were identified by 2-dimensional fluorescence difference gel electrophoresis, and validated by IHC on a tissue array containing 83 HCC and 68 non-tumor liver tissue cores (Seimiya et al., 2008). CHC, as a member of the clathrin complex, is a ubiquitous protein involved in membrane trafficking and mitosis; however, CHC has also been shown to regulate p53 function, and is a gene fusion partner in several human tumor types (Ohmori et al., 2008; Blixt & Royle, 2011). FTCD, a bifunctional enzyme that couples histidine degradation to folate metabolism, is also present in every cell type but most abundantly in the liver (Mao et al., 2004). CHC was found to be upregulated and FTCD downregulated in early HCC relative to the surrounding parenchyma (Seimiya et al., 2008). Although the sensitivity of either CHC or FTCD alone was not sufficiently high for the detection of HCC (52% and 61%, respectively), a sensitivity of 81%, beside a specificity of 94%, could be

Recent Advances in the Immunohistochemistry-Aided Differential Diagnosis of Benign Versus
Malignant Hepatocellular Lesions

79

achieved by combining the two. The authors reported additional gains in efficacy when combining the novel markers with GPC3, and their findings were further evaluated in respect with CHC by Di Tommaso et al. (2011) who tentatively added CHC to the widely accepted 3-marker panel GPC3 + GS + HSP70 (see below).

GPC3 + EZH2 + HSP70. This panel of markers was recently shown to discriminate needle-biopsied benign and malignant nodules with a sensitivity of 81% and a specificity of 100% when cases with 2 positive markers out of 3 were regarded as malignant (Cai et al., 2011). This efficacy was significantly superior to that of any single marker alone, and better than the standard 3-marker panel with GS in the place of EZH2 (see below).

GPC3 + GS + HSP70: the standard 3-marker panel and its derivates. Combination of these three markers was first proposed by the Roncalli group (Di Tommaso et al., 2007), and has been quickly acknowledged as the best IHC panel for the discrimination of early HCC against benign nodules (International Consensus Group, 2009; Roncalli et al., 2011). With any 2 of the 3 markers being unequivocally positive, early HCC could be distinguished from HGDN with 72% sensitivity and 100% specificity in resected specimens, and 59% sensitivity and 100% specificity in needle core biopsies (Di Tommaso et al., 2007, 2009). In both cases, sensitivity and specificity were significantly improved as compared to the application of any of the three markers alone. Recently, inspired by the results of Seimiya et al. (2008), the group tested the added value of including CHC (see under 2.2) as a fourth marker into the diagnostic panel (Di Tommaso et al., 2011). Extension of the 3-marker panel to a 4-marker panel by the inclusion of CHC was shown to yield a further gain in diagnostic efficacy. E.g., by taking 2 positive markers out of the 4 as indicative of HCC, sensitivity of detection of sHCC in core biopsies was improved from 47% to 64%. To the same end, Longerich et al. (2011) complemented the 3-marker panel with ANXA2 (see under 2.2), and achieved 74% sensitivity coupled with 100% specificity in discriminating any benign lesion from HCC in resected specimens.

GPC3 + phenol sulfotranferase 1 (SULT1A1). SULT1A1 is a xenobiotic metabolic enzyme selected by 2-dimensional polyacrylamide gel electrophoresis and confirmed as HCC marker by Western blotting and IHC (Yeo et al., 2010). By IHC, SULT1A1 was found to be downregulated in roughly half of HCCs. By combining the results of GPC3 and SULT1A1 (the IHC-based diagnosis is HCC if GPC3 is positive or SULT1A1 is negative), sensitivity could be improved from 72% (GPC3 alone) to 79%. SULT1A1 was shown to differentiate between LGDN and HCC, but its utility was not specifically addressed in the discrimination of HGDN vs. sHCC.

3. Differentiation of HCC from benign liver tumors

3.1 Focal nodular hyperplasia and hepatocellular adenoma: Entities with distinct pathogenesis and clinical behavior

Focal nodular hyperplasia (FNH), as also suggested by its name, is not a true neoplastic lesion; rather, it is a polyclonal hyperplastic, tumor-like reaction to an intrahepatic vascular malformation or alteration (Schirmacher & Longerich, 2009). With an incidence of 3% in the total population, FNH is the second most common benign liver tumor after hemangioma. Classical morphologic features of FNH include a central stellate scar with abnormal arteries, and surrounding nodules separated by fibrous septa and florid ductular reaction. FNH, unlike HCA, is not prone to malignant transformation or hemorrhage; however, its differential diagnosis by contrast-enhanced imaging techniques may be difficult under certain circumstances, making resection and pathologic examination necessary.

Hepatocellular adenoma (HCA) is 10 times less frequently encountered than FNH; it may nevertheless call for urgent attention due to the risk of hemorrhage and, especially in the β-catenin-mutated subtypes, transformation into HCC. Molecular classification of HCA has led to the identification of three groups: 1) classical HCA with inactivating mutation of hepatocyte nuclear factor 1α (HNF1α); 2) 'atypical' HCA with activating mutation of β-catenin; and 3) inflammatory HCA with inflammatory infiltrate and occasional activating mutation of β-catenin (Bioulac-Sage et al., 2007a). Less than 10% of all HCAs lack any characteristic profile and hence remain unclassified. Inflammatory HCA presents the highest risk of bleeding, while β-catenin-mutated HCA harbors a strong tendency toward malignant transformation, and approx. 40% of cases actually progress to HCC (Schirmacher & Longerich, 2009).

Current recommendations on IHC-assisted pathologic differential diagnosis of FNH and HCA have recently been covered by Bioulac-Sage et al. (2011); the present discussion is mostly based on this excellent review.

3.2 Individual markers and their combinations for the discrimination of HCC vs. benign liver tumors

Agrin. (See section 2.2 for introduction.) Agrin, just like CD34, is diffusely positive over the entire vascular network of HCCs, whereas the expression of agrin is more restricted than that of CD34 in HCAs lacking significant atypia. Thus, agrin IHC is more selective in discriminating typical HCA from HCC when compared to CD34. Strong and ubiquitous vascular agrin immunostaining was present in 26/27 HCCs but only 7/30 HCAs, with 3 of the 7 diffusely agrin-positive HCAs exhibiting marked to severe atypia (Tátrai et al., 2009). By quantitative evaluation of agrin immunostaining, HCA could be distinguished from HCC with a sensitivity of 80% and a specificity of 89%.

Annexin A2 (ANXA2). (See section 2.2 for introduction.) ANXA2 alone did not work as accurately in the discrimination of HCA and HCC as in the differentiation of benign vs. malignant nodules: the vascular network of 6/19 (32%) of HCAs showed diffuse ANXA2 immunostaining (Longerich et al., 2011). However, when combined with the 3-marker panel GPC3 + GS + HSP70, false positives could be eliminated, and satisfactory diagnostic efficacy was obtained (all benign lesions vs. HCC, sensitivity: 74%, specificity: 100%).

β-Catenin is the major target of Wnt signaling and a key transcriptional regulator with well-known functions in hepatic oncogenesis (reviewed by Dahmani et al., 2011). Activation of the β-catenin pathway may accompany both benign and malignant hepatocytic proliferation; mutations of β-catenin, however, are specifically found in the high-risk subtypes of HCA, as well as in up to 50% of HCCs. Overactivation of the β-catenin pathway is hallmarked by aberrant nuclear and/or cytoplasmic β-catenin immunostaining. Such positive nucleocytoplasmic β-catenin staining is absent from FNH but, although often weakly and focally, found in β-catenin-mutated HCA and HCC.

CD34. (See section 2.2 for introduction.) In both FNH and HCA, some sinusoids experience altered perfusion, and a shift toward arterial supply favors the neoexpression of CD34. CD34-positive, arterialized sinusoids are seen to radiate away from portal tract-like structures in FNH, and surround small tumor-supplying arteries in typical HCA

(Theuerkauf et al., 2001). On the other hand, in the majority of HCCs, and also in some cases of 'atypical' HCA (i.e., HCA showing marked cytologic and/or architectural atypia), the entire capillary network of the tumor is diffusely CD34-positive. Although not sufficiently specific on its own, the above features make CD34 a useful ancillary marker when applied in combination (see *Glypican-3* in this section).

C-reactive protein (CRP) and serum amyloid A (SAA) are acute phase proteins upregulated in inflammatory HCA, and as immunomarkers they have been shown to specifically identify this subtype of HCA (Bioulac-Sage et al., 2007b). Both are absent from FNH and non-inflammatory HCA, and only rarely positive in HCC.

Glutamine synthetase (GS). (See section 2.2 for introduction.) GS immunostaining, restricted to 1-2 cell thick hepatocyte plates around hepatic venules in the normal liver, is greatly broadened in FNH, resulting in a map-like pattern of large anastomosing immunopositive areas (Bioulac-Sage et al., 2009). Hepatocytes in the immediate vicinity of fibrous septa and arteries usually remain unstained. Although this is a typical finding, it may be less evident in rare cases with excessive steatosis or sinusoidal dilation. As a contrast, GS immunostaining is either missing or reminiscent of the normal liver in β-catenin non-mutated HCA, and diffusely present over the entire area of both β-catenin-mutated HCA and HCC. Thus, large, contiguous bands of strong GS immunopositivity with interspersed negative areas, together forming a map-like pattern, are indicative of FNH, whereas diffuse GS labeling, either homogeneous or heterogeneous, suggests β-catenin-mutated HCA or HCC.

Glypican-3 (GPC3). (See section 2.2 for introduction.) When evaluating tumors developed in the non-cirrhotic liver, sensitivity issues regarding GPC3 come to the foreground. HCCs that arise in a cirrhotic background, especially those reaching a progressed stage, are overwhelmingly (in up to 90% of cases) GPC3-positive, whereas 36% of HCCs discovered in normal livers were found to be GPC3-negative (Wang et al., 2006). A significant proportion (up to 50%) of well-differentiated HCCs are actually devoid of any GPC3-staining, which calls for extreme caution in the interpretation of GPC3 results, and warns against overestimation of its potency as a single marker in the HCA vs. HCC problem (Shafizadeh et al., 2008). Diffuse GS staining often observed in β-catenin-mutated HCA further obscures the fuzzy borderline between atypical HCA and well-differentiated HCC, and makes the 3-marker panel GPC3 + GS + HSP70 which is so helpful in cirrhosis virtually useless in this situation. Coston et al. (2008) proposed that GPC3 should be combined with CD34 to help identify HCCs with no or little GPC3 positivity but complete CD34 labeling of the vasculature; however, atypical HCAs, too, may show complete CD34-positive pattern.

Liver fatty acid binding protein (LFABP) is a target gene of the liver-specific transcription factor HNF1α (Akiyama et al., 2000); consequently, its expression is practically lost in classical HCAs that harbor biallelic inactivating mutations of HNF1α (Bioulac-Sage et al., 2007b). LFABP, on the other hand, is produced by normal hepatocytes, and its expression is retained in both FNH and HCC. Therefore, negative LFABP staining of a tumor against a background of LFABP-positive liver parenchyma is highly indicative of classical HCA.

4. Conclusion

IHC markers discussed so far are summarized in **Table 1** (DNs vs. sHCC) and **Table 2** (benign hepatocellular tumors vs. HCC).

Like in many other situations, biology knows no black and white, but the pathologist must come up with 'yes' or 'no'. There may be cases, both small nodules and large tumors, that do not embarrass a liver specialist who spends his whole life with examining hepatocellular lesions, but may perplex a less trained observer. For the latter, IHC markers, and marker panels in particular, which are unambiguous to interpret and offer clear guidance, may be invaluable. Moreover, cumbersome cases always turn up that puzzle even the most experienced specialist, who must then seek for external confirmation of his intuition.

Marker	Labeled structure in HCC	Typical pattern		Sens. / Spec.
		Non-malignant nodules	Small HCC	
α-SMA	wall of unpaired arteries	no or few unpaired arteries	many unpaired arteries	ND
agrin	blood vessel walls	ductular reaction positive; sinusoids negative	all blood vessels positive	resected: 87% / 97%
ANXA2	tumor hepatocytes and endothelial cells	proliferating hepatocytes positive	endothelium also positive	resected: 84% / 100%
CD31/34	endothelium	most sinusoids negative, unpaired arteries positive	all blood vessels positive	ND
CAP2	tumor hepatocytes	smooth muscle cells positive, hepatocytes negative	tumor cells positive	ND
CK7/19	none	inner / outer ductular reaction (DR) positive	missing DR in and around the nodule	resected: 83% / 98%; needle: 95% / 90%
EZH2	tumor hepatocytes	few hepatocytes positive	most tumor cells positive	needle: 78% / 93%
GS	tumor hepatocytes	positive staining restricted to periportal and pericentral areas	diffuse positive staining	resected: 70% / 94%; needle: 59% / 98%
GPC3	tumor hepatocytes	hepatocytes negative	tumor cells positive	resected: 74-77% / 96%; needle: 71-83% / 94-100%
HSP70	tumor hepatocytes	bile ducts/ductules positive, hepatocytes negative	tumor cells positive	resected: 78% / 95%; needle: 48% / 94%

ND, not determined

Table 1a. Individual markers for the discrimination of benign vs. malignant nodules in cirrhosis. See text for abbreviations and references.

Recent Advances in the Immunohistochemistry-Aided Differential Diagnosis of Benign Versus
Malignant Hepatocellular Lesions

83

Marker panel	Spec. / Sens.
agrin + CD34	resected: 87% / 100%
CHC + FTCD	tissue array: 81% / 94%
GPC3 + EZH2 + HSP70	needle: 81% / 100%
GPC3 + GS + HSP70	resected: 72% / 100%; needle: 59% / 100%
GPC3 + GS + HSP70 + CHC	needle: 64% / 100%
GPC3 + GS + HSP70 + ANXA2	resected: 74% / 100%
GPC3 + SULT1A1	resected: 79% / ND

ND, not determined

Table 1b. Marker panels for the discrimination of benign vs. malignant nodules in cirrhosis. See text for abbreviations and references.

Marker	Typical pattern		
	FNH	HCA	HCC
agrin	sinusoids negative	vascular network: no or incomplete positivity	vascular network: complete positivity
ANXA2	ND	vascular network: focal positivity	vascular network: complete positivity
β-catenin	no aberrant staining in hepatocytes	nucleocytoplasmic staning in β-catenin-mutated HCA	nucleocytoplasmic staning in β-catenin-mutated HCC
CD34	aberrant arteries in scar positive; some sinusoids positive	sinusoids in arterial inflow areas positive	entire vascular network positive
CRP / SAA	negative	positive in inflammatory HCA; negative in others	rarely positive
GS	positive in map-like pattern	negative, or positive in restricted areas only	diffusely positive
GPC3	negative	negative	positive in tumor hepatocytes
LFABP	positive	negative in HNF1α-mutated HCA; positive in others	positive

Table 2. Markers for the discrimination of benign vs. malignant liver tumors. See text for abbreviations and references.

Optimally, an IHC marker of HCC should show an unequivocal and consistent staining pattern, either positive or negative, throughout the entire malignant lesion, and thus produce a sharp contrast against the non-malignant background. Also, optimal sampling should cover a representative area of the lesion, include some surrounding tissue for reference and, of course, provide high-quality tissue. Although no individual marker meets these strict criteria, and sampling is not always ideal, combining IHC markers has been shown to increase diagnostic success rates even in needle core biopsies where both sample size and quality are limiting. The 3-panel marker consisting of GPC3, GS and HSP70 proved to be a powerful tool in the discrimination of HGDN and early HCC, and extension of the panel with additional markers such as ANXA2, CHC, or EZH2, has been shown to further improve diagnostic accuracy. Conventional markers such as CD31/CD34 or biliary cytokeratins, as well as emerging candidates like agrin or CAP2, may also find application when any doubt remains. Similarly, a characteristic pattern of IHC markers, some indicating malignant hepatocellular transformation and others reflecting arterialization of tumor sinusoids, may greatly facilitate pathologic differentiation of benign hepatocellular tumors vs. HCC.

However, dubious cases will continue to occur, and no degree of certainty can be too much; hence, the quest for new IHC markers is unlikely to come to an end soon. And, since HGDN and early HCC, just like atypical HCA and well-differentiated HCC, probably lie along a continuum of malignant behavior, the ultimate elimination of the word 'borderline' from our vocabulary may remain a hope.

5. Acknowledgment

Publication of this article was supported by the grants Nos. 67925, 75468, and 100904 from the Hungarian Scientific Research Fund (OTKA).

6. References

Abdul-Al, H. M., Makhlouf, H. R., Wang, G. & Goodman, Z. D. (2008). Glypican-3 expression in benign liver tissue with active hepatitis C: implications for the diagnosis of hepatocellular carcinoma. *Human Pathology*, Vol.39, No.2, (February 2008), pp. 209-212, ISSN 0046-8177

Akiyama, T. E., Ward, J. M. & Gonzalez, F. J. (2000). Regulation of the liver fatty acid-binding protein gene by hepatocyte nuclear factor 1alpha (HNF1alpha). Alterations in fatty acid homeostasis in HNF1alpha-deficient mice. *The Journal of Biological Chemistry*, Vol.275, No.35, (September 2000), pp. 27117-27122, ISSN 0021-9258

Akutsu, N., Yamamoto, H., Sasaki, S., Taniguchi, H., Arimura, Y., Imai, K. & Shinomura, Y. (2010). Association of glypican-3 expression with growth signaling molecules in hepatocellular carcinoma. *World Journal of Gastroenterology*, Vol.16, No.28, (July 28 2010), pp. 3521-3528, ISSN 1007-9327

Anatelli, F., Chuang, S. T., Yang, X. J. & Wang, H. L. (2008). Value of glypican 3 immunostaining in the diagnosis of hepatocellular carcinoma on needle biopsy. *American Journal of Clinical Pathology*, Vol.130, No.2, (August 2008), pp. 219-223, ISSN 0002-9173

Baumhoer, D., Tornillo, L., Stadlmann, S., Roncalli, M., Diamantis, E. K. & Terracciano, L. M. (2008). Glypican 3 expression in human nonneoplastic, preneoplastic, and

Recent Advances in the Immunohistochemistry-Aided Differential Diagnosis of Benign Versus
Malignant Hepatocellular Lesions

85

neoplastic tissues: a tissue microarray analysis of 4,387 tissue samples. *American Journal of Clinical Pathology*, Vol.129, No.6, (June 2008), pp. 899-906, ISSN 0002-9173

Bioulac-Sage, P., Balabaud, C., Bedossa, P., Scoazec, J. Y., Chiche, L., Dhillon, A. P., Ferrell, L., Paradis, V., Roskams, T., Vilgrain, V., Wanless, I. R. & Zucman-Rossi, J. (2007a). Pathological diagnosis of liver cell adenoma and focal nodular hyperplasia: Bordeaux update. *Journal of Hepatology*, Vol.46, No.3, (March 2007), pp. 521-527, ISSN 0168-8278

Bioulac-Sage, P., Cubel, G., Balabaud, C. & Zucman-Rossi, J. (2011). Revisiting the pathology of resected benign hepatocellular nodules using new immunohistochemical markers. *Seminars in Liver Disease*, Vol.31, No.1, (February 2011), pp. 91-103, ISSN 1098-8971

Bioulac-Sage, P., Laumonier, H., Rullier, A., Cubel, G., Laurent, C., Zucman-Rossi, J. & Balabaud, C. (2009). Over-expression of glutamine synthetase in focal nodular hyperplasia: a novel easy diagnostic tool in surgical pathology. *Liver International*, Vol.29, No.3, (March 2009), pp. 459-465, ISSN 1478-3231

Bioulac-Sage, P., Rebouissou, S., Thomas, C., Blanc, J. F., Saric, J., Sa Cunha, A., Rullier, A., Cubel, G., Couchy, G., Imbeaud, S., Balabaud, C. & Zucman-Rossi, J. (2007b). Hepatocellular adenoma subtype classification using molecular markers and immunohistochemistry. *Hepatology*, Vol.46, No.3, (September 2007), pp. 740-748, ISSN 0270-9139

Blixt, M. K. & Royle, S. J. (2011). Clathrin heavy chain gene fusions expressed in human cancers: analysis of cellular functions. *Traffic*, Vol.12, No.6, (June 2011), pp. 754-761, ISSN 1600-0854

Bruix, J. & Sherman, M. (2005). Management of hepatocellular carcinoma. *Hepatology*, Vol.42, No.5, (November 2005), pp. 1208-1236, ISSN 0270-9139

Cai, M. Y., Tong, Z. T., Zheng, F., Liao, Y. J., Wang, Y., Rao, H. L., Chen, Y. C., Wu, Q. L., Liu, Y. H., Guan, X. Y., Lin, M. C., Zeng, Y. X., Kung, H. F. & Xie, D. (2011). EZH2 protein: a promising immunomarker for the detection of hepatocellular carcinomas in liver needle biopsies. *Gut*, Vol.60, No.7, (July 2011), pp. 967-976, ISSN 1468-3288

Capurro, M., Wanless, I. R., Sherman, M., Deboer, G., Shi, W., Miyoshi, E. & Filmus, J. (2003). Glypican-3: a novel serum and histochemical marker for hepatocellular carcinoma. *Gastroenterology*, Vol.125, No.1, (July 2003), pp. 89-97, ISSN 0016-5085

Chen, Y., Lin, M. C., Yao, H., Wang, H., Zhang, A. Q., Yu, J., Hui, C. K., Lau, G. K., He, M. L., Sung, J. & Kung, H. F. (2007). Lentivirus-mediated RNA interference targeting enhancer of zeste homolog 2 inhibits hepatocellular carcinoma growth through down-regulation of stathmin. *Hepatology*, Vol.46, No.1, (July 2007), pp. 200-208, ISSN 0270-9139

Christa, L., Simon, M. T., Flinois, J. P., Gebhardt, R., Brechot, C. & Lasserre, C. (1994). Overexpression of glutamine synthetase in human primary liver cancer. *Gastroenterology*, Vol.106, No.5, (May 1994), pp. 1312-1320, ISSN 0016-5085

Chuma, M., Sakamoto, M., Yamazaki, K., Ohta, T., Ohki, M., Asaka, M. & Hirohashi, S. (2003). Expression profiling in multistage hepatocarcinogenesis: identification of HSP70 as a molecular marker of early hepatocellular carcinoma. *Hepatology*, Vol.37, No.1, (January 2003), pp. 198-207, ISSN 0270-9139

Coston, W. M., Loera, S., Lau, S. K., Ishizawa, S., Jiang, Z., Wu, C. L., Yen, Y., Weiss, L. M. & Chu, P. G. (2008). Distinction of hepatocellular carcinoma from benign hepatic mimickers using Glypican-3 and CD34 immunohistochemistry. *American Journal of Surgical Pathology*, Vol.32, No.3, (March 2008), pp. 433-444, ISSN 0147-5185

Couvelard, A., Scoazec, J. Y. & Feldmann, G. (1993). Expression of cell-cell and cell-matrix adhesion proteins by sinusoidal endothelial cells in the normal and cirrhotic human liver. *American Journal of Pathology*, Vol.143, No.3, (September 1993), pp. 738-752, ISSN 0002-9440

Dahmani, R., Just, P. A. & Perret, C. (2011). The Wnt/beta-catenin pathway as a therapeutic target in human hepatocellular carcinoma. *Clinics and Research in Hepatology and Gastroenterology*, (July 2011), doi:10.1016/j.clinre.2011.05.010, ISSN 2210-741X

Di Tommaso, L., Destro, A., Fabbris, V., Spagnuolo, G., Laura Fracanzani, A., Fargion, S., Maggioni, M., Patriarca, C., Maria Macchi, R., Quagliuolo, M., Borzio, M., Iavarone, M., Sangiovanni, A., Colombo, M. & Roncalli, M. (2011). Diagnostic accuracy of clathrin heavy chain staining in a marker panel for the diagnosis of small hepatocellular carcinoma. *Hepatology*, Vol.53, No.5, (May 2011), pp. 1549-1557, ISSN 1527-3350

Di Tommaso, L., Destro, A., Seok, J. Y., Balladore, E., Terracciano, L., Sangiovanni, A., Iavarone, M., Colombo, M., Jang, J. J., Yu, E., Jin, S. Y., Morenghi, E., Park, Y. N. & Roncalli, M. (2009). The application of markers (HSP70 GPC3 and GS) in liver biopsies is useful for detection of hepatocellular carcinoma. *Journal of Hepatology*, Vol.50, No.4, (April 2009), pp. 746-754, ISSN 0168-8278

Di Tommaso, L., Franchi, G., Park, Y. N., Fiamengo, B., Destro, A., Morenghi, E., Montorsi, M., Torzilli, G., Tommasini, M., Terracciano, L., Tornillo, L., Vecchione, R. & Roncalli, M. (2007). Diagnostic value of HSP70, glypican 3, and glutamine synthetase in hepatocellular nodules in cirrhosis. *Hepatology*, Vol.45, No.3, (March 2007), pp. 725-734, ISSN 0270-9139

International Consensus Group for Hepatocellular Neoplasia (2009). Pathologic diagnosis of early hepatocellular carcinoma: a report of the international consensus group for hepatocellular neoplasia. *Hepatology*, Vol.49, No.2, (February 2009), pp. 658-664, ISSN 1527-3350

Khalil, A. A., Kabapy, N. F., Deraz, S. F. & Smith, C. (2011). Heat shock proteins in oncology: Diagnostic biomarkers or therapeutic targets? *Biochimica et Biophysica Acta*, Vol.1816, No.2, (May 2011), pp. 89-104, ISSN 0006-3002

Libbrecht, L., Desmet, V. & Roskams, T. (2005). Preneoplastic lesions in human hepatocarcinogenesis. *Liver International*, Vol.25, No.1, (February 2005), pp. 16-27, ISSN 1478-3223

Libbrecht, L., Severi, T., Cassiman, D., Vander Borght, S., Pirenne, J., Nevens, F., Verslype, C., van Pelt, J. & Roskams, T. (2006). Glypican-3 expression distinguishes small hepatocellular carcinomas from cirrhosis, dysplastic nodules, and focal nodular hyperplasia-like nodules. *American Journal of Surgical Pathology*, Vol.30, No.11, (November 2006), pp. 1405-1411, ISSN 0147-5185

Longerich, T., Haller, M. T., Mogler, C., Aulmann, S., Lohmann, V., Schirmacher, P. & Brand, K. (2011). Annexin A2 as a differential diagnostic marker of hepatocellular tumors. *Pathology Research and Practice*, Vol.207, No.1, (January 2011), pp. 8-14, ISSN 1618-0631

Mao, Y., Vyas, N. K., Vyas, M. N., Chen, D. H., Ludtke, S. J., Chiu, W. & Quiocho, F. A. (2004). Structure of the bifunctional and Golgi-associated formiminotransferase cyclodeaminase octamer. *EMBO Journal*, Vol.23, No.15, (August 2004), pp. 2963-2971, ISSN 0261-4189

Masaki, T., Tokuda, M., Fujimura, T., Ohnishi, M., Tai, Y., Miyamoto, K., Itano, T., Matsui, H., Watanabe, S., Sogawa, K. & et al. (1994). Involvement of annexin I and annexin

Recent Advances in the Immunohistochemistry-Aided Differential Diagnosis of Benign Versus
Malignant Hepatocellular Lesions

87

II in hepatocyte proliferation: can annexins I and II be markers for proliferative hepatocytes? *Hepatology*, Vol.20, No.2, (August 1994), pp. 425-435, ISSN 0270-9139

Mussunoor, S. & Murray, G. I. (2008). The role of annexins in tumour development and progression. *Journal of Pathology*, Vol.216, No.2, (October 2008), pp. 131-140, ISSN 1096-9896

Newman, P. J. (1997). The biology of PECAM-1. *Journal of Clinical Investigation*, Vol.100, No.11 Suppl, (December 1997), pp. S25-29, ISSN 0021-9738

Nielsen, J. S. & McNagny, K. M. (2008). Novel functions of the CD34 family. *Journal of Cell Science*, Vol.121, No. 22, (November 2008), pp. 3683-3692, ISSN 0021-9533

Ohmori, K., Endo, Y., Yoshida, Y., Ohata, H., Taya, Y. & Enari, M. (2008). Monomeric but not trimeric clathrin heavy chain regulates p53-mediated transcription. *Oncogene*, Vol.27, No.15, (Apr 2008), pp. 2215-2227, ISSN 1476-5594

Osada, T., Sakamoto, M., Nagawa, H., Yamamoto, J., Matsuno, Y., Iwamatsu, A., Muto, T. & Hirohashi, S. (1999). Acquisition of glutamine synthetase expression in human hepatocarcinogenesis: relation to disease recurrence and possible regulation by ubiquitin-dependent proteolysis. *Cancer*, Vol.85, No.4, (February 1999), pp. 819-831, ISSN 0008-543X

Park, Y. N. (2011). Update on precursor and early lesions of hepatocellular carcinomas. *Archives of Pathology & Laboratory Medicine*, Vol.135, No.6, (June 2011), pp. 704-715, ISSN 1543-2165

Park, Y. N., Kojiro, M., Di Tommaso, L., Dhillon, A. P., Kondo, F., Nakano, M., Sakamoto, M., Theise, N. D. & Roncalli, M. (2007). Ductular reaction is helpful in defining early stromal invasion, small hepatocellular carcinomas, and dysplastic nodules. *Cancer*, Vol.109, No.5, (March 2007), pp. 915-923, ISSN 0008-543X

Park, Y. N., Yang, C. P., Fernandez, G. J., Cubukcu, O., Thung, S. N. & Theise, N. D. (1998). Neoangiogenesis and sinusoidal "capillarization" in dysplastic nodules of the liver. *American Journal of Surgical Pathology*, Vol.22, No.6, (June 1998), pp. 656-662, ISSN 0147-5185

Ponsaing, L. G., Kiss, K. & Hansen, M. B. (2007). Classification of submucosal tumors in the gastrointestinal tract. *World Journal of Gastroenterology*, Vol.13, No.24, (June 2007), pp. 3311-3315, ISSN 1007-9327

Roncalli, M., Roz, E., Coggi, G., Di Rocco, M. G., Bossi, P., Minola, E., Gambacorta, M. & Borzio, M. (1999). The vascular profile of regenerative and dysplastic nodules of the cirrhotic liver: implications for diagnosis and classification. *Hepatology*, Vol.30, No.5, (November 1999), pp. 1174-1178, ISSN 0270-9139

Roncalli, M., Terracciano, L., Di Tommaso, L., David, E. & Colombo, M. (2011). Liver precancerous lesions and hepatocellular carcinoma: the histology report. *Digestive and Liver Disease*, Vol.43 Suppl 4, (March 2011), pp. S361-372, ISSN 1878-3562

Sakamoto, M. (2009). Early HCC: diagnosis and molecular markers. *Journal of Gastroenterology*, Vol.44 Suppl 19, (2009), pp. 108-111, ISSN 0944-1174

Schirmacher, P. & Longerich, T. (2009). Hochdifferenzierte Lebertumoren. Neue Entwicklungen und ihre diagnostische Relevanz. *Pathologe*, Vol.30 Suppl 2, (December 2009), pp. 200-206, ISSN 1432-1963

Seimiya, M., Tomonaga, T., Matsushita, K., Sunaga, M., Oh-Ishi, M., Kodera, Y., Maeda, T., Takano, S., Togawa, A., Yoshitomi, H., Otsuka, M., Yamamoto, M., Nakano, M., Miyazaki, M. & Nomura, F. (2008). Identification of novel immunohistochemical tumor markers for primary hepatocellular carcinoma; clathrin heavy chain and formiminotransferase cyclodeaminase. *Hepatology*, Vol.48, No.2, (August 2008), pp. 519-530, ISSN 1527-3350

Shafizadeh, N., Ferrell, L. D. & Kakar, S. (2008). Utility and limitations of glypican-3 expression for the diagnosis of hepatocellular carcinoma at both ends of the differentiation spectrum. *Modern Pathology*, Vol.21, No.8, (August 2008), pp. 1011-1018, ISSN 1530-0285

Shibata, R., Mori, T., Du, W., Chuma, M., Gotoh, M., Shimazu, M., Ueda, M., Hirohashi, S. & Sakamoto, M. (2006). Overexpression of cyclase-associated protein 2 in multistage hepatocarcinogenesis. *Clinical Cancer Research*, Vol.12, No.18, (September 2006), pp. 5363-5368, ISSN 1078-0432

Tatrai, P., Dudas, J., Batmunkh, E., Mathe, M., Zalatnai, A., Schaff, Z., Ramadori, G. & Kovalszky, I. (2006). Agrin, a novel basement membrane component in human and rat liver, accumulates in cirrhosis and hepatocellular carcinoma. *Laboratory Investigation*, Vol.86, No.11, (November 2006), pp. 1149-1160, ISSN 0023-6837

Tatrai, P., Somoracz, A., Batmunkh, E., Schirmacher, P., Kiss, A., Schaff, Z., Nagy, P. & Kovalszky, I. (2009). Agrin and CD34 immunohistochemistry for the discrimination of benign versus malignant hepatocellular lesions. *American Journal of Surgical Pathology*, Vol.33, No.6, (June 2009), pp. 874-885, ISSN 1532-0979

Theuerkauf, I., Zhou, H. & Fischer, H. P. (2001). Immunohistochemical patterns of human liver sinusoids under different conditions of pathologic perfusion. *Virchows Archiv*, Vol.438, No.5, (May 2001), pp. 498-504, ISSN 0945-6317

Wang, F. H., Yip, Y. C., Zhang, M., Vong, H. T., Chan, K. I., Wai, K. C. & Wen, J. M. (2010). Diagnostic utility of glypican-3 for hepatocellular carcinoma on liver needle biopsy. *Journal of Clinical Pathology*, Vol.63, No.7, (Jul 2010), pp. 599-603, ISSN 1472-4146

Wang, X. Y., Degos, F., Dubois, S., Tessiore, S., Allegretta, M., Guttmann, R. D., Jothy, S., Belghiti, J., Bedossa, P. & Paradis, V. (2006). Glypican-3 expression in hepatocellular tumors: diagnostic value for preneoplastic lesions and hepatocellular carcinomas. *Human Pathology*, Vol.37, No.11, (November 2006), pp. 1435-1441, ISSN 0046-8177

Xiao, Y. (2011). Enhancer of zeste homolog 2: A potential target for tumor therapy. *International Journal of Biochemistry and Cell Biology*, Vol.43, No.4, (April 2011), pp. 474-477, ISSN 1878-5875

Yeo, M., Na, Y. M., Kim, D. K., Kim, Y. B., Wang, H. J., Lee, J. A., Cheong, J. Y., Lee, K. J., Paik, Y. K. & Cho, S. W. (2010). The loss of phenol sulfotransferase 1 in hepatocellular carcinogenesis. *Proteomics*, Vol.10, No.2, (January 2010), pp. 266-276, ISSN 1615-9861

Yu, G. R., Kim, S. H., Park, S. H., Cui, X. D., Xu, D. Y., Yu, H. C., Cho, B. H., Yeom, Y. I., Kim, S. S., Kim, S. B., Chu, I. S. & Kim, D. G. (2007). Identification of molecular markers for the oncogenic differentiation of hepatocellular carcinoma. *Experimental & Molecular Medicine*, Vol.39, No.5, (October 2007), pp. 641-652, ISSN 1226-3613

Zhu, Z. W., Friess, H., Wang, L., Abou-Shady, M., Zimmermann, A., Lander, A. D., Korc, M., Kleeff, J. & Buchler, M. W. (2001). Enhanced glypican-3 expression differentiates the majority of hepatocellular carcinomas from benign hepatic disorders. *Gut*, Vol.48, No.4, (April 2001), pp. 558-564, ISSN 0017-5749

Zucman-Rossi, J., Benhamouche, S., Godard, C., Boyault, S., Grimber, G., Balabaud, C., Cunha, A. S., Bioulac-Sage, P. & Perret, C. (2007). Differential effects of inactivated Axin1 and activated beta-catenin mutations in human hepatocellular carcinomas. *Oncogene*, Vol.26, No.5, (February 2007), pp. 774-780, ISSN 0950-9232

5

Differential Diagnosis of Hepatocellular Carcinoma on Computed Tomography

Kristina Zviniene
Lithuanian University of Health Sciences
Lithuania

1. Introduction

Focal liver lesions (FLL) are common pathological findings in patients investigated for different gastrointestinal and other diseases. After detecting FLL radiologically, their clinical differential diagnosis is very important.

The precise identity and description of blood circulation of FLL is essential for differential diagnosis by computer tomography (CT). This is why the evaluation of the effectiveness of CT diagnostic criteria in diagnosing FLL is a relevant problem of theoretical and practical radiology, gastroenterology, surgery and oncology.

Multislice spiral CT is a perfect imaging modality to evaluate large area in a short time and visualize lesion optimally with an injection of contrast media (c/m). Scanning may include unenhanced images (without c/m), arterial, portal venous and delayed phases. The speed of contrast injection and optimal scanning protocol are crucial to separate all phases, what is very important in differential diagnostics of FLL.

It is important to optimize scanning time delay in order to achieve qualitative liver CT images. This can be achieved in few ways, including fixed time delay, "bolus" test and automatic scanning technology. In most hospitals and clinics contrast enhanced CT is performed simultaneously with the same scan delay .

To evaluate focal liver lesions Foley and Mallisee suggested triphasic multislice CT. When the whole liver is scanned in 10 sec. or even less, it's possible to achieve different liver CT images in particular time. In arterial phase (25-30 sec. after c/m injection) you can see the ramification of arteries without portal blood addition, contrary in portal veinous phase c/m flows into portal vein. This phase is in 45-50 sec. after the c/m injection starts.

In daily practice additional venous phase images are not necessary, however it could help in doubtful cases. This phase starts in about 70-120 sec. after IV "bolus" injection. As concentration of non-ionic c/m, including iodine, inside and outside the artery is probably the same, some FLL have tendency to "disappear" in this phase. Despite that, this phase is very useful in differentiating cholangiocarcinoma (I-CCC) from other FLL. Delayed phase is important in differential diagnosis of cholangiocarcinoma and hemangioma.

Murakami et al. described double CT scanning in arterial phase. Analyzing early and delayed arterial phase CT images, the so called pseudo-tumours can be found that is a great problem for the patients with liver cirrhosis. But the importance of this method is controversial nowadays, so it is not included into the CT scanning protocols.

In contrast enhanced CT, faster injection (4-5 ml/sec.) is recommended, which guarantees earlier and brighter peak of enhancement in the arteries, and also improves temporal separation of arterial, portal veinous and venous phases.

Concentration of c/m is also very important in contrast enhanced CT. Data from few sources confirms the hypothesis that the concentration of c/m improves greater enhancement and hypervascular liver lesions diagnostics.

Multislice spiral CT has a few advantages in abdominal imaging: gradual and minor inspiration and breath hold decrease body movements and ensure higher quality of the images. With improvement of CT scanners optimization of scanning is necessary to maximize the ability of getting new CT images.

Few studies suggest that multiple-phase CT scans are useful in differentiation and blood supply evaluation of solitary liver lesions. This is why CT scans should be evaluated separately in all phases.

There are multiple FLL types. Even such condition as fatty liver degeneration which is not considered as tumour should be differentiated. This is the reason why all FLL must be classified to make their diagnosis as objective and precise as possible.

Based on the literature, incidentally found <2.0 cm liver lesions of unknown origin, are benign in 75% of all cases, but USA scientists say, it is only about 50%. Scientists from Italy state that <1.5 cm FLL, diagnosed in people with extra-hepatic malignant process are benign in 80% of all cases.

From radiological point of view FLL are classified to hyper- and hypovascular, and also cystic and solid.

The aim is to describe the most important contrast enhanced CT diagnostic criteria for differentiating solid FLL.

2. Most common benign focal liver lesions

Liver cysts are the most common FLL, and they are usually detected incidentally during common follow-up. Liver cysts have specific US, CT and MRI features, so the radiological diagnosis is always clear, usually not complicated and it is not a medicine practice problem. This is why the diagnostics of liver cysts is not discussed in this paper. The diagnostics of non-cystic lesions is much more important and topical.

2.1 Liver hemangioma

Liver hemanioma is the most common (after liver cysts) benign liver lesion presenting 0.4-20% of all liver tumours. Normally it is solitary, well-defined vascularized lesion that can reach 20.0 cm in size. Hemangioma is composed of multiple vascular channels surrounded by endothelium cells with thin fibrotic stroma. Large hemangiomas are usually detected in older patients, with an average age of 54 years. Giant hemangiomas have non-homogenous structure because of fibrosis, necrosis, and cystic zones.

On unenhanced CT scans hemangiomas are hypodense with well-defined boarders. Calcification is rare (10-20%) and usually detected occasionally. Calcifications have rarely been reported in sclerosed or hyalinized and giant hemangiomas. The calcifications can be marginal or central; large and coarse; or multiple, small, and punctuate (e.g. phleboliths). Massive calcification of hemangiomas is extremely rare. The finding of a non-enhancing liver tumour with calcification should not preclude the diagnosis of hemangioma.

Performing contrast enhanced CT (in 2-15 min. after the injection of contrast media) peripheric nodular enhancement with centripetal fill in is observed. An early enhancement of FLL even before contrast media appears in the aorta is typical for hemangioma. According to several authors, globular enhancement in hemangiomas is seen with 88% of sensibility and 84-100% specificity. The lesion is filled-in with c/m depending on the size of hemangioma (fig.1).

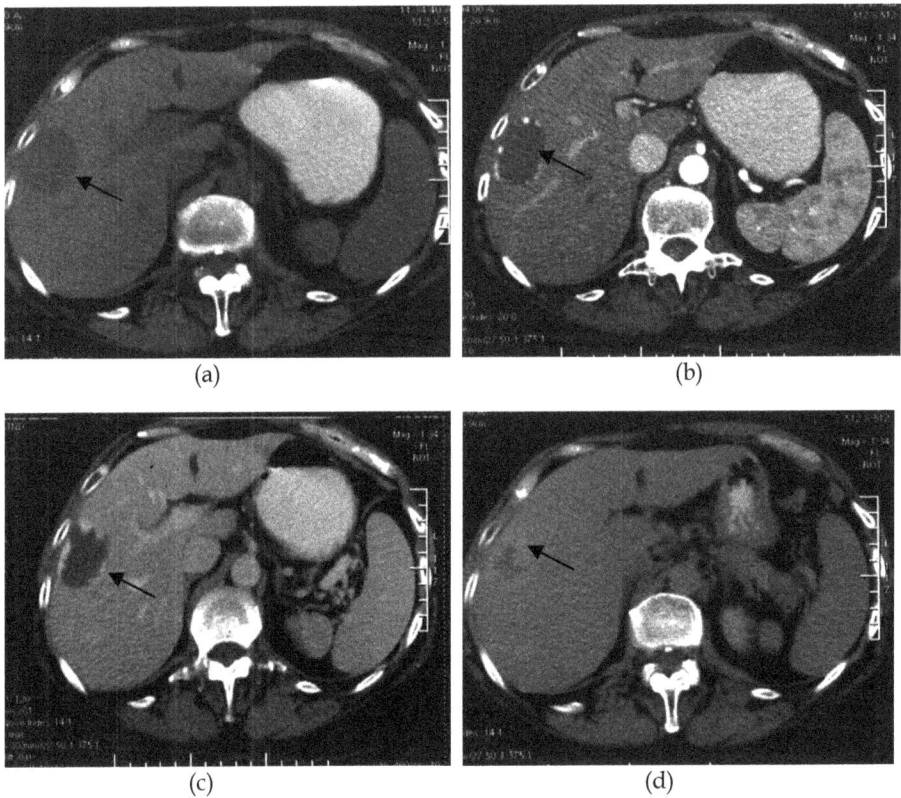

(a)   (b)

(c)   (d)

Fig. 1. Typical hemangioma. (a) Precontrast axial CT images demonstrate a hypodense lesion in the right hepatic lobe. (black arrow) (b,c) Arterial-phase and venous-phase images show progressive, peripheral nodular enhancement of the lesion with centripetal fill in. (arrow) (d) Delayed-phase images show that the lesion is isodense compared to the surrounding liver parenchyma an appearance that suggest persistence of contrast material within the lesion. (arrow)

Small hemangiomas (42% of hemangiomas are <1 cm) enhance rapidly and intensively in an early arterial phase (about 16% of all hemangiomas). The smaller the lesion, the faster it fills in with c/m.

This sign makes it more difficult to differentiate hemangiomas from other hypervascular tumours: islet cell metastases, small HCC, etc. Small hypodense hemangiomas are particularly problematic in patients with underlying malignancy. Some metastases can also have peripheral globular enhancement. Leslie et al. noticed that up to 8% of all cases metastases can show the same enhancement pattern. Another important differential diagnostic sign of hemangioma is attenuation equivalent to that of the aorta during all CT phases. Another valuable sign in differential diagnosis of hemangioma and malignant liver lesion is peripheric hypodense rim at the periphery of the mass. It indicates malignant neoplasm and is never seen in hemangiomas.

Large hemangiomas usually look like heterogenic lesions that enhance normally, however large hemangiomas with scar tissue do not enhance gradually, thus, there are non-enhanced areas.

In the late phase (10 min. after injection of contrast media) hemangiomas become isodense to surrounding liver parenchyma. This is one of the most important signs in differential diagnostics of hemangioma (fig.2)

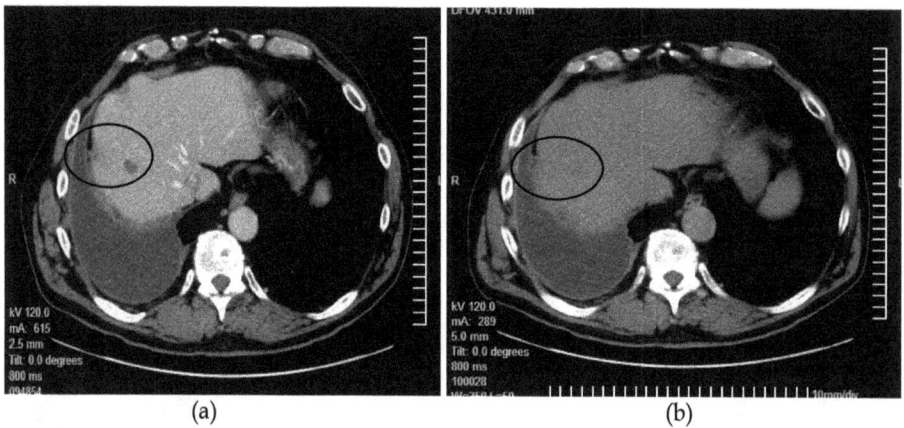

(a)   (b)

Fig. 2. Atypical hemangioma. (a) Portal venous- phase; there is no visible enhancement in the lesion (b) Delayed-phase CT image shows that the lesion is isodense compared to the liver (circle).

Sometimes in the late phase slight peripheral enhancement may be seen. This way of contrast uptake is typical of hialinized hemangioma that, according to some authors, is the last stage of the development of hemangioma. These hemangiomas must be differentiated from malignant tumours of the liver. Percutaneous biopsy is indicated in these cases. In the late phase small hemangiomas (<1 cm) are still slightly hypodense, but hypervascular metastases become contrast-free.

In case of liver steatosis hemangiomas are usually iso- or hyperdense. On unenhanced CT images hemangiomas are isodense to hepatic vessels. Thrombosed, fibrosed or degenerated areas are specific to large hemangiomas and are hypodense compared to hepatic vessels.

Though centripetal fill in is specific to hemangiomas, this finding is not pathognomic; sometimes hepatocellular carcinoma (HCC), cholangiocarcinoma or even liver metastases may have the same features. What is more, early peripheral nodular enhancement can be found in some focal nodular hyperplasia or vascular abnormalities.

Liver hemangiomas are differentiated from focal nodular hyperplasia (FNH) in up to 23% of all cases, however two or more different lesions may be found in the same liver. 33% of multiple FNH should be differentiated with hemangioma. When the tumours have typical CT features, the diagnosis can be made with confidence.

Large heterogeneous hemangiomas must be differentiated from all liver lesions that have scars: FNH, hepatocellular adenoma (HCA), hepatocellular carcinoma (HCC), intrahepatic cholangiocarcinoma. Large hemangiomas usually demonstrate cleft-like central or eccentric areas of scarring that constitute areas of fibrosis, sclerosis (i. e. hyalinization), cystic degeneration, or thrombosis. These areas have variable shape and size and usually do not demonstrate delayed contrast enhancement (fig.3).

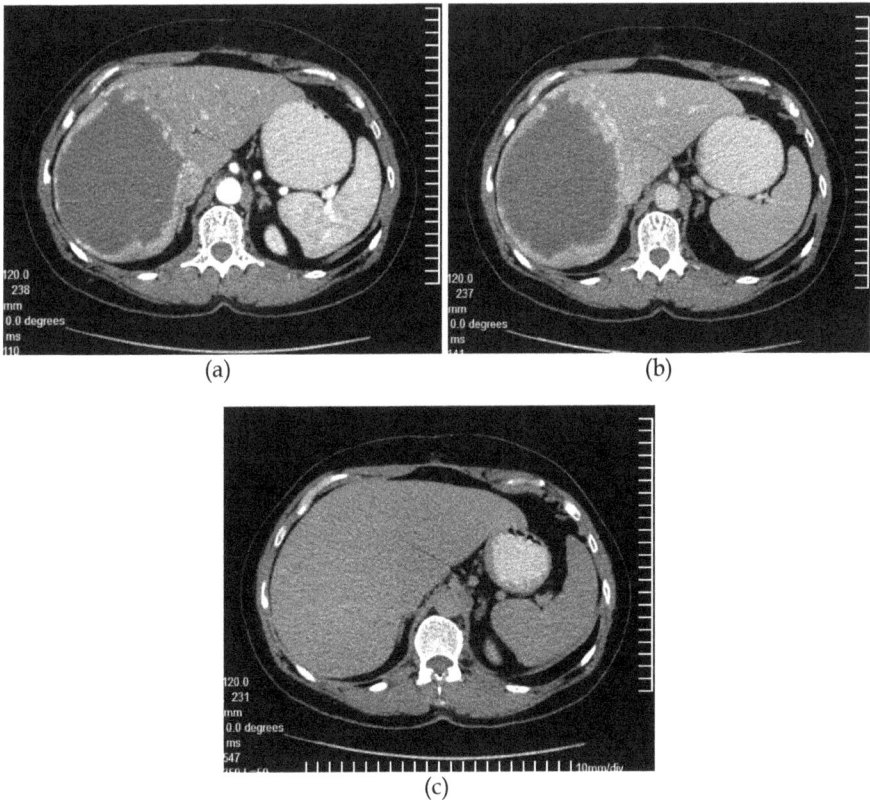

(a)   (b)

(c)

Fig. 3. Large hemangioma. Contrast-enhanced CT images show the typical enhancement pattern of hemangioma.

The essential criteria of evaluation of liver hemangiomas CT images are as follows: hypodense or isodense lesion on precontrast CT images;early peripheral nodular ring enhancement in arterial phase with centripetal fill-in in portal venous phase; and isodense lesion in the delayed phase. Based on these criteria our study shows that CT scanning is 91 % sensitive and 93 % specific.

2.2 Focal nodular hyperplasia

Focal nodular hyperplasia (FNH) is the hyperplasic process of liver, characterized by normal histological view of liver structure, but abnormal arrangement of it. FNH accounts for 1-8% of all primary liver tumours and it is the second most common benign liver neoplasm (after hemangiomas). FNH is diagnosed mostly in women (80-90%) in their twenties-fifties. Oral contraceptives are very important for the development of FNH, particularly the growth of it, but not formation de novo. In men FNH can be diagnosed in those taking anabolic steroids or having testicular tumour.

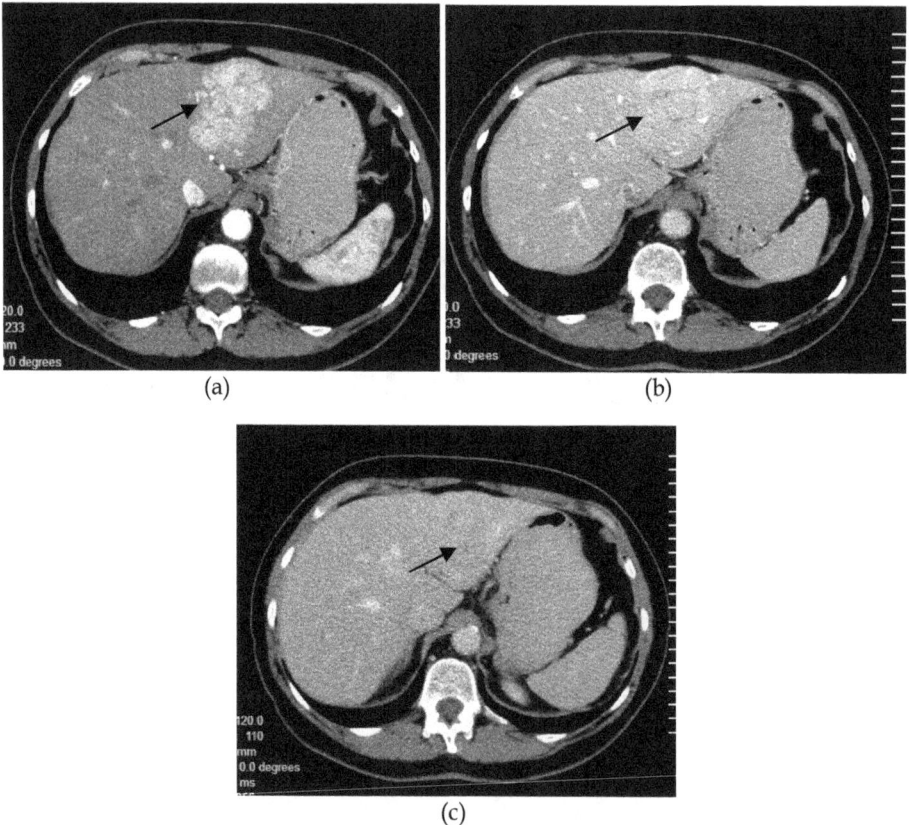

(a)   (b)

(c)

Fig. 4. Focal nodular hyperplasia with deformation of the liver margin . (a) In the arterial phase the hypervascular lesion with a hypodense central scar appears. (b,c) In the portal venous phase CT image FNH is iso- or hypodense to the liver. (arrow)

Etiology and pathogenesis of FNH are unclear. Histologically it is characterized as neoplasm with star-shaped central scar, surrounded with nodules of hyperplastic liver cells and minor ile ducts. In 95% of cases FNH is well-defined solid tumour with clear margins and central scar with blood vessels coming from it. Normally FNH is less than 5.0 cm in diameter and they are usually diagnosed not smaller than 3.0 cm.

On non-enhanced CT images FNH appears as hypodense (42-57%) or isodense (40-48%) lesion without well-defined borders and sometimes with more intensive hypodense central zone. If the lesion is isodense, the 'mass' effect may be the only criteria for detecting FNH. In 15-33% of patients, unenhanced CT images show the hypoattenuating stellate central scar with a central core and radiating fibrous septa. FNH is often subcapsular and that can complicate the course of adjacent vessels.

One third of FNH grows exophyticly and deforms contours of the liver (fig.4).

In arterial phase FNH enhances rapidly and becomes hyperdense (89-100%) because of vascularization of hepatic arteries (entering the FLL). In this situation hypodense central scar is seen clearly .

In portal venous phase the difference between FNH and normal liver parenchyma decreases, and later lesion becomes hypodense except for the central scar which is hyperdense in this phase (usually this scar is formed of efferent central vein) (fig.5).

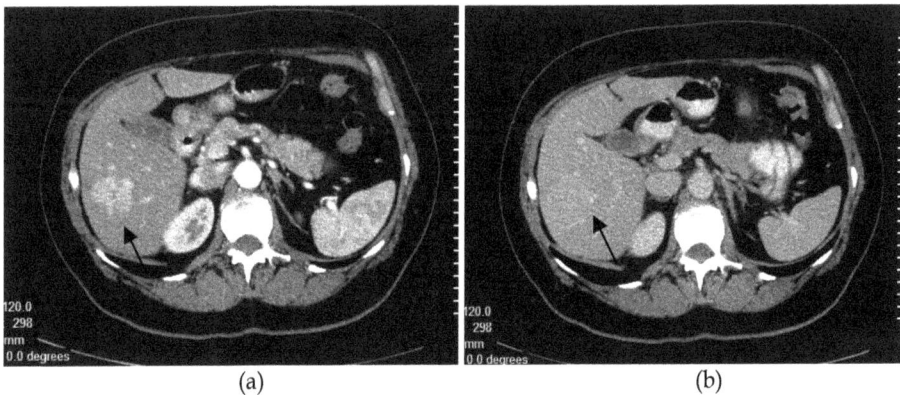

(a)   (b)

Fig. 5. Focal nodular hyperplasia. (a) Arterial phase CT image shows homogeneous enhancement of the lesion, except for the central scar. (arrow) (b) Contrast-enhanced CT image on the portal venous phase shows isoattenuating enhancement of the lesion compared to the liver. (arrow).

Although the typical CT features of FNH are characteristic, atypical features may be seen in more than half of cases. Multiple focal nodular hyperplasias occur in about 20% of patients. Atypical FNH may show less intense enhancement, unusual appearance on non-enhanced central scar and pseudocapsular enhancement on delayed images. In these cases it is very difficult to differentiate FNH from other benign and malignant lesions, such as HCA, HCC, hypervascular liver metastases of FLC.

A central scar is histologically present in almost all patients with FNH. However, it may be subtle and extremely small and is identified with the use of CT in 30%–50% of cases.

Presence of a central scar is clearly related to the size of the lesion. 35% of small FNH (<3 cm) and 65% of large FNH (>3 cm) demonstrated central scar. FNH lesions smaller than 3 cm in size may be more difficult to distinguish from other hypervascular lesions. The scar is typically thin and small and is hypodense compared with the rest of the FNH on unenhanced images, hepatic arterial and portal venous phase images. On delayed phase images, the scar often becomes hyperdense because of retention of contrast media (fig.6).

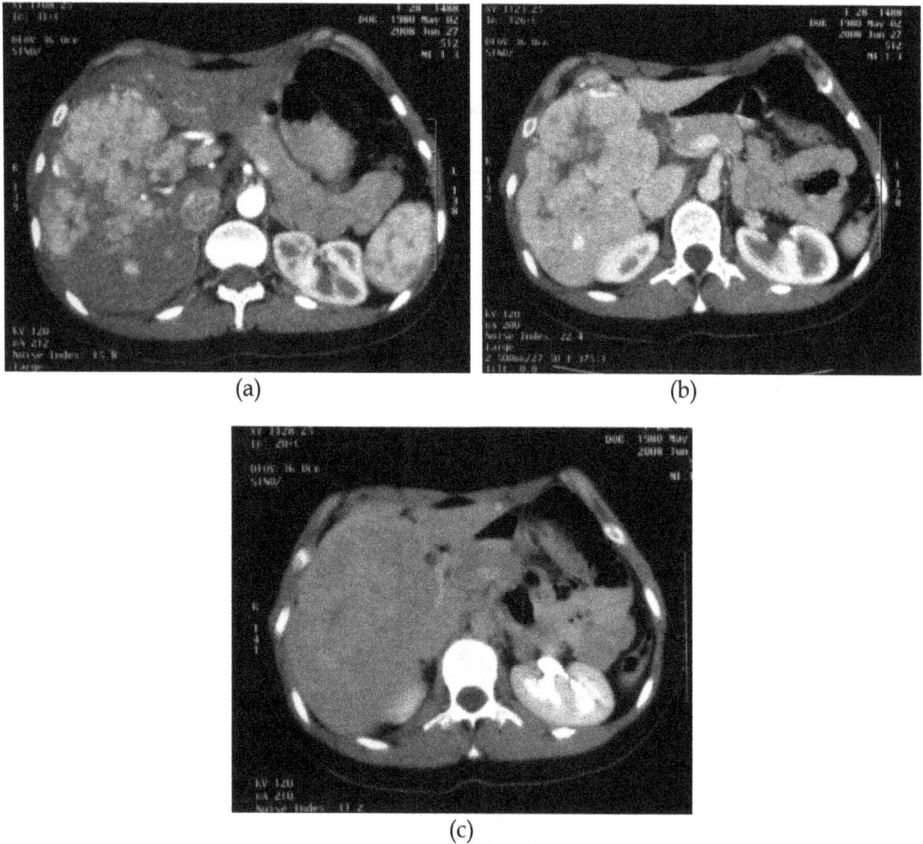

(a)   (b)

(c)

Fig. 6. Large atypical focal nodular hyperplasia. (a) Arterial phase CT image shows lobulated enhancement with a thick irregular scar of the lesion. (b,c) In the portal venous phase, FNH is slighthy hypodense to the liver. The central scar shows contrast enhancement. Pseudocapsule is evident.

Although central scar is very specific for FNH, it can also be seen in other atypical malignant liver lesions, such as gigantic liver hemangioma.

Pseudocapsule is one of atypical FNH signs (8% of cases), which is usually seen in liver steatosis because of the peripheral fibrosis of liver under pressure. Pseudocapsule may be more dense than the liver or FNH. Pseudocapsule should not be regarded as a sign of malignancy.

Internal haemorrhage or necrosis is seen in less than 6% of all cases. Calcification, fatty or necrotic zones are not common findings in FHN.

In some patients with hepatic steatosis, FNH is still isodense or hypodense on non-enhanced CT images; in rare cases, this may be due to fatty infiltration of FNH. Hypothetically, intralesional steatosis in focal nodular hyperplasia can be expected in several types of hepatic injury associated with steatosis, such as alcoholic toxicity, obesity, diabetes, malnutrition, and protein malabsorption.

FNH-like nodules in the cirrhotic liver are usually hypervascular, and they can mimic HCC. Although CT images give you precise diagnosis of FNH in most cases, rarely, a false-positive diagnosis of FNH occurs in cases of fibrolamellar hepatocellular carcinoma, as well as in cases involving other well-differentiated variants of hepatocellular carcinoma. The essential FNH criteria of evalution are as follows: slightly hypodense lesion with brighter low density zone in the centre on unenhanced CT images; strongly homogenous enhancement with hypodense central zone in the arterial phase; and isodense zone with central hyperdense zone in the venous phase. CT scanning is 78% sensitive and 89% specific.

2.3 Hepatocellular adenoma

Hepatocellular adenoma (HCA) is a rare benign liver lesion, which in 80% of cases is a solitary well defined tumour with a capsule. Oral contraceptives and steroids are one of the reasons of HCA development. HCA are more common in women in their twenties-forties. The difficulty of differential diagnosis of FNH and HCA is further compounded by the fact that both types of lesion typically occur in fertile women with a history of oral contraceptive use, who may be asymptomatic. People with glycogen metabolism disorders and haemosiderosis, as well as anabolic steroids taking males, are at a greater risk of HCA development. By the way pregnancy is one of the HCA risk factors. Normally HCA are 8-10 cm sized; in 70-80% of cases they are solitary tumours, however multiple adenomas can occur (sometimes >10 cm). HCA are difficult to differentiate from other hypervascular liver tumours.

Adenomas are more likely to contain areas of heterogenicity, fat, necrosis, hemorrhage and calcification rather than FNH. Adenomas are well defined (85% of cases), non-lobulated (95%), sometimes encapsulated (30%) and rarely calcified (10%).

While adenomas are also benign, they have a low-grade-malignancy potential, may bleed spontaneously, and are usually resected if they are large or if the diagnosis is doubtful. The diagnosis of this benign tumour is important as there is a possibility of rupture. Approximately 50% of tumours demonstrate intratumoural haemorrhage and can present with haemoperitoneum followed by hypotension and shock.

HCA can transform into hepatocellular carcinoma.

Adenomas consist almost entirely of uniform hepatocytes and a variable number of Kupffer cells, most of the adenomas in our experience are nearly isodense compared to normal liver on unenhanced images, portal venous, and delayed-phase images.

Diagnosis of HCA based only on CT scans is complicated, although a few specific HCA signs can be described. On precontrast CT images fatty HCA inserts may look like hypodense areas, and acute subcapsular haemorrhage looks like hyperdense areas. Necrosis and haemorrhage are detected in nearly 25% of HCA.

On contrast enhanced CT images in arterial phase you can see intensive peripheral contrast enhancement, which is caused by subcapsular vessels of the lesion. Central part of the lesion is filled with contrast media (cm) pretty fast as well. The lesion becomes hyperdense, however we can see washout and in portal-venous and late phases HCA becomes isodense. HCA showed more wash-out in the portal phase and 22% of the HCA may be hypodense (fig. 7).

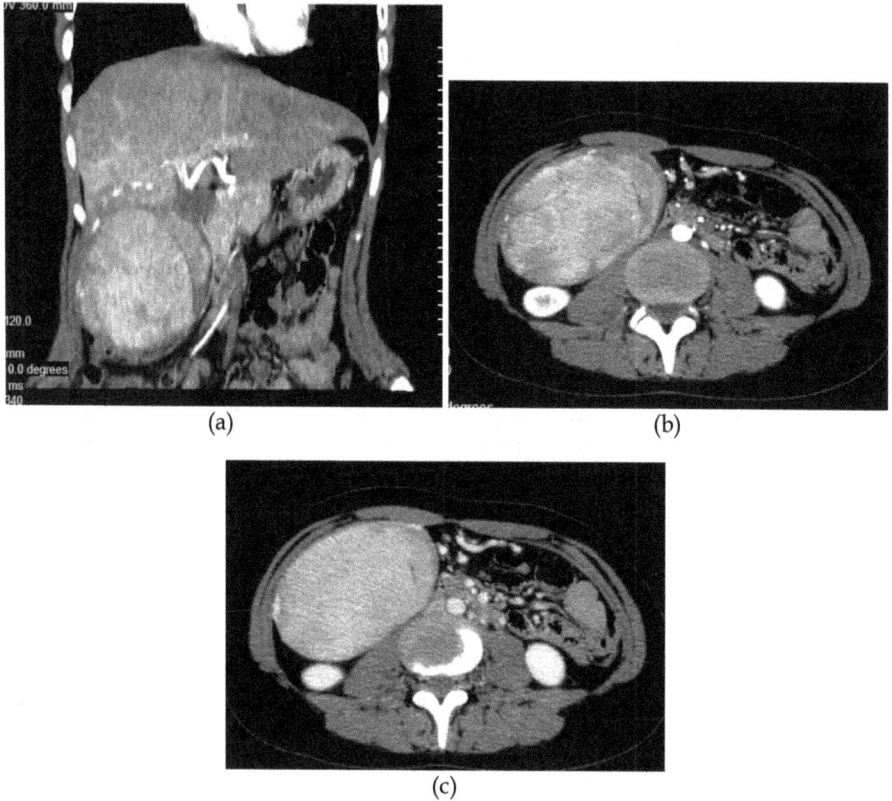

(a)   (b)

(c)

Fig. 7. CT images of large hepatocellular adenoma. A big lesion is seen in S6, deformes hepatic inferior border and goes down up to the level of the right kidney (a) Coronal image. (b,c) Axial images. Hepatic CT arterial phase (a,b) shows slightly heterogeneous enhancement of the tumor. (c) Portal venous CT phase: tumor becomes isointense and homogenous.

These features are typical to the lesions that are smaller than 3.0 cm in size. In some cases a thin capsule can be identified. Small adenomas enhance faster than normal liver tissue. In about 80% of cases HCA demonstrated homogeneous or nearly homogeneous enhancement, except for the acute or previous haemorrhage or fatty tissue in it.

In patients with liver steatosis HCA is hyperdense in all phases.

The differentiation of adenoma from hypervascular metastases may be difficult or even impossible. Most hypervascular metastases are multiple and will manifest as lesions or portions of lesions that are hypoattenuating or hypodense compared to normal liver parenchyma on unenhanced images, portal venous, and late-phases. It is crucial to identify if there is a primary tumour, for example, pancreatic or kidney carcinoma. In the age group of women, who are usually diagnosed with HCA, breast or thyroid carcinomas are the most likely to be the primary tumours.

The essential HCA diagnostic criteria are as follows: isodense lesion on unenhanced CT images; diffuse homogenous enhancement in arterial phase; isodense lesion in venous phase. Contrast enhanced CT shows 71% sensitivity and 93% specificity.

2.4 Rare benign focal liver lesions

2.4.1 Angiomyolipoma

Aniomyolipoma is a benign mesenchymal tumour that usually involves the kidney and rarely the liver. Lipomas or angiomyolipomas have been found in 10% of patients with tuberous sclerosis but can occur in patients without the disease. Angiomyolipomas can be diagnosed in patients of different age and sex, but are more common in women. The lesion can be of different size and may be solitary or multiple. Extremely rare cases of hepatic angiomyolipomas with spontaneous rupture, tumor recurrence, and vascular invasion were reported.

Hepatic angiomyolipomas are composed of varying portions of fat, epithelioid and spindled smooth muscle cells, and thick-walled blood vessels. The imaging features of hepatic angiomyolipomas depend on the relative proportions of the tumour components. It is difficult to diagnose hepatic AMLs with low fat content. Occasionally, it is difficult to distinguish hepatic AMLs from other fat-containing hepatic tumours, such as HCC with fatty metamorphosis, lipoma, and liposarcoma. The feeding blood vessels can be seen in other hypervascular lesions such as HCC and FNH, but the vessels in those cases usually are located in the periphery of the lesion.

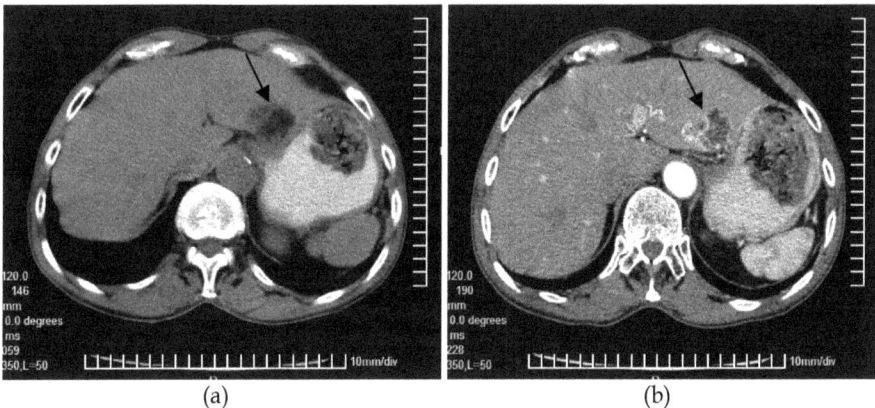

(a)   (b)

Fig. 8. Angiomyolipoma in S2 of the liver. (a) Nonenhanced CT scan shows a hypoattenuating fat-containing lesion in the left liver lobe. (arrow) (b) Arterial phase CT image shows slightly heterogeneous hyperenhancement in the vascular area of the lesion. (arrow)

On contrast enhanced CT images, hepatic angiomyolipomas strongly enhance in the arterial phase and enhancement persists in the venous phase, depending on the vascularisation of the tumour. Such hepatic angiomyolipomas should be differentiated from HCCs and cavernous hemangiomas (fig. 8).

2.4.2 Liver hamartoma

Liver hamartoma is a benign mesenchymal cystic tumour, consisting of gelatinous mesenchymal tissue with cyst formation and remnants of normal hepatic parenchyma. The tumour may have either mesenchymal predominance (a solid appearance) or cystic predominance (multiloculated cystic masses). On CT images mesenchymal hamartoma is a well defined lesion with hypodense central part and septa. Both solid and cystic areas are seen (fig.9).

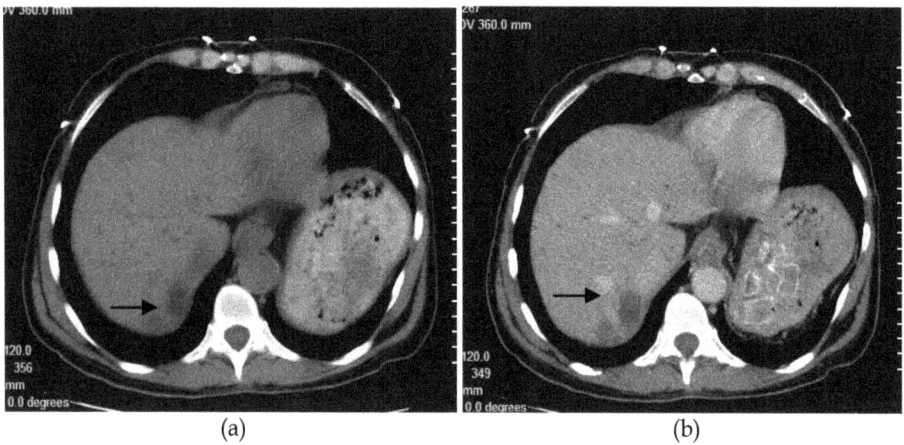

(a)   (b)

Fig. 9. Mesenchymal hamartoma of the liver. (a) unenhanced CT images: we see cystic lesions in S7 (b) enhancement of the septa in portal venous phase. (arrow)

2.4.3 Liver TB granuloma

Liver TB granuloma is the most common manifestation of upper abdominal parenchymatous organ tuberculosis and its incidence has also been increasing. There are three morphological types of liver TB: miliary tuberculosis of the liver associated with generalized miliary tuberculosis, primary miliary tuberculosis of the liver and primary tuberculoma or abscess of the liver. More than half of the patients present with hepatomegaly.

Radiological findings of hepatic tuberculosis are not specific. On CT images liver tuberculoma appears as an unenhancing, central, low density lesion due to cessation necrosis with a slightly enhancing peripheral rim corresponding to surrounding granulation tissue. Calcification can also be observed. TB granuloma should be differentiated from necrotic tumours, such as metastatic carcinoma and hepatocellular carcinoma (fig. 10).

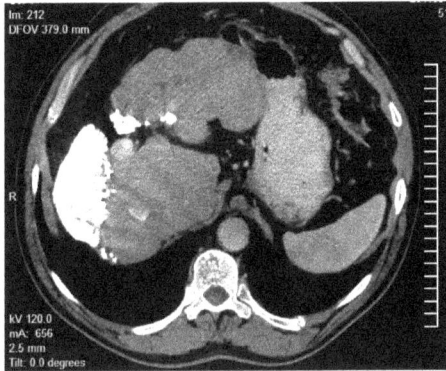

Fig. 10. Liver tuberculosis. Contrast enhanced CT image shows a large irregular miliary confluent calcification. The liver is dicreased in size with irregular margins.

3. Most common malignant focal lesions

Malignant liver tumours are one of the most common oncological diseases all over the world.

It is still unknown why some of the liver cells become malignant; however it is well-known that people with differently damaged liver are at a greater risk of developing liver cancer. The highest risk of liver damage is for those infected with hepatitis B and C viruses. These and other diseases can cause liver cirrhosis, which induces scarring of liver tissue. When the tumour develops in cirrhotic liver, patient's survival and recovery rates are tragically low; and the only treatment option in this situation is liver transplantation.

Malignant liver tumours are more common in men than women (2.7:1) (based on USA data).

According to American Cancer Association (ACA) in 2007 liver tumours were diagnosed de novo in 13650 males and 5510 females.

ACA says liver tumours are among 20 most common oncological diseases in the USA. Though World Health Organization (WHO) states that liver cancer is the third most common mortality reason.

In Japan since 1995 the incidence of liver tumours has also been rising, and mortality from liver tumours is up to 30/100000. About 30000 Japanese people die from liver cancer annually .

In some African and Eastern Asian countries liver cancer is the most common type of malignancy.

According to Lithuanian Cancer Registration Department the rate of liver cancer was 132/100000 in 2001 and 162/100000 in 2005. Primary data on liver cancer in 2010 shows general morbidity of 142/100000: among them 94/100000 – males, 48/100000 – females.

In 2005 liver cancer caused 174/100000 deaths, 89/100000 of them – males and 85/100000 – females.

3.1 Hepatocellular carcinoma

Hepatocellular carcinoma (HCC) is the most common malignant liver lesion caused by hepatocytes damage. Very often HCC is diagnosed in patients who already have some underlying liver disease, such as chronic viral hepatitis, alcoholic cirrhosis, haemochromatosis, etc. With growing population of people with hepatitis C and the disease's tendency to become chronic or cause liver cirrhosis, there is no doubt hepatitis C will become the most important HCC risk factor.

HCC is more common in males than females (4:1) in their fifties-seventies. In some African and Asian countries HCC rate reaches its maximum at 40 yrs.

When the fibrosis is concentrated focally, a finding, often referred to as a focal confluent fibrosis, can create mass lesions that simulate tumours on cross sectional images. These lesions often radiate from the porta hepatis and are wedge-shaped and widest at the capsular surface. The most common sites for confluent fibrosis are the anterior and medial segments of the liver, but it can be present anywhere else. The reliable finding in differentiation of confluent fibrosis from HCC is associated atrophy of hepatic parenchyma with capsular retraction (fig.11).

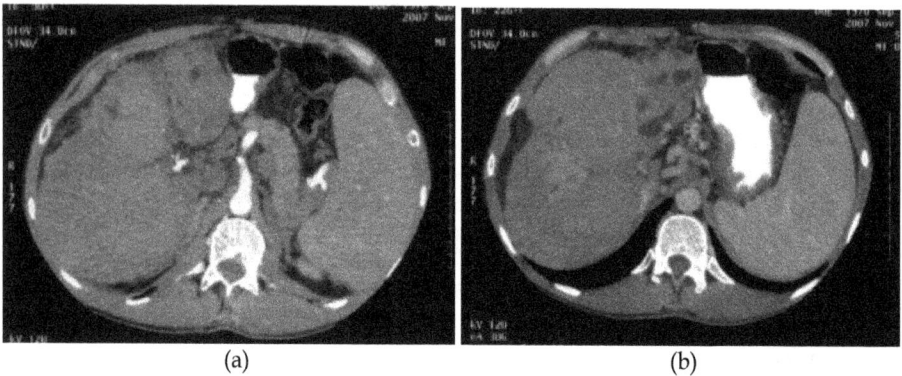

(a)   (b)

Fig. 11. Liver fibrosis. (a) Arterial phase CT image shows heterogeneous area in the right liver lobe, liver capsule retraction. (b) The portal venous phase CT image shows a hyperenhancement of the fibrotic area. Dilated bile ducts in the left liver lobe.

HCC can be solitary, multifocal or diffusely infiltrating, what is least common. Multifocal HCC may look like multiple small foci or one dominant large tumour with multiple satellite nodules. HCC classification can also be based on its growth characteristics. Highly differentiated tumour grows slowly, meanwhile tumour with low grade of differentiation demonstrate aggressive growth patterns.

HCC has a tendency to spread locally involving portal (30-60%) and other hepatic veins (15%). Portal vein is usually involved when the tumour is infiltrative. Intravenously growing tumour must be differentiated from thrombi, based on HCC arterial or venous signal depending on recanalization.

Serum AFP levels are often elevated in patients with large tumours, and the serum AFP level is frequently normal in patients with small tumours.

CT is highly accurate in the staging of HCC, as the number of lesions, segmental anatomy, regional adenopathy, vascular tumour invasion and metastases can be detected easily.

On unenhanced CT images HCC looks like a hypodense lesion. It often happens that small HCCs are not detected on precontrast CT. In HCC, however, there may be metamorphosis, necrosis, periodic changes or haemorrhage; therefore, it is usually heterogeneous attenuation, especially in large HCCs. Fatty metamorphism usually occurs in high grade differentiated HCC and on unenhanced images it looks as a hypodense lesion. In some instances, increased attenuation within the HCC may be due to haemorrhage or calcifications.

Focal hyperdense fragments (calcification areas) or diffuse hyperdense changes (iron accumulations) inside the neoplasm are extremely rare (5-10%).

Optimal liver CT scanning protocol is based on accumulation of contrast substance in arterial, portal vein and venous phases during spiral CT.

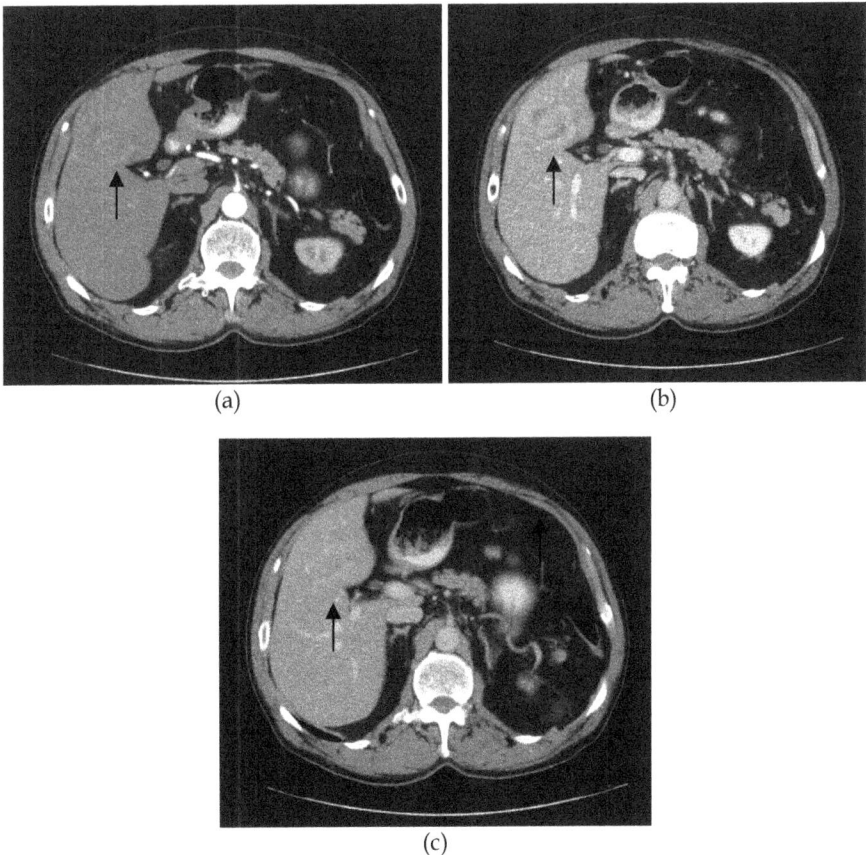

(a)   (b)

(c)

Fig. 12. Hepatocellular carcinoma. (a) Arterial phase CT image shows a typical hyperenhancement of the lesion. (arrow) (b,c) HCC shows washout in portal venous phase. Pathologic diagnosis of this tumor was moderately differentiated hepatocellular carcinoma. (arrow)

The most common HCC sign in arterial phase is enhancement or persistent enhancement and wash-out in portal veinous and venous phases on CT or MRI (fig.12).

Intensive enhancement in HCC is caused by a good vascularization of the tumour. In early arterial phase, the lesions enhance homogeneously or heterogeneously, while most of the small HCC lesions enhance homogeneously. Areas of internal necrosis or fat may remain hypodense.

In the portal venous and equilibrium phases, the contrast media is moving from the intravascular to the intercellular space. The wash-out is rapid because HCC contains less intercellular space than the surrounding liver parenchyma.

The imaging characteristics of HCC vary greatly with the size of the lesion.

Diffusely infiltrating HCCs may be difficult to detect on CT during any enhancement phase (fig.13).

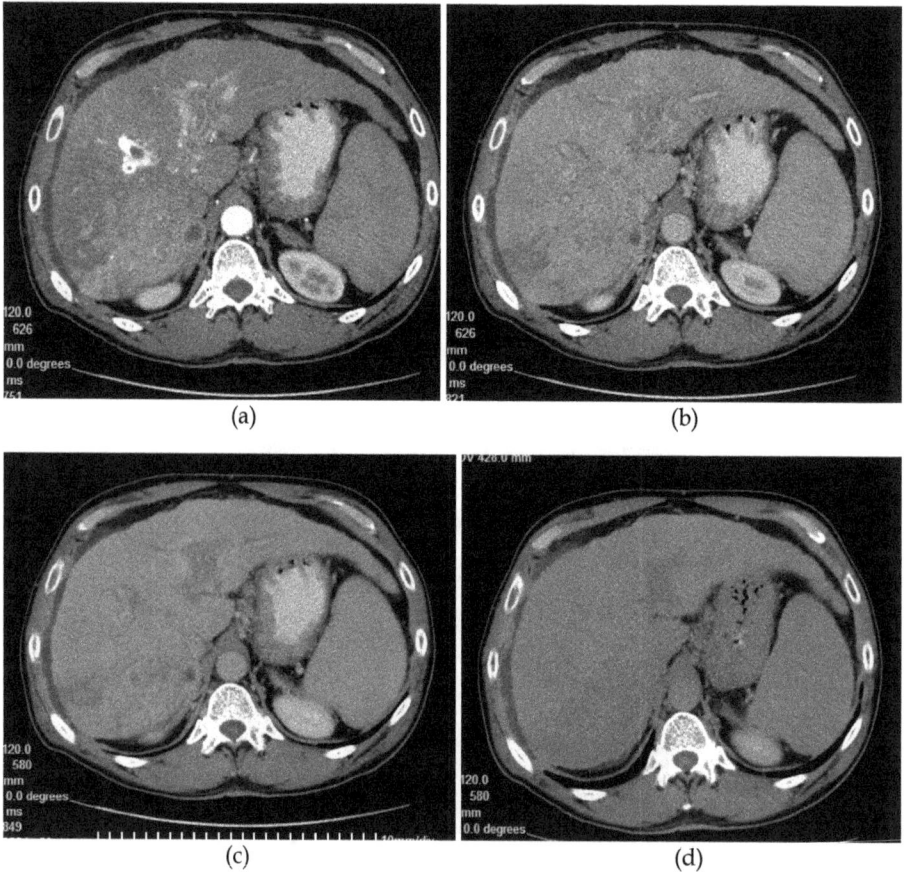

Fig. 13. Diffusely infiltrating hepatocellular carcinoma. (a) Hepatic arterial phase CT image shows slighly heterogeneous mass in the right lobe of the liver and hyperattenuating enhancement of the hepatic parenchyma. (b,c) In the portal venous phase and delayed phase CT images, the tumor shows washout.

Pathologic diagnosis of the tumor was diffusely infiltrating hepatocellular carcinoma.

Well-differentiated and small HCCs more often had atypical enhancement features.

Small HCC (<3 cm) can be hypovascular, do not enhance intensively or show no enhancement at all in arterial phase. In 10% of all cases enhancement is not intensive due to high differentiation degree of HCC. In this situation HCC is easier to identify in portal veinous and venous phases, when hypodense HCC foci are seen due to contrast wash-out (fig. 14).

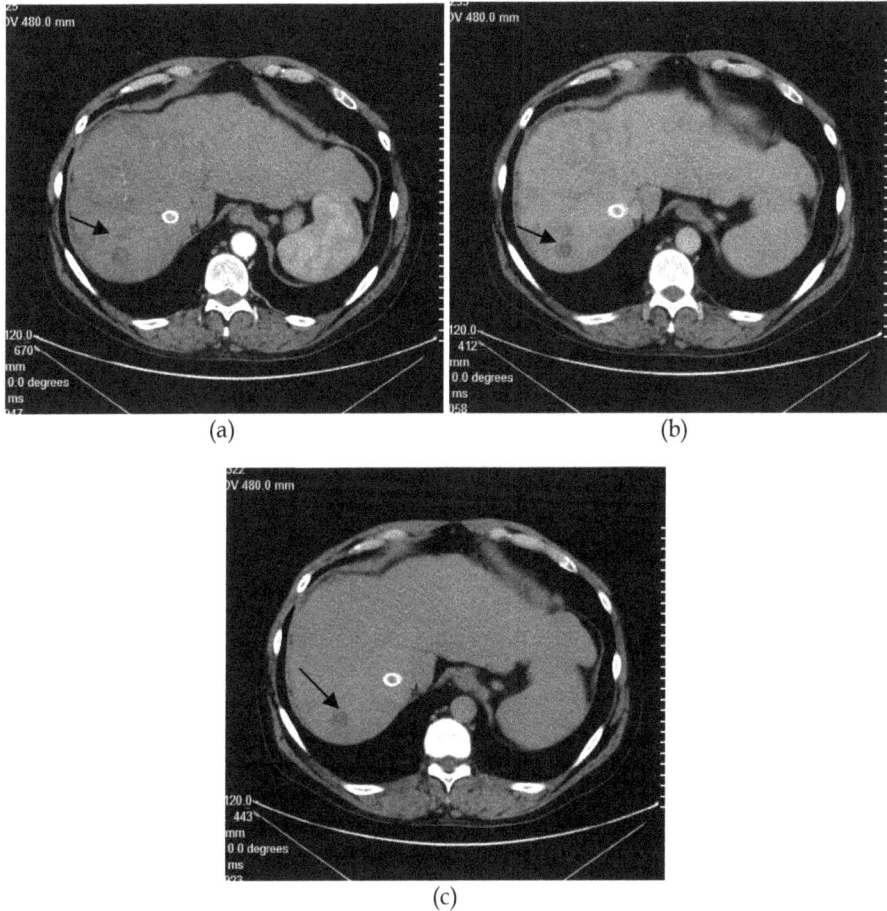

(a)   (b)

(c)

Fig. 14. Atypical hepatocellular carcinoma. (a,b) Arterial and portal venous phase show an atypical finding with no enhancement in the lesion. (arrow) (c) Delayed phase image shows no visible enhancement of the tumor. (arrow)

If HCC is big (> 5 cm), it is identified as a heterogeneous tumour in arterial phase. In these cases additional diagnostic criteria can be identified, it helps to diagnose HCC: in 40-60% of HCC cases a picture of mosaic tumour is seen; lesions of portal or hepatic veins, characterized by defects of vascular lumen filling, are seen in 33-48% of all cases; central scar consisting of collagen, fibrotic and sclerotic tissue and internal fatty components are seen in 2-21% of all cases (fig. 15).

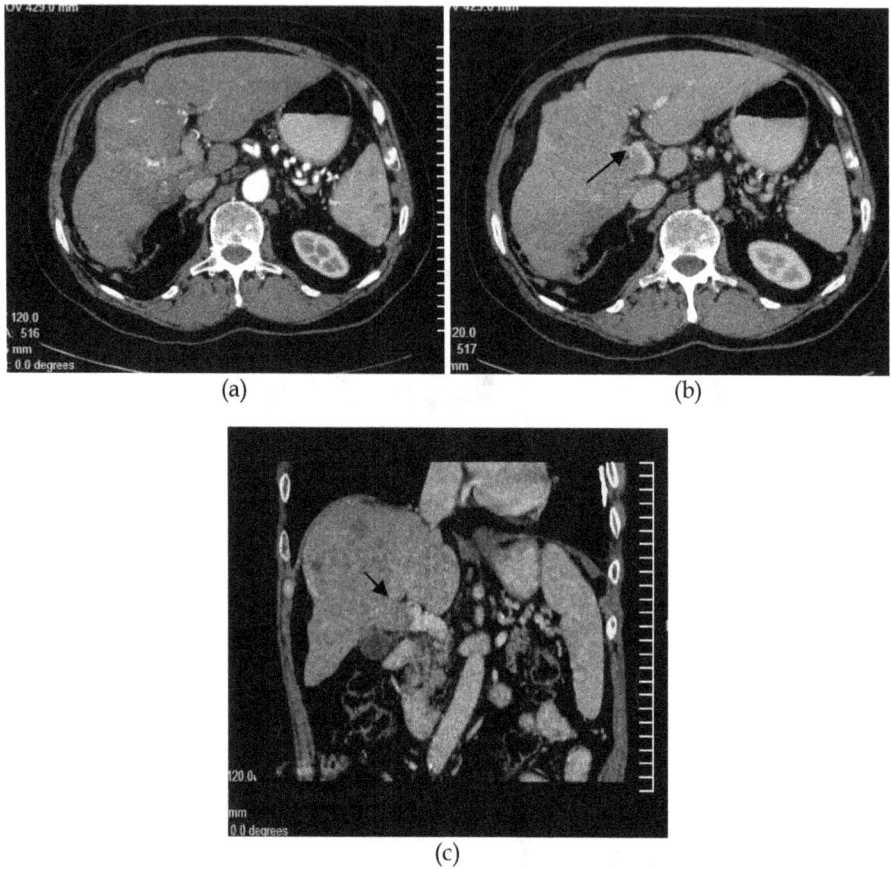

(a)   (b)

(c)

Fig. 15. Hepatocellular carcinoma with portal vein invasion. (a, b) Contrast-enhanced CT image shows the typical enhancement pattern of hepatocellular carcinoma. Invasion of the right portal vein is confirmed. (arrow) (c) On the coronal CT reconstruction, the portal vein is filled with hypodense tumor thrombus, which demonstrates a small amount of enhancement. (arrow)

The capsule, limiting all of the tumour or a part of it, is identified in 30-67% of HCC cases. The capsule is seen as hypodense rim in arterial phase, it enhances in late venous phase. Capsule is more common for the tumours with lower differentiation than those highly differenciated; it is also more common for medium sized (3-10 cm) tumours. Peripheral enhancement in solitary hepatocellular carcinoma (>3.0 cm in diameter) is also uncommon in images obtained by helical CT. Firstly, encapsulated carcinoma pseudocapsule usually shows an enhanced rim, arterioportal shunting around the lesion usually shows very dense, wedge shaped or triangular, peripheral enhancement in hepatic arterial phase and less enhancement in portal venous phase. This sort of enhancement should be differentiated from other focal liver lesions, such as hepatic metastases, hepatic abscess, hepatic inflammatory pseudotumour and hepatic cavernous hemangioma (fig.16).

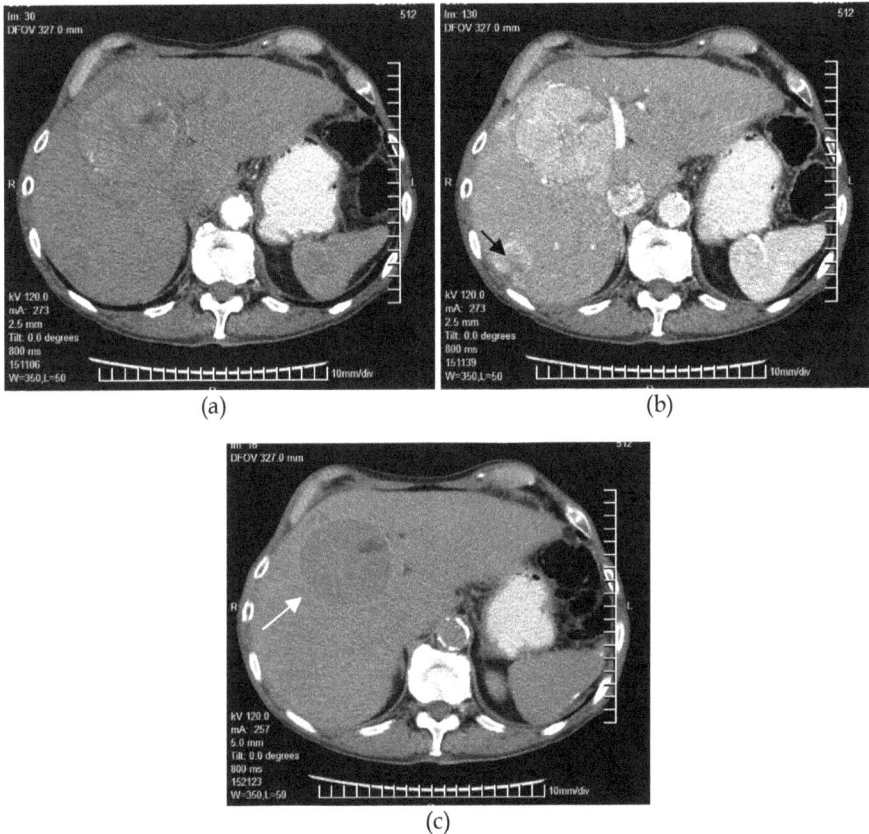

(a)   (b)

(c)

Fig. 16. Hepatocellular carcinoma with satellite nodule. The large tumor is defined on the right liver lobe and small satellite nodule in S7, with capsule retraction. (arrow) (a,b) Contrast enhanced CT images show the typical enhancement pattern of hepatocellular carcinoma. (c) Delayed phase image shows washout of contrast media. A hyperdense rim (white arrow) is present at the periphery of the tumor.

Quick contrast wash out from HCC increases the specificity of CT and allows distinguishing HCC from hemangiomas, hypervascular dysplastic nodules, small arterial portal shunts, which mimics HCC because of contrast uptake in arterial phase. Small hemangiomas can appear with flash filling during the arterial phase and thus simulate HCC. These lesions always show enhancement on delayed-phase images, whereas HCC exhibits a washout of the contrast material, becoming either isoattenuating or hypoattenuating relative to liver tissue.

CT has some lack of specificity in distinguishing HCC from tumours such as metastases, focal nodular hyperplasia, and hepatic adenomas. In general the clinical and radiographic setting indicates which of these is likely in a given patient, as these tumours are rare in cirrhotic liver and HCC is uncommon in the healthy liver.

The essential HCC diagnostic criteria on CT images are as follows: hypodense area on unenhanced CT images; homogenous or heterogeneous enhancement in arterial phase; rapid wash-out in venous phase. Based on these criteria CT is 84% sensitive and 93% specific.

3.2 Intrahepatic cholangiocarcinoma

Intrahepatic cholangiocarcinoma (I-CCC) is a malignant tumour of bile ducts' epithelium, which affects minor branches of intrahepatic bile ducts.

Usually I-CCC is a disease of young people that can be caused by primary sclerosing cholangitis, secondary cholangitis, congenital liver cirrhosis, Caroli disease etc. There is no

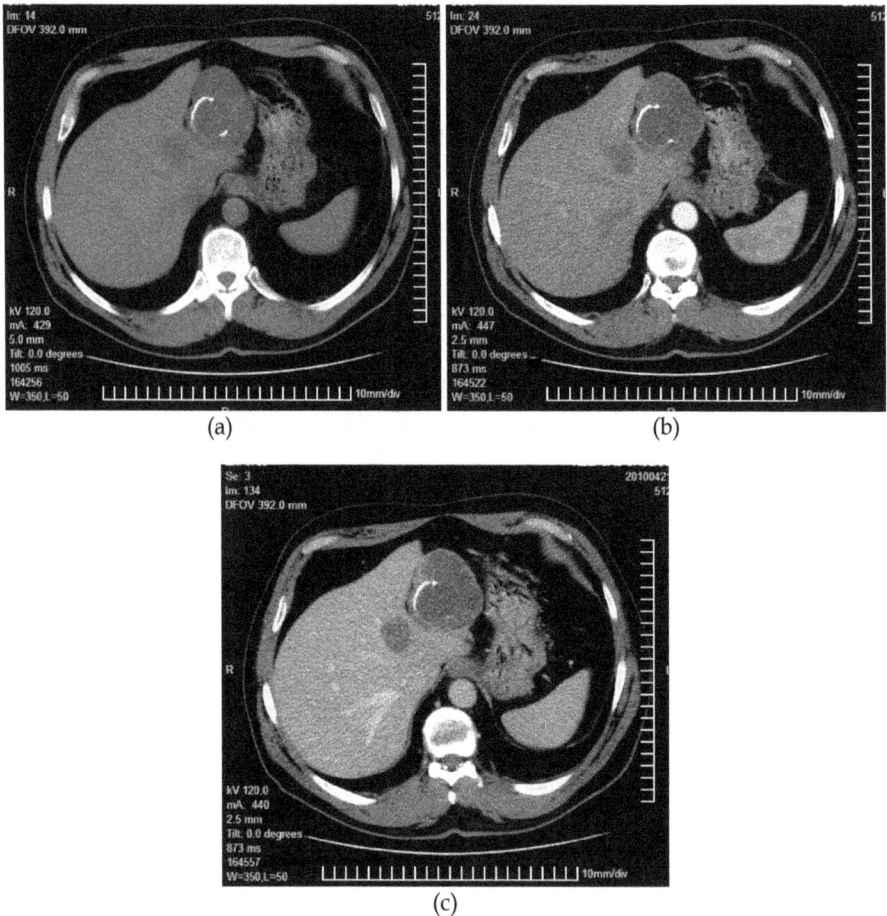

(a)   (b)

(c)

Fig. 17. Intrahepatic cholangiocarcinoma. (a) Unenhanced CT image shows well defined hyhpodense lesion with calcification. Sattelite nodule is also seen. Atrophy of the left liver lobe. (b) Arterial phase CT image shows poorly enhancement of the lesion; tiny septations show enhancement. (c) Portal venous phase shows increased and persistent enhancement of the lesion.

strong evidence that intrahepatic stones can or cannot cause I-CCC, however this disease can be caused by recurrent cholangitis that leads to mucosal hyperplasia, adenomatous changes or carcinoma. I-CCC represents about 15% of all primary liver tumours. By growth types cholangiocarcinoma is classified into mass-forming, periductal infiltrating and intraductal.

On unenhanced CT images I-CCC is seen as solitary not encapsulated hypodense lesion with irregular margins. Hyperdense areas inside the lesion look like calcification (fig.17).

In both arterial and portal venous phases the most important sign is the enhancement of the capsule limiting jagged edges of the tumour. The tumour itself enhances very slowly. This is why CT imaging in arterial and venous phases shows no difference. Tumour tissue enhances only in delayed phase. Deformation of tumour capsule can be seen in 20% of all cases, dilatation of intrahepatic bile ducts is seen in 20-60% of cases (fig.18).

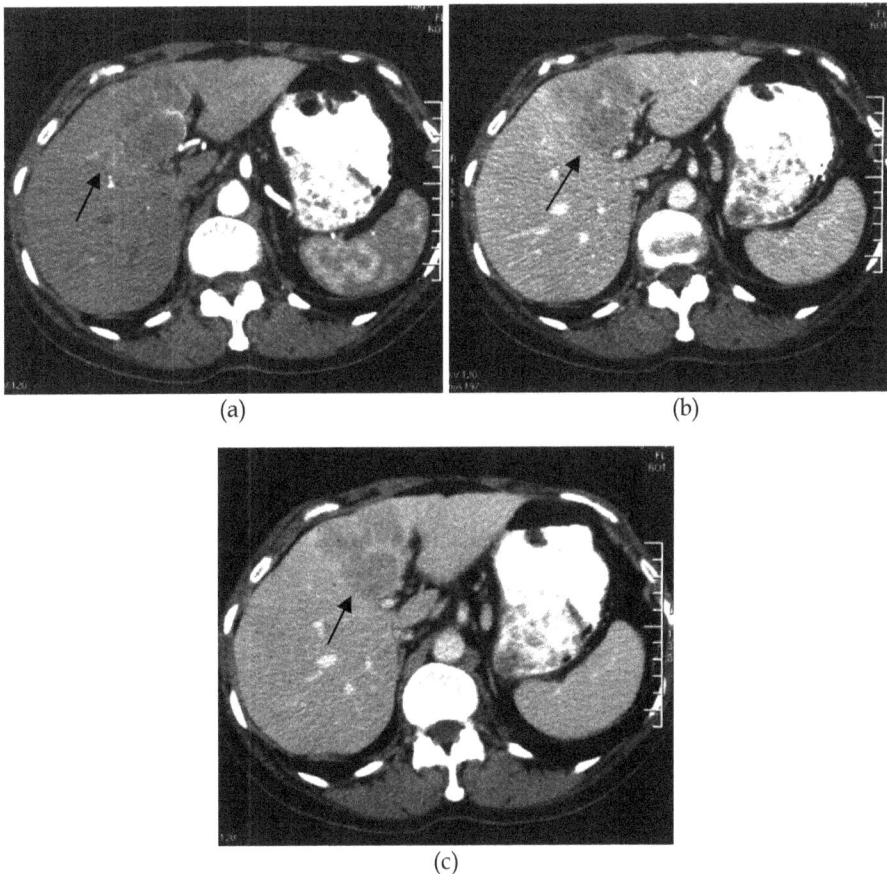

(a)   (b)

(c)

Fig. 18. Mass forming intrahepatic cholangiocarcinoma. (a) the lesion enhances hetreogeneously in arterial phase;(b,c) persistent enhancement is seen in portal venous phase. (arrow)

Mass-forming cholangiocarcinoma is characterized by a homogeneous sclerotic mass with an irregular lobulated margin, typically in the absence of haemorrhage or central necrosis. Uptake of c/m in the late phase is closely related to the amount of interstitial space in the fibrous stroma. Peripheral masses are sometimes associated with capsular retraction. About 80% of all lesions enhance in the late phase.

Diffuse periductal thickening and increased enhancement due to tumour infiltration, with an abnormally dilated or irregularly narrowed duct and peripheral ductal dilatation is typical for periductal infiltrative type. This is one of the least common types of cholangiocarcinoma. Most of hilar cholangiocarcinomas are of this type. Periductal cholangiocarcinoma tends to be localized to one segment or lobe and manifests with ductal dilatation, a finding that is indicative of biliary disease. This is a very important sign differentiating this type of cholangiocarcinoma from periportal lymphangitic metastasis or from the extrahepatic tumour. Metastases are usually localised in a few liver lobes and do not cause ductal dilatation (fig.19).

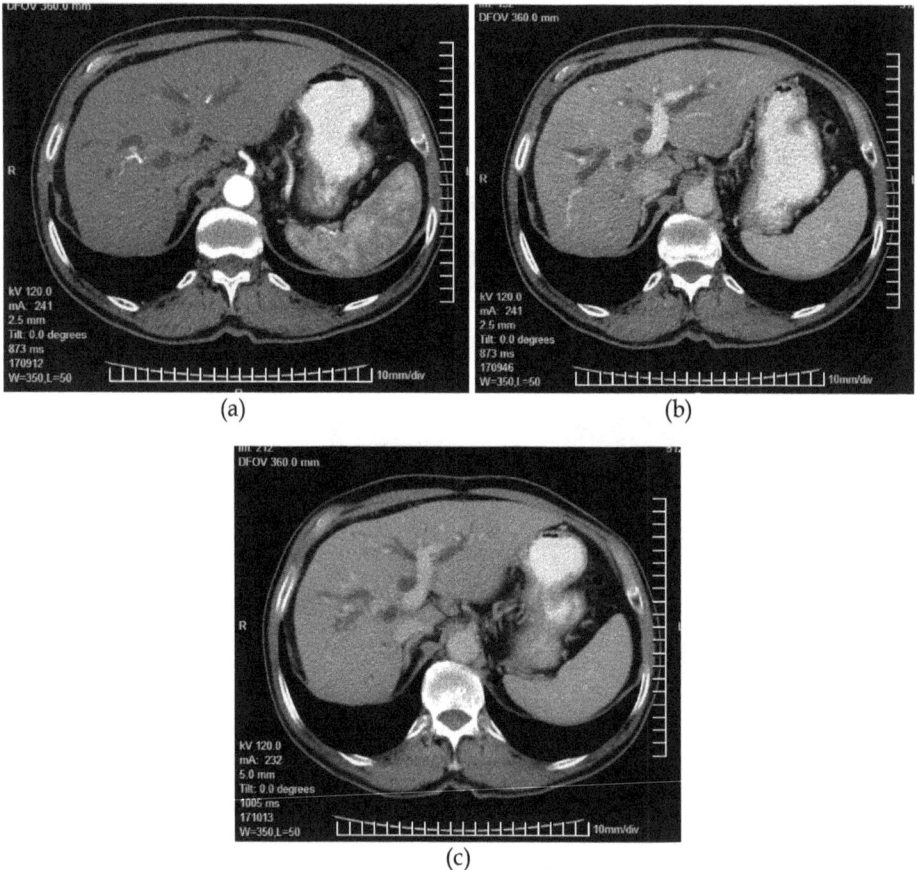
(a)   (b)

(c)

Fig. 19. Intraductal infiltrating cholangiocarcinoma. CT scan images show diffuse ductal dilatation in the both hepatic lobes with no visible intraductal mass.

On precontrast CT images intraductal cholangiocarcinomas appear as a lesion within the dilated bile duct that is hypo- and isodense compared to surrounding liver tissue. After administration of contrast media, the intraductal tumour shows enhancement. This type of tumour can be distinguished from HCC invading the bile duct on the basis of identification of the mass outside the ductal system, hypervascularity at dynamic imaging, the presence of a prominent fibrous capsule or pseudocapsule, and other imaging features favouring HCC. This type of intraductal tumour may also be confused with an intraductal mass-like stone. The absence of enhancement and the high attenuation on unenhanced CT images are useful in making the diagnosis of an intraductal mass-like stone, whereas an enhancing polypoid mass with asymmetric adjacent bile duct wall thickening is suggestive of an intraductal tumour (fig.20).

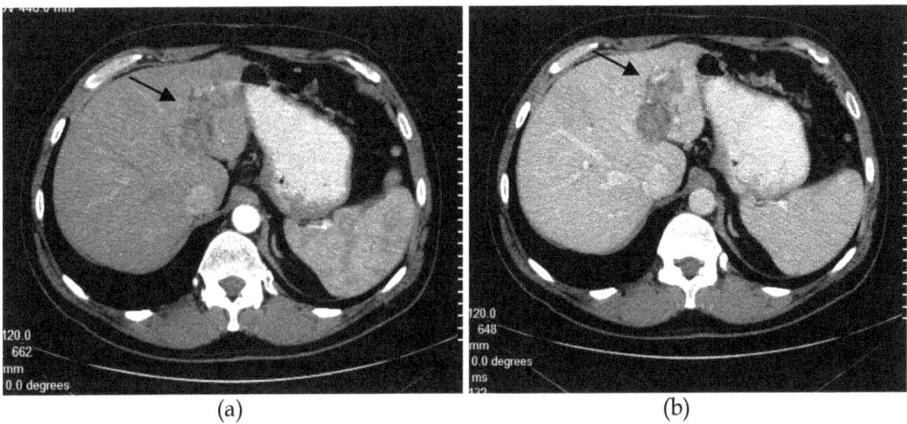

(a)   (b)

Fig. 20. Intrahepatic stone disease. (a,b) Arterial and portal venous phase CT images show dilated intrahepatic bile ducts in the left liver lobe with hepatolithiasis (arrow).

The diagnostic criteria of I-CCC on CT images are as follows: hypodense or isodense lesion on unenhanced CT images; slight peripheral enhancement in arterial phase; that emerges in venous phase. Based on these criteria CT imaging is 78% sensitive and 89% specific.

3.3 Metastases

Liver is the second most common (after lymph nodes) organ, where different malignant tumours metastasize. 80% patients with extrahepatic tumour are expected to have liver metastases. Multiple hepatic metastases are way more common (>90%) than solitary ones (<10%). Both liver lobes are more likely to be affected (77%) than the right one (20%) or the left one (31%) alone. Lesions may be infiltrative, expansive or miliary. Liver metastases may be hypovascular or hypervascular (fig. 21).

Few lesions may look completely different in one patient due to variations in cellular differentiation, fibrosis, necrosis, haemorrhage, and blood supply. This is typical for metastases from renal cell carcinoma, carcinoid, choriocarcinoma and some types of lung cancer. Majority of authors differentiate hypervascular liver metastases from FNH and HCC. Primary tumours that are the most likely to metastasise to the liver are ophthalmic and pancreatic (70-75%), breast, gall-bladder and extrahepatic bile ducts, colon and rectal (about 60%), and stomach (about 50%).

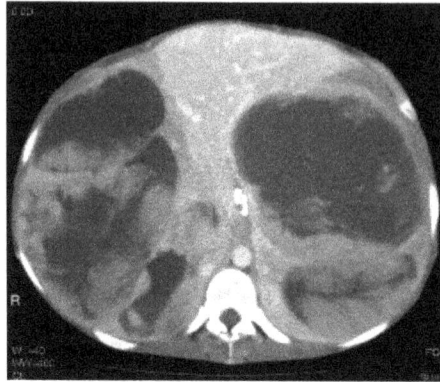

Fig. 21. Hepatic metastases from GIST. Multiple large masses show heterogeneous enhancement, intralesional irregular necrotic areas are seen.

On contrast enhanced CT images characteristic of enhancement of liver metastases is determined by the primary tumor. Most liver metastases are hypovascular. This is why they look hypodense on CT images, especially in portal venous phase compared to normal liver parenchyma. Central hypodense area caused by tissue necrosis may be seen on CT images (fig.22).

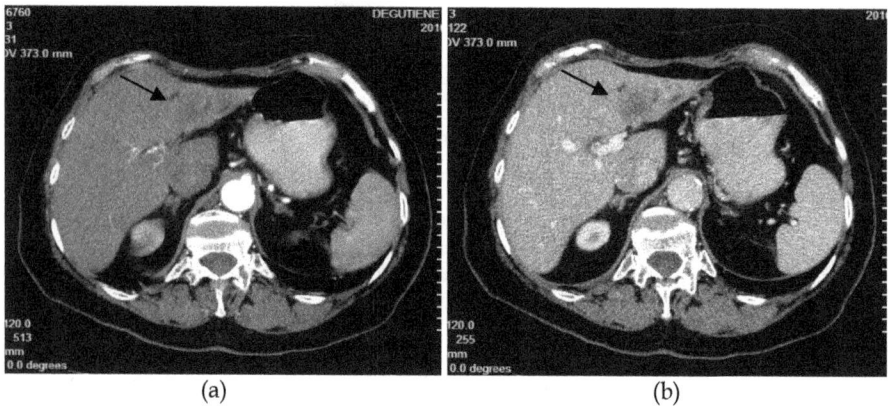

(a)   (b)

Fig. 22. Hepatic metastasis from colon carcinoma. (a) Arterial phase CT image shows a hypodense lesion with biliary duct dilatation in the left liver lobe (arrow). (b) Portal venous phase image: the lesion is hypodense to the surrounding liver parenchyma (arrow).

Peripheral hyperdense border rim can be visualized due to peripheral afferent blood vessels or hyperemia of liver tissue. The borders of metastases may be sharply defined, ill-defined, or nodular, and their shape may be ovoid, round, or irregular.

Hipervascular metastases (RCC, pancreatic carcinoma, sarcoma or melanoma) enhance more or less homogenously intensively in arterial phase. Normally arterial phase is crucial in evaluation of metastases as hyperenhancement is caused by hepatic artery supplying blood to the tumor (fig. 23).

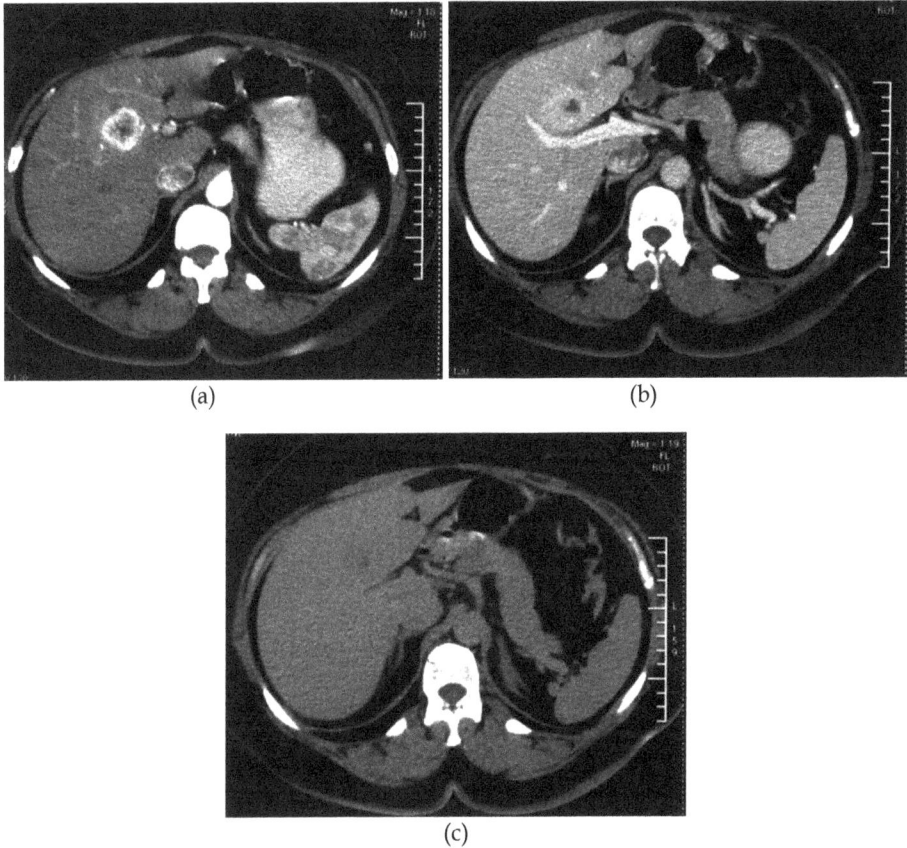

(a)   (b)

(c)

Fig. 23. Hepatic metastasis from renal cell carcinoma. a) Arterial phase CT image shows peripheral contrast enhancement, with hypodense centre of the lesion. (b) Portal venous phase CT image shows a slightly hyperenhancement of the lesion. (c) Delayed phase image - metastatic lesion is hypodense. Central part of the lesion shows necrosis.

However, sometimes metastases can enhance atypically.

In Van Leeuwen study, 11% of colorectal metastases enhanced heterogeneously, and about 60% of metastases from hypervascular tumours did not enhance at all. Metastases may develop calcification that is detectable by CT in the presence of mucin, necrosis, and phosphatase activity (fig.24).

This is typical for metastases from mucin adenocarcinoma, such as colon, pancreatic, and stomach cancer. Sometimes in case of mucin producing tumour cystic metastases may be found in the liver. On CT images they look like foci with peripheral ring enhancement. In all unclear cases differentiation from common liver cysts is required (fig. 25).

It is very important to differentiate peripheral enhancement in FLL, especially metastases, from nodular peripheral enhancement in first few seconds of arterial phase that gradually becomes more intensive in portal venous, venous and delayed phases. This character of enhancement is typical for liver hemangiomas. It is a reliable sign of non-malignant lesion.

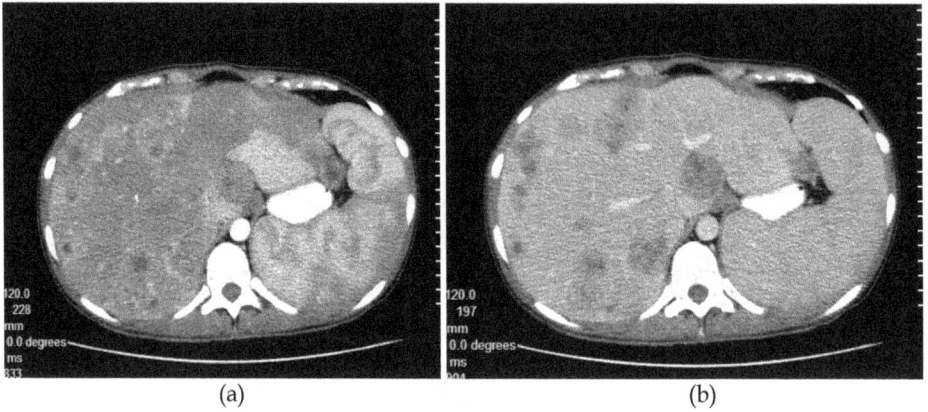

(a)   (b)

Fig. 24. Metastatic melanoma. (a) Contrast-enhanced CT image during hepatic arterial phase shows a multiple hyperattenuating hepatic metastases. (b) On portal venous phase we see washout of contrast media.

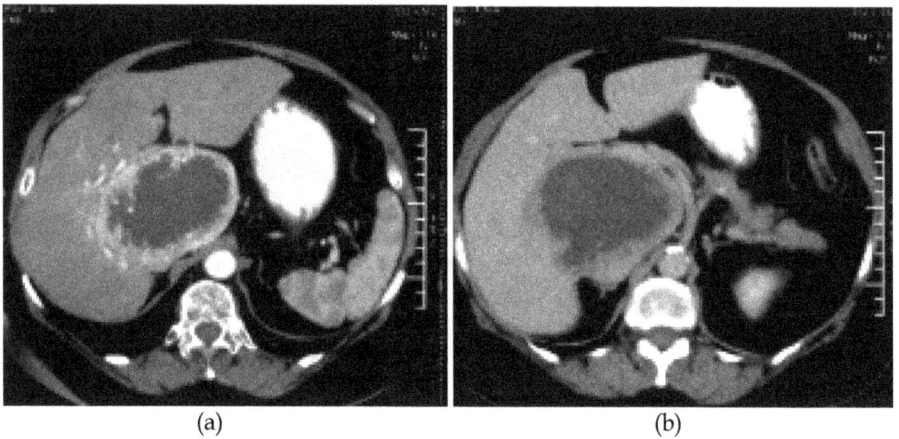

(a)   (b)

Fig. 25. Hepatic metastasis of neuroendocrine tumor. (a) On arterial CT phase, a large hypervascular tumor is seen as hyperattenuating mass with central necrosis. (b) In the portal venous phase tumor becomes isodense to surrounding liver parenchyma; necrosis remains hypodense.

Arterial-venous shunts, liver perfusion abnormalities and focal or diffuse fatty degeneration can also mimic metastases, so radiological differential diagnostic with these lesions is necessary.

In differential diagnostics of HCC and metastases it is very important to identify the following CT diagnostic criteria of hypervascular areas: hypodense lesion on unenhanced

CT images; intensive enhancement in arterial phase and rapid wash-out (hypodense lesion) in venous phase. Based on these criteria CT scanning is 85% sensitive and 86 % specific.

3.4 Rare malignant tumours

Even though these tumours are relatively rare FLL, they also should be differentiated radiologically. These are fibrolamellar carcinoma (FLC), epithelioid haemangioendothelioma (EHE), primary liver lymphoma and biliary cystadenocarcinoma.

3.4.1 Fibrolamellar carcinoma

Fibrolamellar carcinoma (FLC) presents only 2% of all liver tumours and is mostly diagnosed in young women without chronic liver disease. According to available sources, FLC should be differentiated from benign FNL, such as FNH, large haemangioma, and sometimes – HCA. It is challenging to differentiate FLC from HCC when the lesion enhances heterogeneously. This is why the late phase is so important: it visualises hypodense homogenous FLC.

Fibrolamellar carcinoma is another hypervascular tumour occurring in young adults and it usually contains a fibrotic scar. However it is not difficult to differentiate it from FNH. FLC is usually a large (>10-cm), heterogeneous, lobulated mass with broad central or eccentric scars and radiating septa. Calcifications are found in 68% of FLC, and obvious signs of malignancy such as lymphadenopathy (65%), metastases, and biliary and vascular invasion are found in the majority of cases. Calcification is typical of FLC, with a reported incidence of 35–68%. Calcifications may be punctate, nodular, or stellate and are usually small (<5 mm), few (one to three in number), and almost always located near the centre of the tumour. FLC demonstrates a central scar in up to 20–71% of cases. It is typically large and may be broad or stellate, eccentric or central. Invasion of the hepatic vessels or bile ducts was also found to be an important differentiating feature, but it may be seen in less than 5% of cases of FLC.

3.4.2 Epithelioid haemangioendothelioma

Epithelioid hemanioendothelioma (EHE) is a rare and highly malignant tumour with vascular component that develops from epithelioid endothelium cells. On unenhanced CT images epithelioid hemangioendothelioma is hypodense compared to normal hepatic parenchyma. EHE usually localises in lateral liver parts and is formed of fibrotic hypovascular central nucleus and peripheral hypervascular rim that is still seen in the late phase. Capsular retraction is frequently present, and calcification is occasionally seen.

3.4.3 Lymphoma

Primary hepatic lymphoma is an exceptionally rare disease, representing less than 1.0 % of all extranodal lymphomas. Lymphoma of the liver is considered primary in the absence of extra-hepatic involvement or in cases of predominant hepatic presentation. Hepatic lymphoma is more commonly encountered in patients with cirrhosis, mostly secondary to hepatitis C, AIDS, systemic lupus erythematosus and in transplant recipients being treated with immunosuppressive drugs. The prognosis appears to be favourable in patients diagnosed and treated early, unless there is an underlying disease. In 57% of all cases primary liver lymphoma is solitary tumour. On CT images it is seen as hypodense homogenous lesion of variable size and enhancement. Secondary lymphoma tends to present as multiple lesions in most cases, but can also show a single lesion or diffusely infiltrate the liver. CT features of hepatic lymphoma are non-specific and do not allow differentiation from other solitary or multicentric hepatic tumours (fig.26).

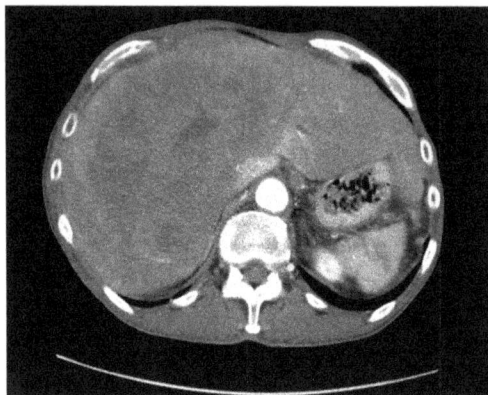

Fig. 26. B cell lymphoma. Arterial phase CT image shows a large heterogeneous tumor in the right lobe with hypodense central necrosis.

3.4.4 Billiary cystadenocarcinoma

Billiary cystadenocarcinoma is a malignant tumour, developed from billiary cysadenoma (fig. 27).

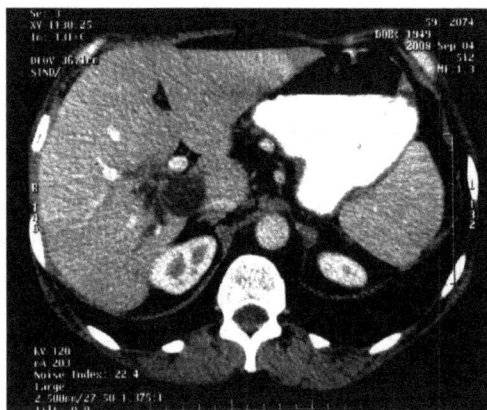

Fig. 27. Biliary cystadenoma in S1 with biliary ductal dilatation. Contrast-enhanced CT image shows a hypodense lesion in the liver without contrast enhancement. A partial septation of the lesion is present.

It is a large cystic tumour that is usually septated, but may be unilocular. The cystic spaces contain mucinous or serous fluid. On CT images both cystadenoma or cystadenocarcinoma are well defined cystic lesions that do not enhance. We can see an enhancement of the wall and septa of the tumour. Calcifications and soft tissue components are possible.

4. Conclusion

Contrast enhanced CT is a powerful imaging technique for the accurate diagnostics of HCC. Arterial and portal venous phases are important in evaluation of FLL. Delayed phase is essential in differential diagnosis of benign and malignant lesions. These imging techniques should be optimized for the evaluation of suspected HCC. Typical CT features may help in differentiating HCC from other liver lesions.

Contrast enhanced CT is important technique for the accurate diagnosis of HCC. Optimal scanning protocol is essential. Delayed phase should be always included in scanning protocol.

5. Acknowledgment

I am particularly indebted to all the radiologist of our department of Radiology in Lithuanian University of Health Sciences Kaunas Clinics for their help in gathering CT images of interesting and extremely rare cases.

6. References

Albrecht T., Hohmann J., Oldenburg A., Skrok J., & Wolf KJ. (2004). Detection and characterisation of liver metastases. Europen Radiology, Vol.14,suppl 8, pp. 25-33, ISSN 0938-7994.

Albrecht T., Thorelius L., Solbiati L., Cova L., & Frauscher F. (2005). Contrast-enhanced ultrasound in clinical practice. Springer-Verlag Italia, Milan, ISBN 88-470-0304.

Anderson SW., Kruskal JB., & Kane RA. (2009). Benign hepatic tumors and iatrogenic pseudotumors. Radiographic, Vol. 29, pp. 211-229, ISSN 0271-5333.

Appelbaum L., Lederman R., Agid R., & Libson E. (2005). Hepatic lymphoma: an imaging approach with emphasis on image-guided Needle biopsy. IMAJ, Vol. 7, pp. 19-22, ISSN 1565-1088.

Arab M., Mansoori D., Abbasidezfouli A., Shadmehr M. & Afsari M. (2002). Splenic tuberculosis: a case report. Acta Medica Iranica, Vol. 40, No.1, pp. 26-28, ISSN 1560-8239.

B. E. Van Beers. (2008). Diagnosis of cholangiocarcinoma. Review article. HPB, Vol. 10, pp. 87-93, ISSN 1365-182X print/ISSN 1477-2574 (online).

Banshodani M., Ishiyama K., Amano H., Tashiro H., Arihiro K., Itamoto T., & Ohdan H. (2009). Hepatic angiomyolipoma with minimal intratumoral fat content. Case reports in Gastroenterology, Vol. 3, pp. 324-331, ISSN 1662-0631.

Basaran C., Karcaaltincaba M., Akata D., Karabulut N., Akinci D., Ozmen M., & Akhan O. (2005). Fat-containing lesions of the liver: cross-sectional imaging findings with emphasis on MRI. AJR, Vol.184, pp.1103-1110, ISSN 1844-1103.

Blachar AB., Federle MP., Ferris JV., Lacomis JM., Waltz JS., Armfield DR., Chu G., Almusa O., Grazioli L., Balzano E., & Li W. (2002). Radiologists' performance in the diagnosis of liver tumors with central scars by using specific CT criteria. Radiology, Vol. 223, pp. 532-539, ISSN.0033-8419.

Brancatelli G., Federle MP., Blachar A., & Grazioli L. (2001). Hemangioma in the cirrhotic liver: diagnosis and natural history. Radiology, Vol. 219, pp. 69-74, ISSN. 0033-8419.

Brancatelli G., Federle MP., Grazioli L., Blachar A., Peterson MS., & Thaete L. (2001 b). Focal nodular hyperplasia: CT findings with emphasis on multiphasic helical CT in 78 patients. Radiology, Vol. 219, pp. 61–68, ISSN 0033-8419.

Carlson SK., Johnson C.D., Bender C.E., & Welch TJ. (2000). CT of focal nodular hyperplasia of the liver. Pictorial essay. AJR, Vol. 174, pp. 705-712, ISSN 1743-705.

Caturelli E., Pompili M., Bartolucci F., Siena DA., Sperandeo M., Andriulli A., & Bisceglia M. (2001). Hemangioma-like lesions in chronic liver disease: diagnostic evaluation in patients. Radiology, Vol. 220, pp. 337-342, ISSN 0033-8419

Cha E-Y., Kim KW., Choi YJ., Song JS., Cho KJ., & Lee M-G. (2008). Multicystic cavernous hemangioma of the liver: ultrasonography, CT, MR appearances and pathological correlation. The British Journal of Radiology, Vol. 81, pp. 37-39, ISSN 0007-1285.

Chuan-Miao XIE., Lie Zheng., Yun-Xian MO., Li Li., Chao-Mei Ruan Yan-Chun LU., & Pei – Hong WU. (2007). Helical double-phase CT scan imaging features of hepatocellular karcinoma and pathology of false-positive lesions. Chinese Journal of Cancer, Vol. 26, No. 1, pp.1-6, ISSN 16735269.

Chung YE., Kim M-F., Park YN., Choi F-Y., Pyo FY., Kim YC., Cho HF., KimK A., & Choi SY. (2009). Varying appearances of cholangiocarcinoma: radiologic-pathologic correlation. Radiographics, Vol. 29, pp. 683-700, ISSN 0271-5333.

Eldad S.Bialecki & Adrian M. Di Bisceglie. (2005). Diagnosis of hepatocellular carcinoma. HPB, Vol. 7, pp. 26-34, ISSN 1365-182X print/ ISSN 1477-2574 (online).

Foley WD., Mallisee TA., Hohenwalter MD., Wilson CR., Quiroz FA. & Taylor AJ. (2000). Multiphase hepatic CT with a multidetector CT scanner. Am J Roentgenol, Vol. 175, pp. 679-685, ISSN 1753-679.

Goshima S., Kanematsu M., Kondo H., Yokoyama R., Miyoshi T., Kato H., Hoshi H., Onozuka M., & Moriyama N. (2006). MDCT of the liver and hypervascular hepatocellular carcinomas: optimizing scan delnys for bolus-tracking techniques of hepatic arterial and portal venos phases. AJR, Vol. 187, pp. W25-W32, ISSN 1871-W25.

Grazioli L., Federle MP., Brancatelli G., Ichikawa T., Olivetti L., & Blachar A. (2001). Hepatic adenomas: imaging and pathologic findings. Radiographics, Vol. 21, pp. 877-894, ISSN 0271-5333.

Grazioli L., Morana G., Kirchin MA., & Schneider G. (2005). Accurate differentiation of focal nodular hyperplasia from hepatic adenoma at Gadobenate Dimeglumine-enhanced MR imaging: prospective study. Radiology, Vol. 236, pp.166-177, ISSN 0033-8419.

Hussain SM., Terkivatan T., Zondervan PE., Lanjouw E., Sjoerd de Rave, IJzermans Jan N.M., & Rob A. de Man. (2004). Focal nodular hyperplasia: findings at state of the art MR imaging, US, CT, and pathologic analysis. Radiographics, Vol. 24, pp. 3-19, ISSN 0271-5333.

Iannaccone R., Piacentini F., Murakami T., Paradis V., Belghiti J., Hori M., Kim T., Durand F., Wakasa K., Monden M., Nakamura H., Passariello R., & Vilgrain V. (2007). Hepatocellular carcinoma in patients with nonalcoholic fatty liver disease: helical CT and MR imaging findings with clinical-pathologic comparison. Radiology, Vol. 243, No. 2, pp.422-430, ISSN 0033-8419.

Ichikawa T., Federle MP., Grazioli L., & Nalesnik M. (2000). Hepatocellular adenoma: multiphasic CT and histopathologic findings in 25 patients. Radiology, Vol. 214, pp. 861-868, ISSN 0033-8419.

Yoon SH., Lee JM., So YH., Hong SH., KimS J., Han JK., & Choi BI. (2009). Multiphasic MDCT enhancement pattern of hepatocellular carcinoma smaller than 3 cm in diametre: tumor size and cellular differentiation. AJR, Vol. 193, pp.W482-W489, ISSN 1936-W482.

Jacomina W. Van den Esschert, Thomas M. van Gulik, & Phoa S.S.K.S. (2010). Imaging modalities for focal nodular hyperplasia and hepatocellular adenoma. Digestive Surgery, Vol. 27, pp.46-55, ISSN 0271-0046.

Jang H-J., KimT K., Lim HK., Park SJ., Sim JS., Kim HY., & Lee J-H. (2003). Hepatic hemangioma: atypical appearances on CT, MR imaging, and sonography. Pictorial essay. AJR, Vol. 180, pp.135-141, ISSN 0361-803X.

Jeong YY., Yim NY., & Kang HK. (2005). Hepatocellular carcinoma in the cirrhotic liver with helical CT and MRI: imaging spectrum and pitfalls of cirrhosis-related nodules. AJR, Vol. 185, pp. 1024-1032, ISSN 1854-1024.

Jeong MG., Yu JS., & Kim KW. (2000). Hepatic cavernous hemangioma: temporal peritumotal enhancement during multiphase dynamic MR imaging. Radiology, Vol. 213, pp. 692-697, ISSN 0033-8419.

Karcaaltincaba M., & Sirlin CB. (2010). CT and MRI of diffuse lobar involvement pattern in liver pathology. Diagnostic and interventional radiology, Vol.5, pp. 1-8, ISSN 21053176.

Ke-guo ZHENG, Jing-xian SHEN, Gen-shu WANG & Da-sheng XU. (2007). Small hepatocellular carcinoma with peripheral enhancement: pathological correlation with dual phase images by helical CT. Chinese medical Journal, Vol. 120, No.18, pp.1583-1586, ISSN: 0366-6999.

Kim HG. (2006). Biliary cystic neoplasm: biliary cistadenoma and biliary cystadenocarcinoma. Korean Journal of Gastroenterology, Vol. 47, No. 1, pp. 5-14, ISSN 1598-9992.

Kim KW, Kim AY., KimT K., Kim SY., Park M-S., Park SH., Lee KH., Kim JK., Kim P-N., Ha HK., Lee M-G. (2006). Hepatic hemangiomas with arterioportal shunt: sonographic appearances with CT and MRI correlation. AJR, Vol.187, pp. 406-414, ISSN 0361-803X pint/ISSN 1874-W406 (online).

Kim KW., Kim MJ., Lee SS., Kim HJ., Shin YM., Kim P-N., & Lee M-G. (2008). Sparingo f fatty infiltration around focal hepatic lesions in patients with hepatic steatosis: sonographic appearance with CT and MRI correlation. AJR, Vol. 190, pp. 1018-1027, ISSN 1904-1018.

Kim S J., Lee JM., Han JK., KimK H., Lee JY., & Choi BI. (2007). Peripheral mass-forming cholangiocarcinoma in cirrhotic liver. AJR, Vol. 189, pp. 1428-1434, ISSN 0361-803X print/ISSN 1896-1428 (online).

Kim T., Federle MP., Baron RL., Peterson MS., & Kawamori Y. (2001). Discrimination of smals hepatic hemangiomas from hypervascular malinant tumors smaller than 3 cm with three-phase helical CT. Radiology, Vol. 219, pp 699-706, ISSN 0033-8419.

Kumar V. & Pandey D. (2008). Isolated hepatosplenic tuberculosis. Hepatobiliary and pancreatic diseases International, Vol. 7, No. 3, pp. 328-330, ISSN 1499-3872.

Lee YH., Kim SH., Cho M-Y., Shim KY., & Kim MS. (2007). Focal nodular hyperplasia – like nodules in alcoholic liver cirrhosis: radiologic – pathologic correlation. AJR, Vol. 188, pp. 459-463, ISSN 1885-W459.

Lee J., Lee WJ., Lim HK., Lim JH., Choi N., Park M., KimS W., & Park CK. (2008). Early hepatocellular carcinoma: three-phase helical CT features of 16 patients. Korean J Radiology, Vol. 9, pp. 325-332, ISSN 1229-6929.

LimA KP., Patel N., Gedroyc WMW., Blomley MJK., Hamilton G., & Taylor-Robinson SD. (2002). Hepatocellular adenoma: diagnostic difficulties and novel imaging techniques. Case report. The British Journal of Radiology, Vol. 75, pp. 695-699, ISSN 0007-1285 print/ ISSN 1748-880X(online).

M.A. Hayat. (2009). Methods of Cancer Diagnosis, Therapy and Prognosis – liver Cancer. Volume 5, Part IV, Part 6. Springer-Science + Business Media B.V., ISBN 978-1-4020-9803-1-P, USA.

Manouras A., Markogiannakis H., Lagoudianakis E., & Katergiannakis V. (2006). Biliary cistadenoma with mesenchymal stroma: Report of a case and review of the literature. World J Gastroenterol, Vol.12, No. 37, pp. 6062-6069, ISSN 1007-9327.

Marchal G., Vogl T.J., Heiken J.P., Rubin G.D. (2005). Multidetector – Row Computed Tomography. (Scaning and contrast protocols). Springer-Verlag, ISBN 88-470-0305-9, Milan, Italy.

Masood A., Kairouz S., Hudhud K.H. Hegazi A.Z., Banu A., & Gupta N.C. (2009). Primary non-Hodgkin lymphoma of liver. Current Oncology, Vol. 16, No. 4, pp.74-77, ISSN 1718-7729.

Mita K., KimS R., Kudo M., Imoto S., Nakajima T., Ando K., Fukuda K., Matsuoka T., Maekawa Y., & Hayashi Y. (2010). Diagnostic sensitivity of imaging modalities for hepatocellular carcinoma smaller than 2 cm. World J Gastroenterology, Vol. 16, No. 33, pp. 4187-4192, ISSN 1007-9327 (print), ISSN 2219-2840 (online).

Monzawa S., Ischikawa T, Nakajima H., Kitanaka Y., Omata K., & Araki T. (2007). Dynamic CT for detecting small hepatocellular carcinoma: usefulness of delayed pase imaging. AJR, Vol. 188, pp.147-153, ISSN 1881-147.

Mortele KJ., Praet M., H. Van Vlierberghe, Kunnen., & Ros P.R. (2000). CT and MR imaginė findings in focal nodular hyperplasia of the liver: radiologic – pathologic correlation. AJR, Vol.175, pp.687-692, ISSN 1753-687.

Murakami T., Kim T., Takamura M., Hori M., Takahashi S., Federle MP., Tsuda K., Osuga K., Kawata S., Nakamura H. & Kudo M. (2001). Hypervascular hepatocellular carcinoma: detection with double arterial phase multi-detector row helical CT. Radiology, No.218, pp. 763-767, ISSN.0033-8419

Nakanuma Y., Sato Y., Harada K., Sasaki M., Xu J., & Ikeda H. (2010). Pathological classification of intrahepatic cholangiocarcinoma based on a new concept. World J of Hepatology, Vol. 2, No. 12, pp. 419-427, ISSN 1948-5182.

Natsuizaka M., Kudo M., Suzuki M., Takano M., Tsuyuguchi M., Kawamura N., Noguchi S., Wada A., Nakata M., Ogasawara M., Kiyama Y., Asaka M., & Kasai M. (2009). Diffuse large B-cell lymphoma with massive portal vein tumor thrombosis in a patient with alcoholic cirrhosis: a case report and literature review. Internal medicine, Vol. 48, pp.805-808, ISSN 0918-2918.

Nino-Murcia M., Olcott EW., Jeffrey RB., Lamm RL., Beaulieu CF., & Jain KA. (2000) Focal liver lesions: pattern – based classification scheme for enhancement at arterial phase. Radiology, Vol. 215, pp. 746–751, ISSN 1527-1315.

Nouira K., Allani R., Bougamra I., Bouzaidi K., Azaiez O., Mizouni H., Messaoud MB., & Menif E. (2007). Atypical small hemangiomas of the liver: hypervascular hemangiomas. International journal of biomedical science, Vol.3, No.4, pp. 302-304, ISSN 15509702

Numminen K., Isoniemi H., Halavaara J., Tervahartiala P., Makisalo H., Laasonen L., & Hockerstedt K. (2005). Preoperative assessment of focal liver lesions: multidetector computed tomography challenges magnetic resonance imaging. Acta Radiol , Vol. 46, pp. 9-15, ISSN 0284-1851.

Oliva MR., & Saini S. (2004). Liver cancer imaging: role of CT, MRI, US and PET. Cancer imaging, Vol. 4, pp. S42-S46, ISSN 1740-5025.

Outwater EK. (2010). Imaging of the liver for hepatocellular Cancer. Cancer control, Vol. 17, No. 2, pp. 72-82, ISSN 20404790.

Pitton MB., Kloeckner R., Herber S., Otto G., Kreitner KF., & Dueber C. (2009). MRI versus 64-row MDCT for diagnosis of hepatocellular carcinoma. World J Gastroenterology, Vol. 15, No. 48, pp. 6044-6051, ISSN 1007-9327.

Purl A.S., Nayyar A.K. & Vij J.C. (1994). Hepatic tuberculosis. Indian Journal of tuberculosis, Vol.41, pp. 131-134, ISSN 0971-5916.

Quiroga S., Sebastia C., Pallisa E., Castella E., Perez-Lafuente M.,& Alvarez-Castells. (2001). Improved diagnosis of hepatic perfusion disorers: value of hepatic arterial phase imaging during helical CT. Radiographics, Vol. 21, pp. 65-81, ISSN 0271-5333.

Raptopoulos VD., Blake SP., Weisinger K., Atkins MB., Keogan MT., & Kruskal JB. (2001). Multiphase contrast-enhanced helical CT of liver metastases from renal cell karcinoma. Europen Radiology, Vol.11, No. 12, pp. 2504-2509, ISSN 0938-7994.

Ri-Sheng Y., Zhang S-Z., Wu J-J & Li R-F. (2004). Imaging diagnosis of 12 patients with hepatic tuberculosis. World Journal of Gastroenterology, Vol. 10, No. 11, pp. 1639-1642, ISSN 1007-9327.

Robinson PH. (2008). Hepatocellular carcinoma: development and early detection. Cancer imaging, Vol. 8, pp. S128-S131, ISSN 1740-5025.

Ronzoni A., Artioli D., Scardina R., Battistig L., Minola E., Sironi S., & Vanzulli A. (2007). Role of MDCT in the diagnosis of hepatocellular carcinoma in patients with cirrhosis undergoing orthotopic liver transplantation. AJR, Vol. 189, pp. 792-798., ISSN 1894-792.

Ruppert-Kohlmayr AJ., Uggowitzer MM., Kugler C., Zebedin D., Schaffler G., & Ruppert GS. (2001). Focal nodular hyperplasia and hepatocellular adenoma of the liver: differentiation with multiphasic helical CT. AJR, Vol. 176, pp.1493-1498, ISSN 1766-1493.

Saluja SS., Ray S., Pal S., Kukeraja M., Srivastava DN., Sahni P., & Chattopadhyay T. (2007). Hepatobiliary and pancreatic tuberculosis: a two decade experience. Research article. BMC Surgery, pp. 7-10, ISSN 1471-2482.

Sanders LM., Botet JF., Straus DJ., Ryan J., Filippa DA., & Newhouse JH. (1989). CT of primary lymphoma of the liver. AJR, Vol. 152, pp.973-976, ISSN 1525-0973.

Schwarz LH., Gandras EJ., Colangelo SM., Ercolani MC., & Panicek DM. (1999). Prevalence and importance of small hepatic lesions found at CT in patients with cancer. Radiology, Vol. 210, pp. 71-74, ISSN.0033-8419.

Scott DJ., Guthrie JA., Arnold P., Ward J., Atchley J., Wilson D., & Robinson PJ. (2001). Dual-phase helical CT versus portal venous phase CT for the detection of colorectal liver metastases: correlation with intra-operative sonography, surgical and pathological findings. Clinical Radiology, Vol.56, pp. 235-242, ISSN 0009-9260.

Sharma S.K., Smith-Rohrberg D., Tahir M., Mohan A. & Seith A. (2007). Radiological manifestations of splenic tuberculosis: a 23-patient case series from India. Indian J Med Res, Vol. 125, pp. 669-678, ISSN 17642503.

Soyer P, Poccard M, Boudiaf M, Abitbol M., Hamzi L., Panis Y., Valleur P., & Rymer R. (2004). Detection of hypovascular hepatic metastases at triple-phase helical CT: sensivity of phases and comparison with surgical and histopathologic findings. Radiology, Vol. 231, pp. 413-420, ISSN 0033-8419.

Sood D., Kumaran V., Buxi TBS., Nundy S., & Soin AS. (2009). Liver hemangioma mimicking cholangiocarcinoma – a diagnostic dilema. Tropical gastroenterology, Vol. 30, No.1, pp. 44-46, ISSN 0250-636X.

Szklaruk J., & Bhosale P. (2007). Hepatocellular carcinoma: MRI and CT examination. Reviews. IMAJ, Vol. 9, pp.153-155, ISSN 1565-1088.

Takayasu K., Muramatsu Y., Mizuguchi Y., Okusaka T., Shimada K., Takayama T., & Sakamoto M. (2006). CT evaluation of the progression of hypoattenuating nodular lesions in virus-related chronic liver disease. AJR, Vol. 187, pp. 454-463, ISSN 1872-454.

Toriyama E., Nasashima A., Hayashi H., Abe K., Kinoshita N., Yuge S., Nagayasu T., Uetani M., & Hayashi T. (2010). A case of intrahepatic clear cell cholangiocarcinoma. World J of Gastroenterology, Vol. 16, pp. 2571-2576, ISSN 1007-9327.

Tranquart F., Bleuzen A., & Kissel A. (2004). Value of combined conventional and contrast enhanced sonography in the evaluation of hepatic disorders. J Radol., Vol. 85, No.1, pp. 755-762, ISSN 0221-0363.

Vilgrain V., Boulos L., Vullierme M-P., Denys A., Terris B., & Menu Y. (2000). Imaging of atypical hemangiomas of the liver with pathologic correlation. Radiographics, Vol.20, No. 2, pp. 379-397, ISSN 0271-5333

Xu A-M., Cheng H-Y., Chen D., Jis Y-C., & Wu M-C. (2002). Plane and weighted tri-phase helical CT findings in the diagnosis of liver focal nodular hyperplasia. Hepatobilliary & Pancreatic Diseases International, Vol. 1, No. 2, pp. 219-223, ISSN 1499-3872.

Zhao H., Yao J-L., Wang Y., & Zhou K-R. (2007). Detection of smals hepatocellular carcinoma: comparison of dynamic enhancement magnetic resonance imaging and multiphase multirow-detector helical CT scaning. World J Gastroenterology, Vol.13, No.8, pp.1252-1256, ISSN 1007-9327.

Zviniene K., Zaboriene I., Basevicius A., Jurkiene N., Barauskas G., & Pundzius J. (2010). Comparative diagnostic value of contrast-enhanced ultrasonography, computed tomography, ang magnetic resonance imaging in diagnosis of hepatic hemangiomas. Medicina (Kaunas), Vol. 46, No.5, pp. 329-335, ISSN 1010-660X pint/1648-9144 (online)

[http://emedicine.medscape.com/article/368377].
[www.loc.lt].

6

Signal Intensity Characteristics of Liver Masses at Hepatobiliary Phase Images of Gadoxetate-Enhanced MR (EOB-MR): Qualitative Assessment

Keiko Sakamoto, Yoshinobu Shinagawa, Ritsuko Fujimitsu, Mikiko Ida,
Hideyuki Higashihara, Kouichi Takano and Kengo Yoshimitsu*

*Department of Radiology, Faculty of Medicine, Fukuoka University,
Nanakuma, Johnan-ku, Fukuoka
Japan*

1. Introduction

Gadolinium ethoxybenzyl diethylenetriamineoentacetic acid (gadoxetic acid disodium, or Gd-EOB-DTPA, Primovist, BayerSchering, Germany) is a liver cell specific contrast agent, with which dynamic phase images can be obtained to assess arterial blood supply or arterial flow to the liver tumors, in addition to hepatobiliary phase (HBP) images that yields high accuracy in the detection of liver lesions [1-3]. In other words, Gd-EOB-DTPA behaves as non-specific extracellular contrast agent in the early dynamic phase, and as a tissue-specific contrast agent in later phases. Evaluation of vascularity helps in part differentiate various liver lesions, applying our previous experience of Gd-based extracellular contrast medium [4-6]. It is sometimes difficult, however, to make differentiation only from findings of Gd-EOB-DTPA-enhanced MR (EOB-MR) images, because of insufficient arterial enhancement due to small dose of Gd-EOB-DTPA used (25 μ mol/kg), and lack of "equilibrium phase images" in the conventional sense of the word [1].

On HBP images, because most of the liver lesions, except for some hepatocellular lesions, uptake little Gd-EOB-DTPA, they are uniformly considered to present as hypointense areas in contrast to the well-enhanced normal surrounding liver parenchyma [1-6]. However, it has already been reported that most of the liver tumors do enhance on the HBP images [1,5,6] possibly through several different mechanisms. Both liver metastasis and hepatocellular carcinoma (HCC) exhibit 20-30% higher signal intensity on HBP as compared to precontrast images [1,6]; the presumed mechanism for the former is contrast accumulation in the abundant fibrous interstitium or stroma, by similar mechanism as that of conventional extracellular Gd-based contrast medium [7], and that for the latter is either cellular uptake of Gd-EOB-DTPA by the neoplastic cells or interstitial accumulation, or both. Focal nodular hyperplasia (FNH) is well known to show 150% higher signal [1,6] because of

---

* Corresponding Author

the characteristic cellular uptake of Gd-EOB-DTPA by the tumor. Hemangioma becomes 50% higher in signal on HBP [1,6] possibly due to contrast retension in the blood pool in the sinusoidal space in the tumor.

We therefore hypothesized that patterns of signal intensity on HBP images, when assessed in detail, may vary according to the types of liver masses and also that it may be of some help in the characterization of each entity. Thus, we conducted this study to elucidate whether qualitative assessment of signal intensity on HBP of Gd-EOB-DTPA-enhanced MR (EOB-MR) is useful in differential diagnosis of liver masses, in addition to the assessment of patterns of blood supply on the dynamic phase images.

2. Materials and methods

2.1 Patients

Between June 2008 and November 2008, 65 patients underwent Gd-EOB-DTPA enhanced MR in our institute. Medical charts and radiological images, including MR and CT images, were retrospectively reviewed, and liver lesions were recruited according to the inclusion criteria as shown below. Our institutional review board approved this study without requiring specific informed consent for this study because of its retrospective nature.

Inclusion criteria of the lesions are as follows: 1) image quality is not degraded due to any artifacts, 2) confirmation of the etiology of the lesions is obtained either pathologically or clinicoradiologically. Exclusion criteria were: 1) poor image quality due to artifacts, such as motion, respiratoy, or susceptibility artifacts (lesions visualized in the edge slices of the imaging slab where considerable signal drop was noted were also excluded) 2) lack of final confirmation according to our definition as shown below. Clinicoradiological criteria of the liver masses were as follows: hypovascular hepatocellular nodules (group1) were defined as those nodules which were detected on ultrasonography (US) in patients with hepatitis or cirrhosis, and showed no hypervascularity on dynamic MDCT which were obtained within four weeks from EOB-MR, or on dynamic phase of EOB-MR. Hypervascular hepatocellular carcinoma (HCC) (group 2) were defined as lesions which exhibited typical early enhancement and subsequent washout (lower density than the surrounding hepatic tissue on portal venous or equilibrium phase images) [8] on MDCT in patients with hepatitis or cirrhosis, or those which accumulated lipiodol after transcatheter treatment in patients who had previously had pathologically proven HCC. Hemangiomas (groups 3) were defined as those for which conventional MR or dynamic CT had shown typical findings [8,9], and remained unchanged over one year. Metastases (group 4) were defined as those nodules which progressed on the follow-up imaging studies including CT/US in patients with pathologically proven primary malignancies. FNH (group 5) were defined as those nodules which strongly enhances on the arterial phase and becomes similar density on the equilibrium phase images of MDCT, and also associated with at least partial uptake of superparamagnetic ironoxide (SPIO) confirmed on T2- or T2*-weighted MR images [8].

2.2 MR and CT technique

MR examination was performed in a 1.5 T clinical unit (Achieva Nova Dual, Philips Medical Sytems, Netherland). T1-weighted chemical-shift gradient-echo images (CSI) were initially obtained under breath-holding using the following parameters; repetition time (TR) 165 msec, eho-time (TE) 2.3 and 4.6 msec, flip angle (FA) 75 degrees, 256 matrix and slice thickness/gap=7-8/1 mm. Then dynamic scan was performed using three-dimensional (3D) T1-weighted field-echo images with fat suppression (T1-high resolution isotropic volumetric excitation: THRIVE) (TR/TE/FA=4.7 msec/2.3 msec/15 degrees, 4 mm thickness with gap - 2 mm, 224 matrix) and test injection method. First, the injection rate was determined according to each patient as the whole amount of contrast (0.025mmol/kg) was injected at 3 sec (fixed injection time), and additional 0.5 mL Gd-EOB-DTPA was injected at that rate for test injection, followed by an injection of 20 mL saline. Single-level, sequential, axial, turbo filed-echo (repetition time/echo time = 13.4/1.47, 60° flip angle) were performed every 1 second for 60 seconds at the level of the center of the aorta at the level of celiac artery using as large a region of interest as possible. A time-signal intensity curve was generated using the software package on the MR imaging system. The time delay from the commencement of the test injection to the arrival of Gd at the abdominal aorta was recorded as arrival time of the aorta (Tao). According to the previous literature [10,11] and to our personal experience, the optimal arterial dominant phase (T) was roughly calculated using the following formula: T = Tao + 9 – 1/2 (acquisition time). Dynamic MR scanning was performed with THRIVE before and at T, T + 30, 90, and 240 seconds after the beginning of bolus administration of Gd-EOB-DTPA.

Subsequently, two types of T2-weighted images are obtained. First, tubo-spin-echo sequence with breath-holding (TR/TE/echo-train=10000/120/59, slice thickness/gap=7-8/1 mm) and then, 3D T2-weighted imaging with fat saturation (VISTA; TR/TE/echo-train=2000/99/79) was performed with respiratory navigation; slice thickness and gap=3 and -1.5mm, scan time approximately 8 min). Then, diffusion-weighted images were obtained with TR/TE/FA=1500/72/90 degree, b factors 0 and 1000, 3NEX, and respiratory navigation. In 15 minutes, hepatocellular phase images were obtained with THRIVE in the axial and coronal direction, the same sequence as one used for the dynamic study.

CT was obtained with a 64-row multidetector CT (Aquilion 64, Toshiba, Tokyo, Japan) with the following parameters; 120kVp, auto-mAs, 0.5 mmx64, pitch 53, reconstruction 2 mm thickness. After unenhanced scanning of the upper abdomen, 600 mgI/kg iodinated contrast medium (Iopamiron 370, Bayer-Schering, Germany) was injected in 30 sec via superficial venous branches of the upper extremities, and arterial dominant phase (40 sec delay or delay determined by bolus tracking method), portal phase (70 sec delay), and equilibrium phase (240 sec delay) imaged were obtained.

2.3 Assessment

Signal intensity of the liver lesion on HBP was qualitatively graded into five categories using surrounding non-tumorous liver parenchyma and the inferior vena cava (IVC) as reference tissue; H (higher than the surrounding liver), I (similar to the liver), L1 (lower than the liver, and higher than IVC), L2 (similar to IVC), and L3 (lower than IVC). Visual comparison of the mass to IVC was made primarily within the same slice as the target mass is located, but when IVC is too small in size and hard to evaluate its signal intensity at visual inspection, the adjacent slices available were referred to. Two radiologists (SK, KY) interpreted the axial HBP images of 54 patients, and disagreement was resolve by consensus. Signal pattern was compared between the groups using ANOVA with post-hoc test.

In the early stages of multistep hepatocarcinogenesis [12,13], some hepatocelllar nodules including regenerative nodules (RN), dysplastic nodules (DN), early hepatocellular carcinomas (eHCC) or well differentiated hepatocellular carcinomas (wHCC), have been known to exhibit high signal intensity on T1WI, either related or unrelated to fatty metamorphosis [14-17]. Therefore, there could be a hypothesis that signal intensity before contrast administration may influence signal intensity on the postcontrast image. To test this hypothesis, we correlated SI on HBP in groups 1 and 2, namely hypo- and hypervascular hepatocellular nodules, to the incidence of lesions exhibiting high signal intensity (H) on the precontrast THRIVE image using Spearman's rank correlation. Because fat suppression is applied to THRIVE, high signal on precontrast THRIVE indicates non-fatty component with short T1 characteristics, such as copper or iron accumulation [14-16]. Also correlated was to the presence of fat on CSI, namely presence of signal loss on out-of-phase images [17] as compared to in-phase images.

3. Results

Among the 65 patients, 10 patients were excluded because these did not meet the incluson criteria. In one patient, there were a combined-hepatocellular and cholangiocellular carcinoma that were surgically resected and pathologically confirmed, but this was excluded because of its too small number that would not tolerate statistical evaluation. Finally 154 liver nodules in 54 patients consisted the study population for this study. There were 41 men and 13 women, with age ranging from 32 to 92 years old (mean 67). The details of the recruited 154 liver masses are as follows: group1 (n=45) 9 were pathologically proven by biopsy (4 dysplastic nodules, 2 well-differentiated carcinoma, 1 well to moderately differentiated carcinoma) and remaining 37 were clinicoradiologically proven: group 2 (n=78) 10 were pathologically proven either by biopsy or surgery (3 well differentiated carcinoma and 7 moderately differentiated carcinoma) and remaining 68 were clinicoradiologically proven: group 3 (n=13) all lesions were proven clinicoradiologicallly: group 4 (n=17) all were clinicoradiologically proven (primary lesion for 7 masses was colorectal carcinoma, that for 4 was gastrointestinal stromal tumor, that for 3 was breast carcinoma, and that for another 3 was renal cell carcinoma): group 5 (n=2) all FNH nodules were confirmed clinicoradiologically.

The details of signal pattern of the four groups are shown in Table 1. There was significant difference between the groups (p<0.05, Kruscal-Wallis test). The difference was significant between group 5 and other 4 groups (p<0.005, ANOVA with Bonferroni-Dunn's post-hoc test). Namely, the lesions showing high signal intensity on HBP are considered to suggest the diagnosis of FNH. None of the FNH nodules in this series had typical central scar. Using high signal intensity on HBP as a sign of FNH, 100% sensitivity, 97% specificity, 33% positive predictive value, and 100% negative predictive value, were obtained. There were one and two lesions that showed high signal intensity on HBP in groups 1 and 2, respectively. There was no such lesion in groups 3 and 4. Among these nodules, hypovacular hepatic nodule (n=1) can be discriminated from FNH by its hypovascular nature (Fig.2). The two lesions in group 2 (hypervascular HCC) can be discriminated from FNH by the presence of its fibrous capsule and/or nodule-in-nodule appearance (Figs.3 and 4). Thus, combining all findings of EOB-MRI, 100% sensitivity, 100% specificity, 100% positive and negative predictive values, were achieved.

	Group 1 (n=56)	Group 2 (n=78)	Group 3 (n=13)	Group 4 (n=17)	Group 5 (n=2)
H	1	2	0	0	2
I	5	5	3	0	0
L1	19	21	2	9	0
L2	16	31	4	0	0
L3	5	19	4	8	0

Group 1: hypovascular hepatocellular nodules,
Group 2: hypervascular hepatocellular carcinoma,   Group 3: hemangioma,
Group 4: metastasis,   Group 5: focal nodular hyperplasia
H: higher signal than that of the surrounding liver tissue,
I: similar signal intensity as that of the liver,
L1: lower than the liver, but higher than the signal of inferior vena cava (IVC)
L2: similar signal as that of IVC
L3: lower signal than that of IVC
Differences were significant between group5 and groups 1, 2, 3, and 4. ($p<0.005$, ANOVA with
Bonferroni-Dunn's post-hoc test)

Table 1. Signal intensity of various liver lesions on hepatobiliary phase images

4. Discussion

Qualitative diagnosis on EOB-MR is usually achieved by combining information obtained from precontrast conventional MR images (signal intensities on T1WI and T2WI, chemical shift imaging, and diffusion-weighted images), and enhancement pattern on the dynamic phase images [1,2,4-6]. It is sometimes challenging, however, because of insufficient arterial enhancement secondary to the small dose of Gd-EOB-DTPA used (25 μ mol/kg) in contrast to conventional Gd-based extracellular contrast medium (0.1 mmol/kg). In addition, since hepatocellular uptake of Gd-EOB-DTPA occurs shortly after Gd-EOB-DTPA administration [1], there is no "equilibrium phase" images on EOB-MR in its strict sense of the word, which precludes simple application of our previous diagnostic experience based on Gd-based extracellular contrast medium. Our results suggested SI on HBP images may help differentiate FNH from other liver nodules, particularly combining findings on other pulse sequences.

High signal intensity on HBP was suggested to be characteristic to FNH, which is concordant to the previous reports [1,6] (Fig.1). Although few, however, there were several non-FNH nodules that showed high signal intensity on HBP. High signal intensity of one hypovascular hepatocellular nodule may be attributable to high signal intensity on precontrast T1-weighted image, which are sometimes observed in dysplatic nodules or early HCC, due to cooper or iron deposition [12-14] (Fig.2) or fatty metamorphosis [15]. Because EOB uptake have been reported to be almost constant regardless of the grade of HCC, if the precontrast signal intensity is high, that would be directly reflected on the SI on HBP [16]. The differentiation of this nodule from FNH was easy, because of its hypovascular nature as seen on the arterial phase of dynamic study. High SI of two hypervascular HCCs (group 2) on HBP may be attributable to its cellular function of Gd-EOB-DTPA uptake, typically known as green hepatoma [17, 18]. One of these two was easily discriminated from FNH by the presence of fibrous capsule seen as hypointense rim on the arterial phase image or on HBP (Fig.3). The other one was associated with a typical nodule-in-nodule appearance [8], which also helped differentiate this from FNH (Fig.4).

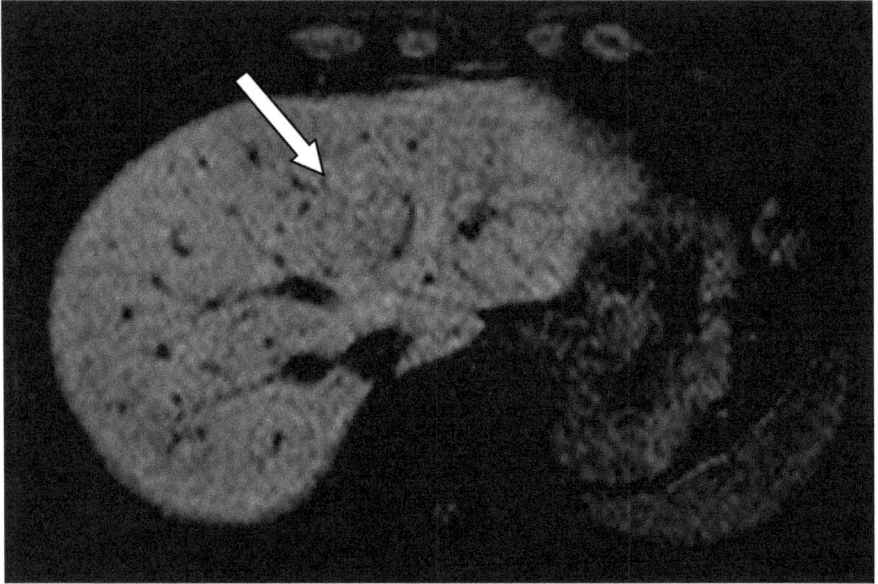

A.

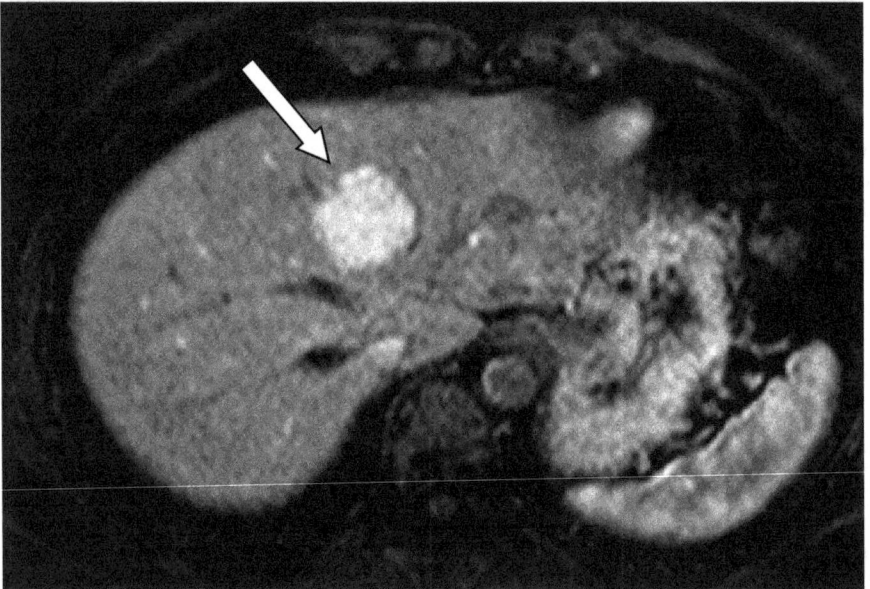

B.

Signal Intensity Characteristics of Liver Masses at Hepatobiliary Phase Images of Gadoxetate-Enhanced
MR (EOB-MR): Qualitative Assessment

129

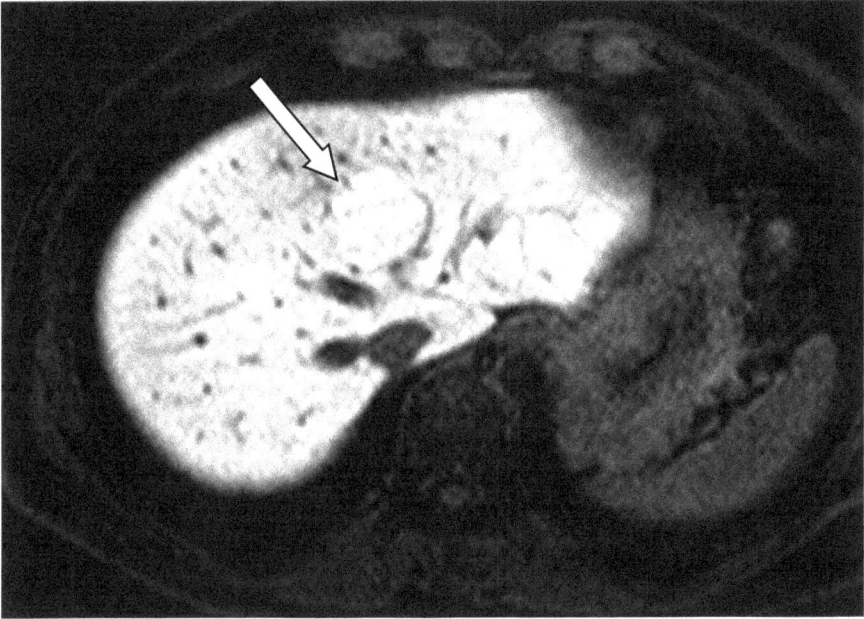

C.

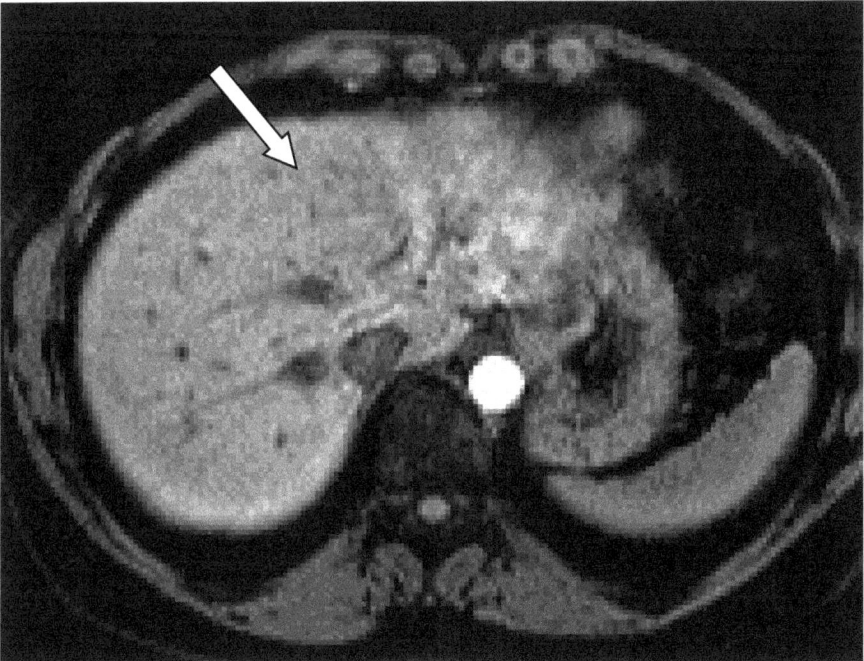

D.

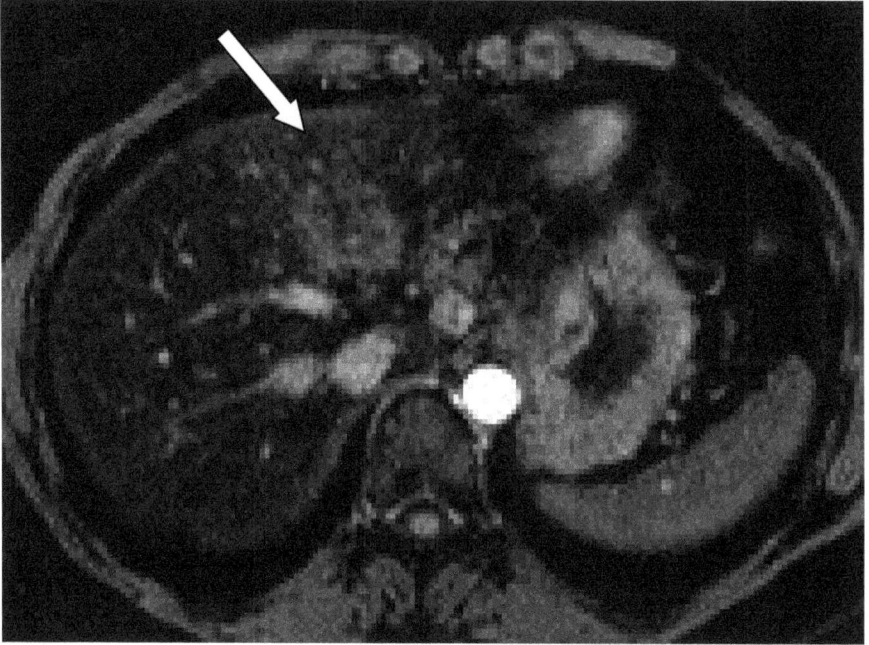

E.

Fig. 1. 43-year-old asymptomatic woman with minimal liver dysfunction. The mass in the left hepatic lobe has remained unchanged for over three years and clinical diagnosis of focal nodular hyperplasia (group 5) is made.

A. Precontrast image of the dynamic study. The lesion exhibited similar or slightly lower signal intensity as compared to the surrounding liver tissue (arrow).

B. Arterial phase image of the dynamic study of gadoxetate (EOB) enhanced MR. The lesion is strongly enhanced (arrow).

C. Hepatobiliary phase image shows homogeneous uptake of EOB within the mass.

D. Precontrast T2*weighted images (TR/ TE/ FA=266msec /9.2msec /30 degrees) revealed an almost isointense or slightly hypointese mass (arrow).

E. T2* weighted images after administration of superparamagnetic iron oxide (SPIO). The signal intensity of the lesion is partially reduced (arrow) suggesting uptake of SPIO.

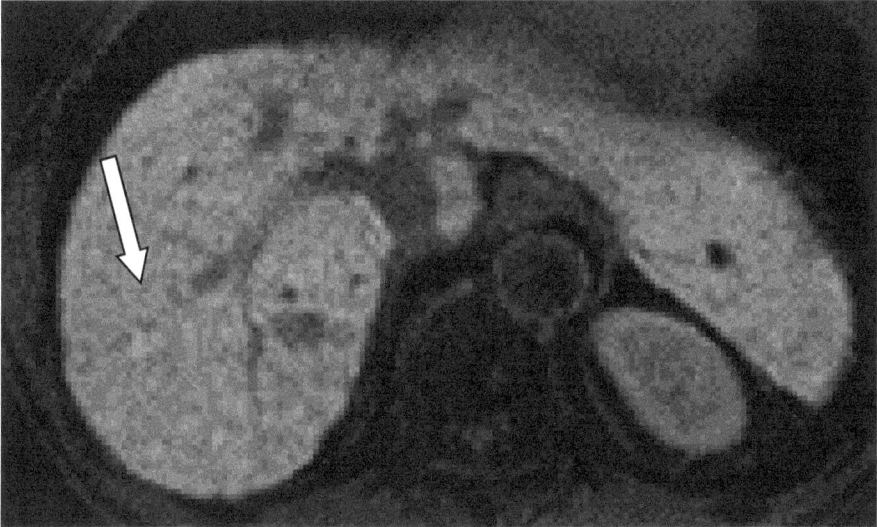

A.

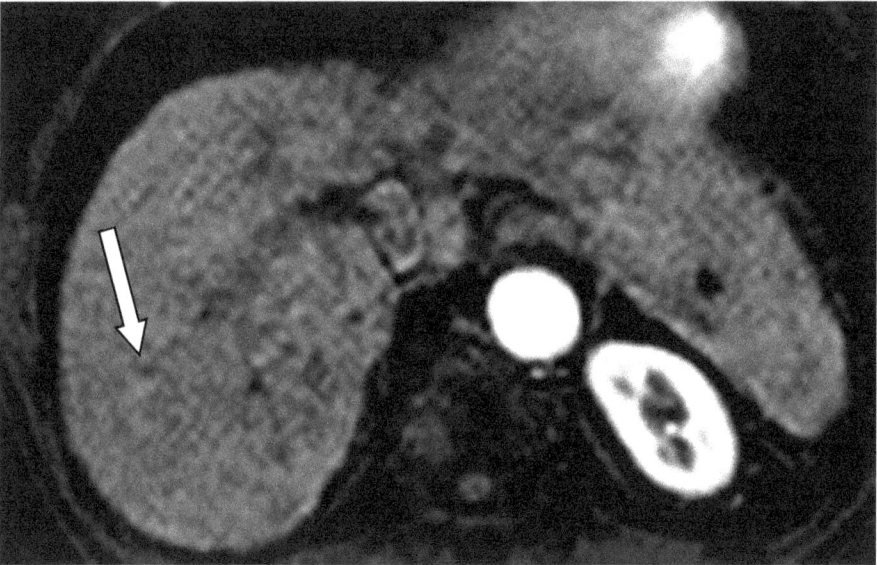

B.

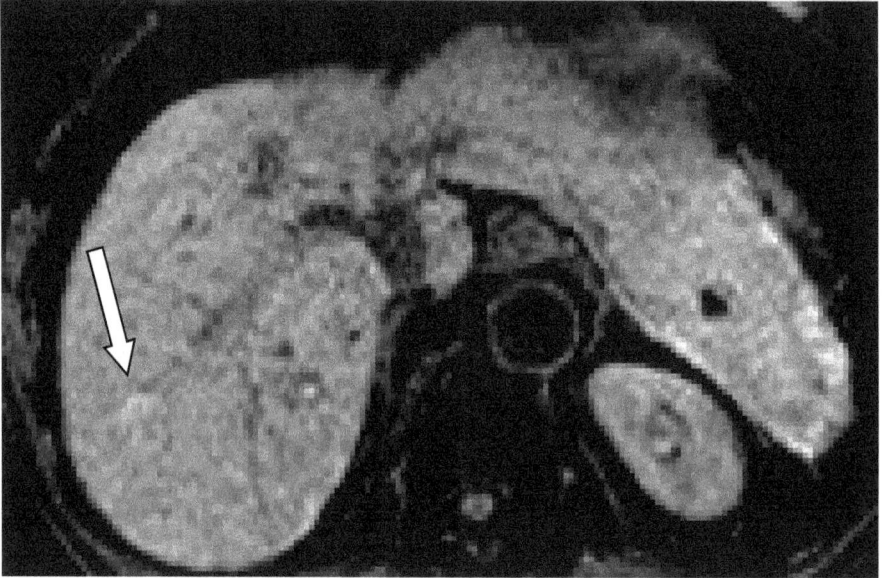

C.

Fig. 2. 58-year-old woman with a histology-proven early hepatocellular carcinoma (group 1) who had been followed up for chronic hepatitis C.

A. Precontrast THRIVE image. A nodule with similar or slightly higher signal as compared to the surrounding liver tissue is seen (arrow).

B. Arterial dominant phase THRIVE image after injection of Gd-EOB-DTPA. No significant enhancement is observed (arrow). MDCT obtained at the same period also fail to show arterial vascularity (not shown).

C. Hepatobiliary phase image of THRIVE image. The nodule exhibit almost similar or slightly lower signal intensity as compared to the surrounding liver tissue (arrow) (I-L1).

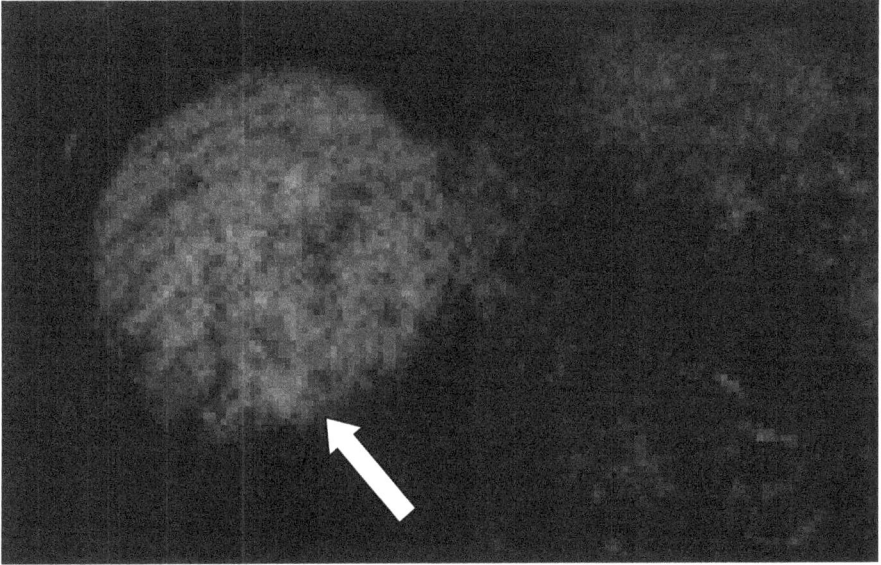

A.

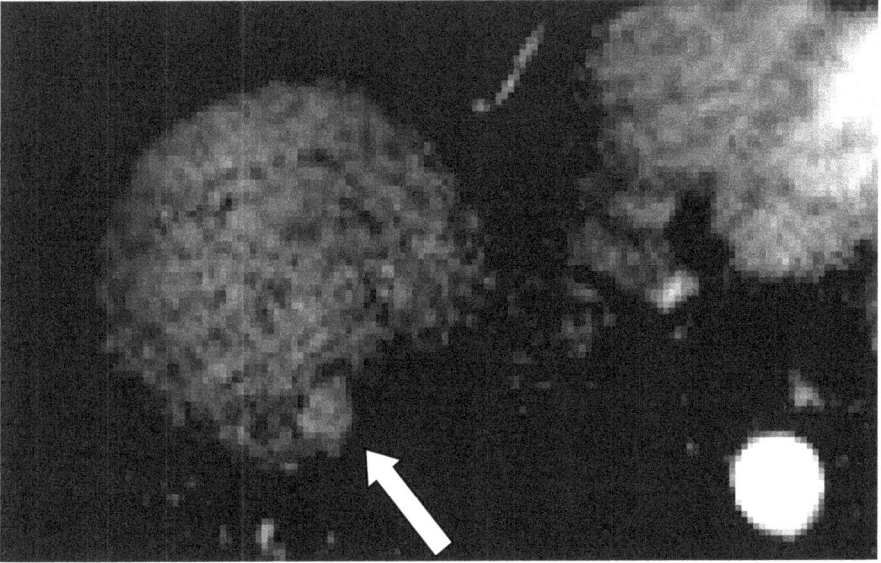

B.

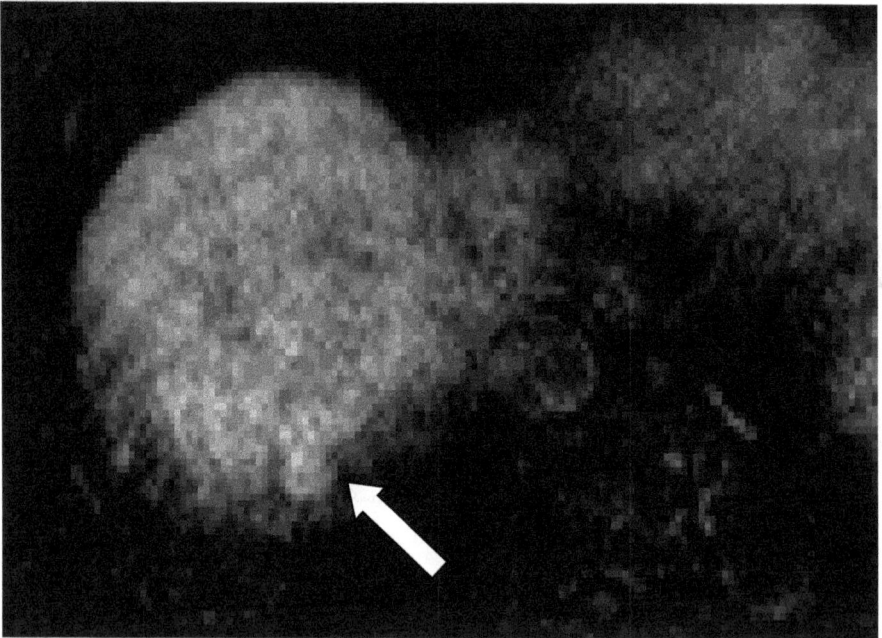

C.

Fig. 3. 54-year-old man with a clinicoradiologically proven hypervascular hepatocellular carcinoma (group 2) which was treated with transarterial chemoembolization.
A. Precontrast THRIVE image. A nodule with similar or slightly higher signal as compared to the surrounding liver tissue is seen (arrow).
B. Arterial dominant phase THRIVE image after injection of Gd-EOB-DTPA. Significant enhancent is observed (arrow). MDCT obtained at the same period also showed arterial enhancement (not shown). Note hypointense fibrous capsule.
C. Hepatobiliary phase image of THRIVE image. The nodule exhibit higher signal intensity than the surrounding liver tissue (arrow) (H). The fibrous capsule is partially seen.

Thus, using combined all findings on EOB-MRI, we could achieve 100% sensitivity, 100% specificity, 100% positive predictive value, and 100% negative predictive value, in discriminating FNH from other lesions. Our results, however, suggest the difficulty in differentiation among other 4 categories using SI on HBP, namely hypovascular hepatocellular lesions, hyper vascular HCC, hemangiomas, and metastasis. For the differentiation among these entities, findings on other sequences, including dynamic phase images, T2-weighted images, diffusion-weighted images, and chemical shift images, may be important.

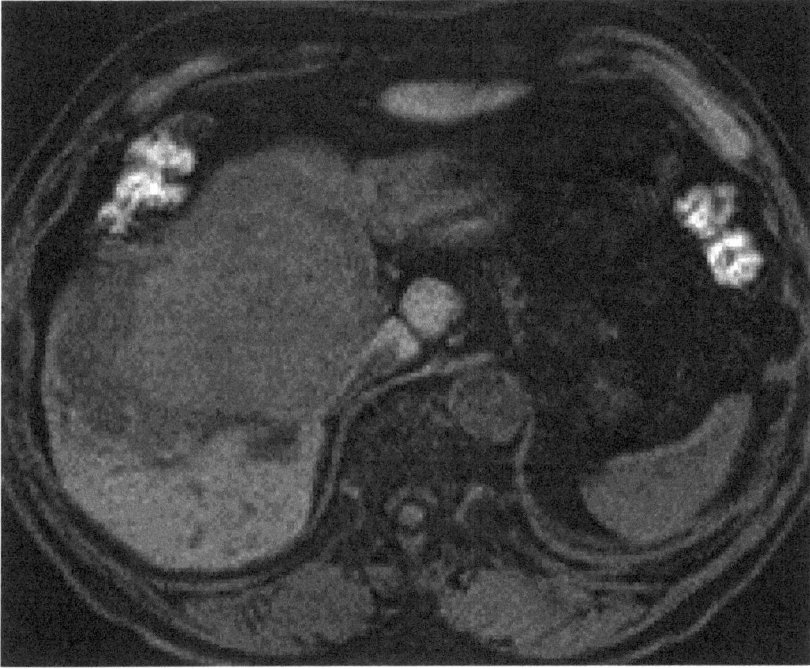

A.

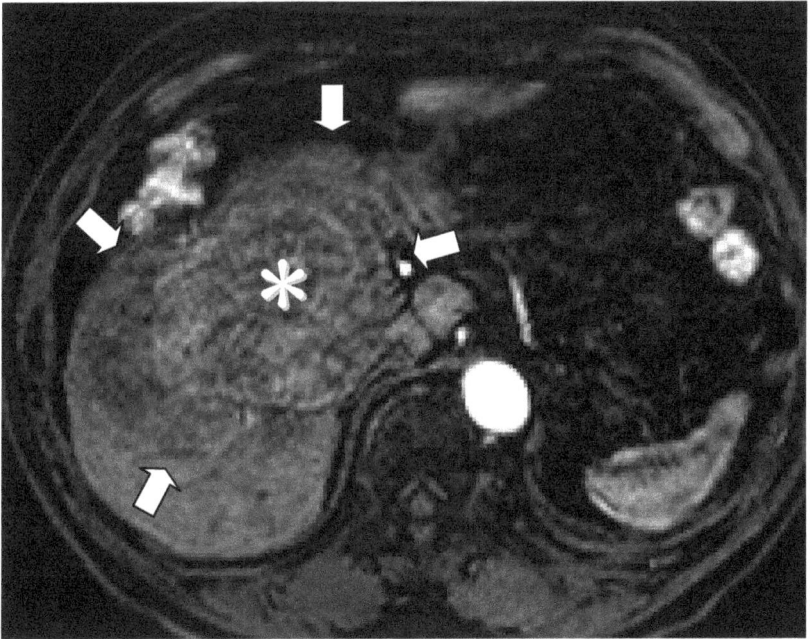

B.

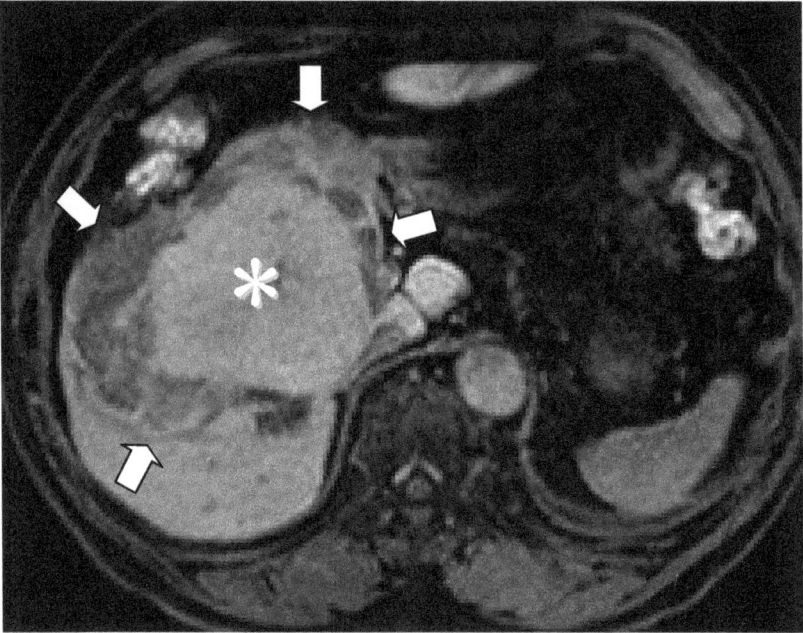

C.

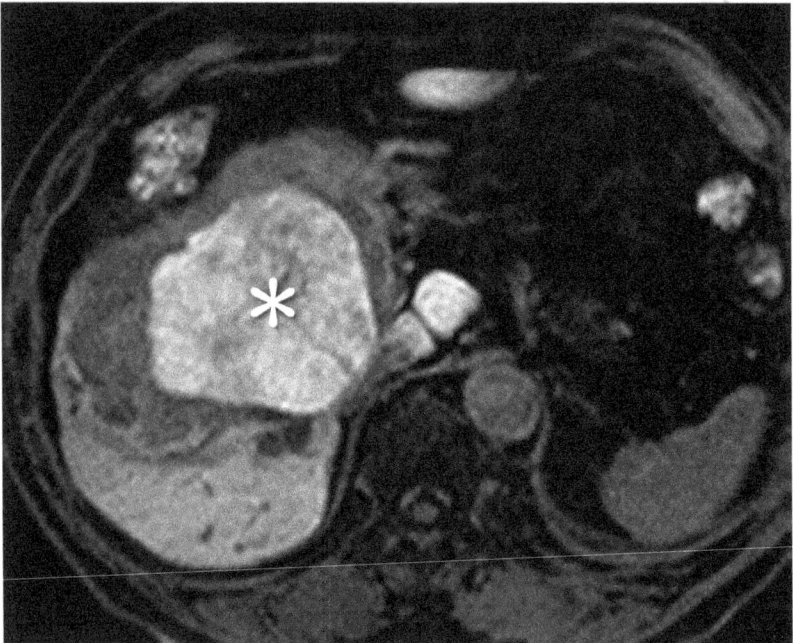

Fig. 4. 75-year-old man with a pathologically proven hypervascular hepatocellular carcinoma (group 2).

A. Precontrast image. A large heterogeneous mass is seen in the right hepatic lobe.
B. Arterial dominant phase image after injection of Gd-EOB-DTPA. Significant enhancement is observed in the central component of the mass (star), whereas peripheral components shows only faint enhancement (arrows).
C. Late phase image of the dynamic phase. Each component of the mass shows various enhancement pattern, resulting in so-called nodule-in-nodule appearance (star and arrows).
D. Hepatobiliary phase image. The predominant central part shows apparent high signal (star) (H).

There are several limitations in our study, in addition to its retrospective nature. First, the biggest limitation is the lack of pathological proof in the majority of the liver masses enrolled in this study. Particularly, lesions in groups 1 and 2 are considered quite heterogeneous: nodules in group 1 may include DN, eHCC, wHCC, and some RNs and mHCC; lesions in group2 may include wHCC, mHCC, and pHCC. The results could have been different if only histology-proven lesions are recruited. Another limitation may be the adequacy of the use of signal intensity of IVC as a reference tissue to assess the relative signal intensity of the liver masses. Because of the possible flow effect, signal intensity of IVC could be inconsistent. We therefore measured SI of IVC in the first several patients and confirmed there are less than 10% signal difference in IVC between the slices except for the edge slices of the scanning slab. This may partly be attributable to the sufficient saturation pulse used in THRIVE sequence we used in this study. One needs to be careful of this issue, therefore, when other sequence is used for HBP images of EOB-MR, in which spatial saturation pulse is insufficient. Other reason for the usage of IVC as reference tissue is that it is almost always visualized in the images of the liver and therefore easy to be used for direct comparison. Ideally speaking, quantitative measurement of enhancement ratio of HBP image vs precotrast images would have been performed, but we preferred practical method to evaluate the HPB images which would help differentiate liver nodules in daily practice. Third, the time delay of 15 minutes for HBP imaging may be somewhat short as compared to the previous reports [1-6]. Because it has been reported that HBP persist from about 10 to 40 minutes after injection of Gd-EOB-DTPA [1,6], and our preliminary assessment revealed no significant difference in the lesion detection between 15 and 20 minutes delay images (unpublished data), we adopted 15 minutes delay for HBP in our institute for clinical demand in terms of patient through-put. It is still possible, however, that different results may be obtained if HBP images were obtained in 20 minutes or even later.

In conclusion, signal patterns on 15-minute-delay HBP images are different between FNH and other liver nodules, including hypovascular hepatocellular nodules, hypervascular HCC, hemangiomas, and metastases, and are useful in differentiating these nodules. Combining all EOB-MR findings, 100% sensitivity, specificity, positive and negative predictive values were achieved in differentiating FNH from non-FNH.

5. Acknowledgement

Authors thank Professor Shotaro Sakisaka, Chair of Department of Gastroenterology and Hepatology, Faculty of Medicine, Fukuoka University, for providing clinical data of the patients.

6. References

[1] Vogl TJ, Kummel S, Hammerfstingl R, et al. Liver tumors: comparison of MR imaging with Gd-EOB-DTPA and Gd-DTPA. Radiology 1996; 200:59-67

[2] Huppertz A, Balzer T, Blakeborough A, et al. Improved detection of focal liver lesions at MR imaging: gadoxetic acid-enhanced MR images with intraoperative findings. Radiology 2004; 230:266-275

[3] Kim SH, Kim SH, Lee J, et al. Gadoxetic acid-enhanced MRI versus triple-phase MDCT for the preoperative detection of hepatocellular carcinoma. AJR 2009; 192:1675-81

[4] Halavaara J, Breuer J, Ayuso C, et al. Liver tumor characterization: comparison between liver-specific gadoxetic acid disodium-enhanced MRI and biphasic CT – a multicenter trial. J Comput Assist Tomogr 2006;30:345-354

[5] Hppeertz A, Haraida S, Kraus A, et al. Enhancement of focal liver lesions at gadoxetic acid-enhanced MR imaging: correlation with histopathologic findings and spiral CT – initial observations. Radiology 2005;234:468-478

[6] Reimer P, Schneider G, Schima W. Hepatoboliary contrast agents for contrast-enhanced MRI of the liver: properties, clinical development, and applications. Eur Radiol 2004;14:559-578

[7] Gabata T, Matsui O, Kadoya M, et al. Delayed MR imaging of the liver: correlation of delayed enhancement of hepatic tumors and pathological appearance. Abdom Imaging 1998;23;309-313

[8] McTabish JD, ROs PR. Hepatic mass lesions. In: Haaga JR, Lanzieri CF, Gilkeson RC, eds. CT and MR Imaging of the Whole Body, 2nd ed. St.Louis, MO: Mosby, 2003;1271-1312

[9] Itai Y, Ohtomo K, Furui S, et al. Noninvasive diagnosis of small cavernous hemangioma of the liver: advantage of the liver. AJR, 1985; 145:1195-1199

[10] Shinozaki K, Yoshimitsu K, Irie H, et al. Comparison of test-injection method and fixed-time method for depiction of hepatocellular carcinoma using dynamic steady-state free precession magnetic resonance imaging. J Comput Assist Tomogr. 2004;28:628-34

[11] Yoshimitsu K, Honda H. Dynamic MR imaging of the upper abdomen: timing optimization and pulse sequence selection. Nippon Igaku Hoshasen Gakkai Zasshi. 2001;61:408-13, in Japanese

[12] Kitagawa K, Matsui O, Kadoya M, et al. Hepatocellular carcinoma with excessive copper accumulation: CT and MR findings. Radiology 1991;180:623-628

[13] Ebara M, Watanabe S, Kita K, et al. MR imaging of small hepatocellular carcinoma: effect of intratumoral copper content on signal intensity. Radiology 1991;180:617-621

[14] Honda H, Kaneko K, Knazawa Y, et al. MR imaging of hepatocellular carcinomas: effect of Cu and Fe contents on signal intensity. Abdom Imaging 1997;22:60-66

[15] Martin J, Sentis M, Zidan A, et al. Fatty metamorphosis of hepatocellular carcinoma: detection with chemical shift gradient-echo MR imaging. Radiology 1995;195:125-130

[16] Kogita S , Imai Y, Okada M, et al. Gd-EOB-DTPA-enhanced magnetic resonance images of hepatocellular carcinoma: correlation with histological grading and portal blood flow. Eur Radiol 2010: 20:2405-2413

[17] Narita M, Hatano E, Arizono S, et al. Expression of OATP1B3 determines uptake of Gd-EOB-DTPA in hepatocellular carcinoma. J Gastroenterol 2009;44:793-798

[18] Asayama Y, Tajima T, Nishie A, et al. Uptate of Gd-EOB-DTPA by hepatocellular carcinoma: radiologic –pathologic correlation with special reference to bile production. EJR 2010 E-pub ahead of print

7

Strategic Assay Developments for Detection of HBV 1762T/1764A Double Mutation in Urine of Patients with HBV-Associated Hepatocellular Carcinomas

Selena Y. Lin[1], Surbhi Jain[1], Wei Song[2],
Chi-Tan Hu[3] and Ying-Hsiu Su[1]
[1]Department of Microbiology and Immunology,
Drexel University College of Medicine, Doylestown, PA
[2]JBS Science Inc, Doylestown, PA
[3]Department of Gastroenterology and Hepatology,
Buddhist Tzu Chi General Hospital and Tzu Chi University, Hualien
[1,2]USA
[3]Taiwan

1. Introduction

Hepatocellular carcinoma (HCC) is the 7th most common cancer worldwide and remains the third leading cause of cancer deaths (Yang and Roberts 2010). It has a 5-year survival rate of less than 11% even in developed nations (Garcia, Jemal et al. 2007). The 5-year survival rate drops from 26% to 2% in patients with localized versus metastasized cancer (ACS, 2010). The poor prognosis is due mainly to late detection with the methods currently available. Thus, a better screening method to detect HCC at its early, curative stage is needed to improve its outcome. One of the major etiological factors associated with HCC development is chronic infection with hepatitis B virus (HBV). In developing countries, 59% of liver cancers are attributable to HBV and, in developed countries, 23% of liver cancers are attributable to HBV (Garcia, Jemal et al. 2007).

The contribution of HBV to the pathogenesis of HCC is believed to be multifactorial including the possible role of HBV mutants. A double mutation—an adenine (A) to thymine (T) transversion at nucleotide position 1762 and a guanine (G) to adenine (A) transition at nucleotide position 1764 (1762T/1764A)—in the HBV genome has been found in 50% to 85% of HCC tumor tissues (Hsia, Yuwen et al. 1996; Baptista, Kramvis et al. 1999; Arbuthnot and Kew 2001; Hannoun, Horal et al. 2002; Kuang, Jackson et al. 2004; Kuang, Lekawanvijit et al. 2005). It has been shown that chronic HBV carriers with the HBV 1762T/1764A double mutation have an elevated risk of HCC and that the risk increases with increasing viral load of the double mutation (Yuan, Ambinder et al. 2009). Thus, the HBV 1762T/1764A double mutation is an important risk factor for HCC for people infected chronically with HBV (Chen, Iloeje et al. 2007; Yuan, Ambinder et al. 2009).

This double mutation appears to be associated with enhanced viral replication and increased severity of liver inflammation, which may contribute ultimately to the development of HCC (Laskus, Rakela et al. 1995; Takahashi, Aoyama et al. 1995; Baptista, Kramvis et al. 1999; Hou, Lau et al. 1999; Pang, Yuen et al. 2004). Furthermore, this mutation has been associated with decreased circulating HBV e antigen (HBeAg) and is thought to trigger the host immune response to HBV infected hepatocytes leading to increased apoptosis and regeneration. This could contribute to host liver injury and progression to HCC (Yang, Yeh et al. 2008). Previous studies have shown that the HBV 1762T/1764A double mutation can be detected in plasma samples from patients with HCC (Zhang, Gong et al. 2002; Kuang, Jackson et al. 2004; Kuang, Lekawanvijit et al. 2005; Yang, Yeh et al. 2008); the results of these studies suggest that the HBV 1762T/1764A double mutation is a potential biomarker for the early detection of HCC in long-term carriers of HBV.

Some of the available methods for detection of this double mutation involve PCR amplification of the target sequence followed by direct DNA sequencing(Baptista, Kramvis et al. 1999), PCR followed by restriction enzyme digestion(Takahashi, Aoyama et al. 1995), mismatched PCR coupled with restriction fragment length polymorphism analysis(Hou, Lau et al. 1999), or short oligonucleotide mass spectra analysis (SOMA) (Kuang, Jackson et al. 2004). These methods are not feasible for clinical use as they are either time-consuming, labor intensive, or insensitive due to the excessive HBV wild type DNA molecules in the sample.

The authors (Su, Wang et al. 2004; Su, Wang et al. 2005; Su, Wang et al. 2008) and other researchers(Botezatu, Serdyuk et al. 2000; Serdyuk, Botezatu et al. 2001; Chan, Leung et al. 2008; Melkonyan, Feaver et al. 2008) have shown that urine contains DNA from the circulation. This circulation-derived urine DNA, transrenal DNA, is fragmented mostly into segments of fewer than 300 base pairs (bp) (designated as low-molecular-weight urine DNA) and can be used to detect tumor-derived genetic mutations. The authors have also shown that the preferential isolation of low-molecular-weight urine DNA from total urine DNA and its use as the substrate enhances the sensitivity and specificity of the urine test for detecting tumor-derived circulating DNA markers (Su, Song et al. 2008). Moreover, the authors have shown that the concentration of circulation-derived DNA in urine is comparable to that in blood (Su, Wang et al. 2008).

As mentioned, the HBV 1762T/1764A double mutation was detected in the plasma of patients with HCC (Kuang, Jackson et al. 2004; Kuang, Lekawanvijit et al. 2005; Yang, Yeh et al. 2008). To the authors' knowledge, none of the previous studies have attempted to detect the HBV 1762T/1764A double mutation in urine. Urine is an advantageous bodily substrate in HCC screening as it proves absolutely noninvasive, opportune for collection in remote geographic areas such as developing countries, and further requires no special facility or equipment apart from sterile collection containers, as compared to the requirements for serum or plasma collection. Thus, it was of interest to see if the HBV 1762T/1764A double mutation sequence could be detected in the urine of patients with HCC who were infected with HBV.

Our study involves development of two PCR-based assays for detecting this HBV 1762T/1764A double mutation. The first assay comprises of a real-time PCR assay (HybProbe_DM) utilizing hybridization probes and an oligonucleotide clamp containing locked nucleic acids (LNAs). This LNA clamp complementary to HBV wild type DNA can reduce interference from HBV wild type to allow for increased sensitivity for detecting the HBV double mutation. However, Sikora et al.(Sikora, Zimmermann et al. 2010) and Shekhtman et al. (Shekhtman, Anne et al. 2009) suggested that polymerase chain reaction (PCR) assays targeting template sequences of 50 nucleotides (nt) or less are necessary to obtain a sensitivity greater than 50% in order to detect DNA of interest in urine derived from the circulation. Thus, a second assay containing a 2-step nested PCR assay (HBVDM_40) with a target template size of 40 bp and incorporation of locked nucleic acid was also developed. Both assays were then tested to detect HBV 1762T/1764A double mutation in urine of HBV-infected patients with HCC. The HBV double mutation was detected in the urine by this two-step PCR assay and suggest that it is necessary to minimize the targeting template size to have sufficient sensitivity to detect circulating DNA markers in urine.

2. Assay design and development

The goal of our study is to develop an assay suitable for urine detection of the HBV 1762T/1764A double mutation. We outline two approaches taken. The first is a real-time PCR-based assay utilizing fluorescent hybridization probes along with a LNA clamp complementary to HBV wild type DNA, as described previously (Ren, Lin et al. 2009). This assay allows real-time quantification of HBV 1762T/1764A double mutation DNA as well as PCR product characterization through melting curve analysis. The LNA clamp increases sensitivity of this assay by inhibiting HBV wild type DNA amplification allowing detection of HBV 1762T/1764A double mutation. However, this assay contains a 133 bp amplicon size and may not be suitable to detect low molecular weight urine DNA. A second assay was developed targeting a template size of 40 bp. This assay does not contain real-time capabilities and is a 2-step nested PCR assay. The use of LNA is also incorporated, but rather than appropriating a wild type clamp LNA was incorporated into the PCR primers to allow for selective amplification of the HBV 1762T/1764A double mutation DNA. The assays' design and development are highlighted below.

2.1 HybProbe_DM assay

This assay was validated by PCR and direct DNA sequencing. The PCR (186 bp) utilized primers SeqFwd and SeqRev that lay outside of HybProbe_DM assay (Fig 1). The HybProbe_DM assay was designed on a LightCycler® 2.0 platform. The sensor and anchor hybridization probe are labelled below. The LNA clamp is a 16 nt oligonucleotide complementary to HBV wild type DNA and contains 10 LNA (Fig 1).

Plasmid containing 186bp segment (from positions 1642 to 1827 of the HBV genome) HBV wild type DNA and 1762T/1764A double mutation were constructed using pPCR-Script AMP SK(+) vector (Stratagene, La Jolla, Ca). The amount of plasmid DNA was determined using a Nanodrop™ 1000 spectrophotometer (Thermo Fisher Scientific, Wilmington, DE) at 260 nm absorbance and confirmed by ethidium bromide staining agarose gel with a known quantity of 100-bp molecular weight DNA standard (New England Biolabs, Ipswich, MA).

These plasmids served as control templates in the testing of these assays. The real time PCR assay was assembled in a final volume of 10 µl containing 1X reaction buffer, 0.5 unit of LightCycler® FastStart Taq polymerase (Roche Applied Science, Indianapolis, IN), 0.4 µM of each PCR primer (LC Fwd and LC Rev), 2.5 mM $MgCl_2$, 500 ng/µl, BSA, 200 µM dNTP, 0.2

uM Sensor, 0.2 uM Anchor, and 2 µM HBV wild type-specific LNA-containing oligonucleotide
(Ren, Lin et al. 2009). The reaction was incubated in the LightCycler II (Roche Applied Science)
at 95°C 10min to activate the Taq polymerase, followed by amplification at 95°C 5 s, 65°C 15 s,
52°C 10 s, and 65°C 10 s for 45 cycles. Both the Sensor and the LNA clamp are phosphorylated
at the 3' end so that they cannot function as primers.

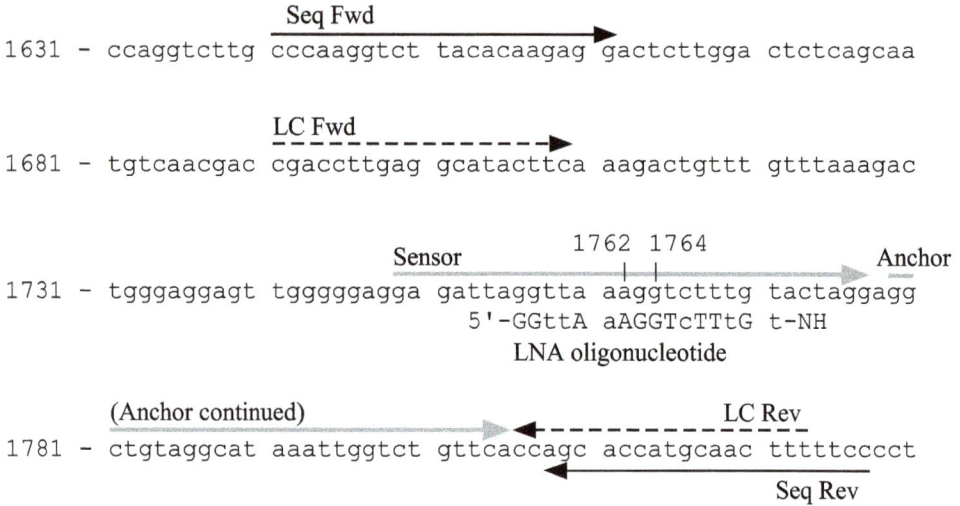

```
                   Seq Fwd
1631 - ccaggtcttg cccaaggtct tacacaagag gactcttgga ctctcagcaa

       LC Fwd
1681 - tgtcaacgac cgaccttgag gcatacttca aagactgttt gtttaaagac

                                      1762 1764
                    Sensor                              Anchor
1731 - tgggaggagt tgggggagga gattaggtta aaggtctttg tactaggagg
                            5'-GGttA aAGGTcTTtG t-NH
                              LNA oligonucleotide

     (Anchor continued)                              LC Rev
1781 - ctgtaggcat aaattggtct gttcaccagc accatgcaac tttttccoct
                                              Seq Rev
```

Fig. 1. HybProbe_DM oligonucleotides design. HBV wild type DNA sequence (GeneBank
Accession #X04615) from positions 1631 to 1830. Positions and direction of oligonucleotides
are denoted by marked arrows and LNA-containing oligonucleotide is listed with LNA
denoted by capital letters.

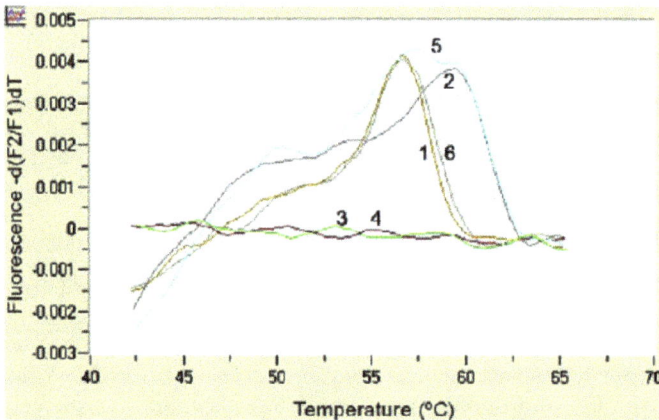

Fig. 2. Differentiation of the HBV 1762T/1764A double mutation from the HBV wild type
DNA by melting curve analysis and the wild type clamp. (1) HBV 1762T/1764A (300
copies); (2) HBV wild type DNA (300 copies); (3) H_2O only; (4) HBV wild type DNA plus
LNA clamp; (5) wild type: HBV 1762T/1764A equal molar mix; (6) wild type: HBV
1762T/1764A mix plus LNA clamp.

Sensitivity was validated using varying ratios of mutant in HBV wild type DNA background in the presence of LNA clamp. A minimum of 10 copies of mutant HBV DNA was detected (Fig. 2) and a mutant/wild type ratio of 1:3000 (Fig. 3).

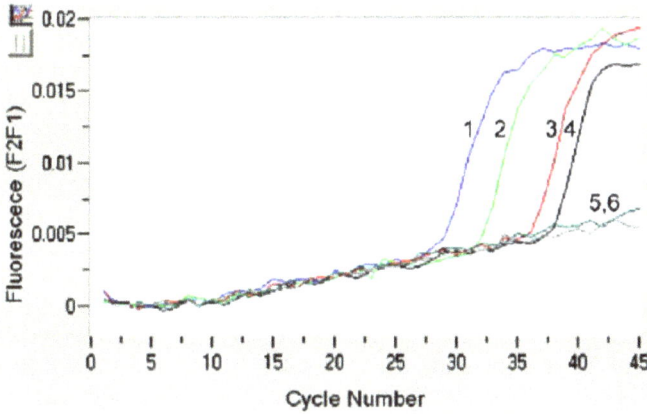

Fig. 3. Sensitivity of LNA-mediated clamped real-time PCR for the detection of HBV 1762T/1764A double mutation. Amplification curves of HBV 1762T/1764A double mutation at (1) 3000 copies; (2) 300 copies; (3) 30 copies; (4) 10 copies; (5) 5 copies; (6) 0 copy (H_2O only). The PCR was carried out in the presence of 30,000 copies of HBV wild type DNA and 2 µM of wild type clamp.

2.2 HBVDM_40 assay

This assay was developed to suit urine detection criterion. To detect HBV double mutation in the small fragmented DNA templates of urine, a two-step nested PCR assay targeting a 40-bp DNA fragment from the nucleotide positions 1743 to 1787 of the HBV genome was developed with the sequences and location of primers displayed in Fig 4. To enhance the amplification specificity of the mutated sequences, two LNAs were incorporated into the forward primer of the first PCR at the mutation sites, positions 1762 and 1764. An artificial tag sequence was added to increase the size of the first amplicon. Thus, the nested primers

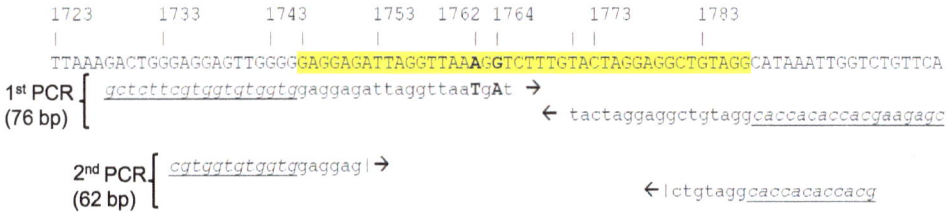

Fig. 4. HBVDM_40 assay showing locations and sequences of the primers for the first and second step PCR reactions. The nucleotide sequence of the HBV wild type genomes (GenBank accession # X04615) from 1723 to 1805 is listed and the target sequence of the assay (40 nt) is highlighted. The LNA nucleotides in the forward primer of the first-step PCR are at positions 1762 and 1764 (indicated by capital letters). The tag sequences of each primer are italicized and underlined.

for the second PCR reaction could be designed to contain most of the tag sequence. DNA isolated from a hepatoma cell line, HepG2 (American Type Culture Collection, Manassas, VA), that is free of any known hepatotropic viruses(Javitt 1990), was used as a negative control for HBV DNA.

To determine the sensitivity and specificity of the HBVDM_40 assay, a serial dilution of HBV 1762T/1764A double mutation positive control plasmid construct ranging from 1,000 copies to 1 copy per µL was prepared. The 1762T/1764A double mutation serial dilution standard, 1,000 copies of wild type plasmid DNA, and 5 ng HBV-negative control HepG2 DNA were then tested using the HBVDM_40 assay. The first PCR was assembled in a final volume of 20 µL containing 0.5 U HotStar Taq (Qiagen, Valencia, CA), 1X PCR buffer, 200 µM dNTPs, 1 µM of each primer, and DNA templates. The cycle profile was 95°C for 15 min to activate the Taq polymerase, followed by 95°C for 30 sec, 62°C for 30 sec, 72°C for 30 sec for 30 cycles, and a final extension for 4 min at 72°C. The PCR product of the first PCR reaction was diluted 1 to 1000, and 1 µL of the dilution was used as the template for the second PCR reaction. For the second step of the PCR reaction, the reaction was assembled in a final volume of 20 µL containing 0.5 U HotStar Taq (Qiagen), 1X PCR buffer, 200 µM dNTPs, 0.5 µM of each primer, and DNA templates. The cycle profile was 95°C for 15 min to activate the Taq polymerase, followed by 95°C for 30 sec, 55°C for 30 sec, 72°C for 30 sec for 35 cycles, and a final extension for 4 min at 72°C. The PCR product was analyzed in a 12% polyacrylamide gel using the TrackIt™ 25 bp DNA Ladder (Invitrogen, Carlsbad, CA).

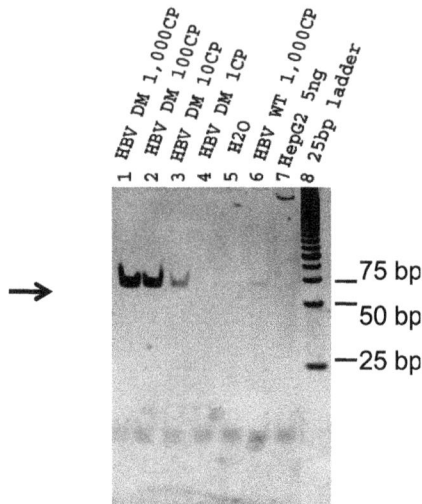

Fig. 5. Sensitivity and specificity of the HBVDM_40 assay. Serial 10-fold dilutions from 1 copy to 1000 copies of HBV 1762T/1764A double mutation positive control plasmid DNA and 1000 copies of the plasmid DNA containing HBV wild type sequences, 5 ng of HepG2 DNA, and H₂O were subjected to the HBVDM_40 assay. PCR products of the second-step PCR were analyzed in 12% polyacrylamide gel, stained with ethidium bromide, and visualized by photographing under a UV-transilluminator. The location of an expected 62-bp amplicon is indicated by the arrow. The TrackIt™ 25 bp DNA Ladder was used to indicate molecular weight markers.

As shown in Fig. 5, this two-step nested PCR assay could detect specifically as few as 10 copies of the HBV 1762T/1764A double mutation. No detectable PCR product was obtained from the water, 1000 copies of HBV wild type plasmid DNA, or 5 ng of HepG2 DNA. Overall, both of these assays display similar sensitivity (10 copies of HBV 1762T/1764A double mutation).

3. Assay comparison in patient testing

The assays were subjected to 15 HCC patient samples. Patient information is listed in Table 1. For a negative control, urine samples from 31 subjects (18 men and 13 women; average

Code	Age	Gender	HBV-infected	HCV-infected	Stage of HCC	Tumor size by Ultrasound or CT	AFP level (ng/mL)
2K	53	M	+	ND	II	5.5 cm	22.04
3K	74	M	-	ND	I	11 cm	12.68
5K	29	M	+	-	II	7 cm	24302
6K	71	F	+	ND	III	3 cm	667.1
7K	65	M	+	-	II	2 cm	6.2
8K	57	M	+	ND	III	16 cm	18032
10K	56	M	+	-	II	2.8 cm	4.68
17K	70	F	-	+	I	2.7 cm	820.6
18K	67	F	+	-	II	5 cm	3.53
19K	64	M	+	ND	III	6 cm	6.98
20K	57	M	+	ND	I	2.5 cm	4.03
21K	64	F	-	+	I	5 cm	6.71
25K	60	M	+	ND	III	5.5 cm	1.78
26K	48	M	+	-	II	3.5 cm	6101
27K	58	F	+	ND	II	2.3 cm	789.8

F, female; HBV, hepatitis B virus; HCV, hepatitis C virus; HCC, hepatocellular carcinoma; M, male; ND, not determined

Table 1. Clinical Information for patients with HCC. Participants with diagnosed HCC were recruited from the National Cheng-Kung University Medical Center liver clinic. Patients with cancer were enrolled from surgical or oncologic services (prior to initiation of chemotherapy, radiation therapy, or surgery). Eligible patients with HCC were tested for detectable hepatitis B surface antigen, and 11 out of 15 patients with HCC were found to be positive. *AFP, alpha-fetoprotein; CT, computerized tomography; F, Female; M, male; HBV, hepatitis B virus; HCC, hepatocellular carcinoma; HCV, hepatitis C virus; ND, not determined*

age, 41 years, range 18–73 years) who were negative for any liver disease, including infection with HBV or hepatitis C virus, were collected. These patient samples were obtained under institutional review board approvals. Total urine DNA from each urine sample was isolated and fractionated for the low molecular weight urine DNA fraction using carboxylated magnetic beads (AgentCourt Bioscience Corporation, Beverly, MA) as described previously(Su, Song et al. 2008). DNA isolated from 15 urine matched HCC tissues was tested for HBV wild type, to confirm the pathological information provided and for the appearance of the 1762T/1764A double mutation.

HBV infection status indicated in the patients' records was confirmed by performing the HybProbe_DM assay with HCC tissue samples, in the absence of the LNA clamp, to allow amplification of both wild type and mutated sequences. The tumor tissue DNA was isolated by proteinase K/SDS treatment followed by phenol/chloroform extraction and ethanol precipitation. As expected, of the 15 HCC tissue samples tested, 4 samples (3K, 8K, 17K, and 21K) did not contain any detectable HBV DNA; this result was consistent with the pathological records provided (Table 1). The tissue DNA was then tested to detect the HBV 1762T/1764A double mutation using the HBVDM_40 assay and the HBV double mutation HybProbe assay. The results are summarized in Table 2.

HybProbe_DM assay detected 8 of 11 (72%) and the HBVDM_40 assay detected 9 of 11 (82%) HBV-infected HCC tissue DNA samples for HBV 1762T/1764A double mutation. This is consistent with previous findings whereby 1762T/1764A double mutation was found in 50% to 85% of HBV-infected HCC tissues (Hsia, Yuwen et al. 1996; Baptista, Kramvis et al. 1999; Arbuthnot and Kew 2001; Hannoun, Horal et al. 2002; Kuang, Jackson et al. 2004; Kuang, Lekawanvijit et al. 2005). Subsequently, the low molecular weight urine DNA isolated from 15 corresponding urine samples was subjected to both the HybProbe_DM and HBVDM_40 assays. As expected, the HBV double mutation HybProbe_DM assay, targeting 133 bp of the region of interest, was not sensitive enough to detect the DNA marker that is within fragmented, circulation-derived transrenal DNA (< 300 bp). Only one urine sample (6K) from the 11 patients with HCC who were infected with HBV was positive for the HBV 1762T/1764A double mutation by the HBV double mutation HybProbe_DM assay (data not shown), whereas 8 HBV-infected HCC urine samples were positive for HBV 1762T/1764A double mutation by the HBVDM_40 assay.

Interestingly, there were two urine samples (5K and 18K) that were HBV 1762T/1764A double mutation positive whose matched tissue samples were negative for HBV 1762T/1764A double mutation. It is possible that the 1762T/1764A double mutation detected in the urine samples was derived from the HCC tissue that was not part of the paraffin-embedded tumor tissue sections obtained.

Although the sensitivities of both the HBV LNA-mediated clamped HybProbe_DM assay and the HBVDM_40 assay are similar, 10 copies per assay, the HBVDM_40 assay is more suitable for detecting HBV 1762T/1764A double mutation when the urine DNA substrate was used, due to the smaller target template size. The maintenance of similar sensitivity in such a short amplicon is attributed to the LNA molecules incorporated at the sites of the mutations in the forward primer to amplify selectively the 1762T/1764A double mutation sequences. This substitutes the role of the 16nt LNA clamp in the HybProbe_DM assay that used in order to inhibit amplification of wild type sequences. Through this approach the target template size can be shortened and suitable for urine detection of circulation derived DNA markers.

Subject	HBV	HBV Double Mutation HybProbe Assay		HBV Double Mutation_40 Assay	
		Tissue	Urine	Tissue	Urine
2K	+	DM	-	DM	DM
3K	-	-	-	-	-
5K	+	WT	-	DM	DM
6K	+	DM	DM	DM	DM
7K	+	DM	-	DM	DM
8K	-	-	-	-	-
10K	+	WT	-	-	-
17K	-	-	-	-	-
18K	+	WT	-	-	DM
19K	+	DM	-	DM	-
20K	+	DM	-	DM	DM
21K	-	-	-	-	-
25K	+	DM	-	DM	-
26K	+	DM	-	DM	DM
27K	+	DM	-	DM	DM

[a]Each DNA sample was tested twice. Positivity is defined as both assays positive.
DM, HBV DNA 1762T/1764A double mutation sequence; WT, wild-type sequence.

Table 2. Detection of HBV double mutations in HCC tissues and matched urine[a]

4. Discussion

Individuals infected with HBV are a high-risk group for developing HCC. They need to be screened regularly for HCC. However, the latent period between contracting HBV infection and developing HCC ranges from a few to 30 years (Kim, Lee et al. 2000). Currently, the alpha-fetoprotein blood test and ultrasonography are the only screening methods available. Given the cost and the technical expertise required for blood collection and ultrasonography, a noninvasive, urine-based screening method is highly preferable and likely to have higher compliance than serum assays or imaging. It has been suggested that the HBV 1762T/1764A double mutation is a potential predictive marker for HCC because of its association with 50% to 85% of HBV-associated HCC and its detection in the circulation of patients infected with HBV who were either diagnosed with HCC at the time the blood was collected or who developed HCC a few years later (Kuang, Lekawanvijit et al. 2005).

To the authors' knowledge, this is the first report of the detection of HBV 1762T/1764A double mutation in the urine of patients with HCC and infected with HBV. This finding was achieved by developing a PCR assay that targets a template size of 40 bp optimized for use with transrenal DNA and is the first step toward developing a urine test for screening for HCC in individuals infected with HBV. The source of the HBV 1762T/1764A double mutation DNA detected in the urine of patients with HCC is unclear. It is possible that the HBV 1762T/1764A double mutation DNA is derived from the breakdown of DNA from the HBV infectious particles in circulation, from the closed circular form of the HBV genome, or from the integrated HBV genome released from infected hepatocytes. Because the DNA substrate is the low molecular weight urine DNA fraction (less than 1 Kb), the authors do not think that the HBV 1762T/1764A double mutation DNA detected was derived from infectious HBV virions in urine or in the circulation. Previous studies by the authors have shown that low molecular weight urine DNA co-migrated with DNA of 1 to 2 nucleosomes isolated in serum, which suggests that the source of this low molecular weight urine DNA is mostly from apoptotic cells (Su, Wang et al. 2004). It has been suggested that the turnover of hepatocytes in liver infected with HBV is increased, mostly by apoptosis. The authors thus speculate that the HBV 1762T/1764A double mutation detected in the urine of patients with HCC who were infected with HBV might originate from apoptotic infected hepatocytes.

In this small pilot study, the association of the detection of HBV double mutation sequences with the size of the tumor (Tables 1 and 2) was not found, perhaps because the sample size was too small. In this cohort, only 1 (20K) of 11 HCCs from patients infected with HBV was a stage I tumor. Interestingly, HBV double mutation was detected in this stage I tumor (20K, tumor size 2 cm), but not in 3 higher stage tumors [10K (stage II, tumor size 2 cm), 19K (stage III, tumor size 6 cm), and 25K (stage III, tumor size 5.5 cm)]. A larger number of samples are needed for this comparison. As discussed earlier, the amount of tumor DNA in urine could be due to the amount of apoptosis of the tumor. With heterogeneity of HCC, the rate of apoptosis might vary from tumor to tumor. Other physiological conditions such as hydration of body could also contribute to the concentration of circulation-derived DNA in urine. Nevertheless, it is encouraging that 9 of 11 urine samples from patients with HCC who were infected with HBV were positive for HBV double mutation by the HBVDM_40 assay, suggesting that this assay could be included in a urine test for HCC screening for patients infected with HBV. The assay developed in this study is not robust enough to be used in clinical settings for routine screenings. Nevertheless, the HBV 1762T/1764A double mutation was detected in the urine by this two-step PCR assay; this study showed that it is necessary to minimize the targeting template size to have sufficient sensitivity to detect the circulating DNA marker in urine. The development of a high-throughput quantitative assay for this marker to translate this finding for clinical use is in progress.

It would be of great interest to compare the detectability of the HBV double mutation DNA in urine with that of the current screening methods, the serum level of alpha-fetoprotein and ultrasound. Although the sample size is small (n=15), 3 (7K, 18K, 20K) of 6 urine samples from AFP-negative (< 20 ng/mL) patients with HCC who were infected with HBV were positive for the HBV double mutation by HBVDM_40 assay. The HBV 1762T/1764A double mutation would need to be evaluated in a large-scale study to determine how early in the disease process of HCC this marker appears in the urine by screening the urine from patients with hepatitis, cirrhosis, or HCC who were infected with HBV. Thus, the specificity and sensitivity of the marker alone for HCC screening can be determined.

The use of urine for cancer detection shows promise for potential clinical applications in HCC screening. Current literature has implicated other HBV mutations as potential HCC screening markers. A mutation in the precore region is of interest. Not only has this mutation been shown to be genotype specific but also to play a role in HBeAg secretion by forming a premature stop codon. Precore variants can be first detected around the time of HBeAg seroconversion and potentially prevent HBeAg synthesis without prohibiting production of infectious HBV virions (Kao 2003; Yang, Yeh et al. 2008). A particular precore region mutation involves position 1896 a G to A substitution (G1896A), however it depends on the nucleotide present at position 1858 as it forms a stem structure. As a result, this G1896A mutation rarely occurs in HBV genotype A due to pairing with dominate C1858 not T1858 as seen in other genotypes. The impact of this mutation is still in question. Studies have shown this mutation to be associated with a more aggressive disease such as reactivation of chronic HBV while others have shown the opposite where there is a better prognosis with the occurrence of this mutation (Kao 2003; Yang, Yeh et al. 2008).

Other mutations at position C1653T in the enhancer II region and position 1753 T to C/A/G in the core promoter region have also been found. However, the mutation at 1753 was not found to be significantly associated with HCC development, but the core promoter mutation at 1753 were found to correlate with HCC development. The C to T mutation at 1653 alters the X protein possibly contributing to hepatocarcinogenesis and shows increased frequency with progression from chronic hepatitis to cirrhosis (Yuen et al., 2008). Although the link between the core promoter mutations and development of HCC is still unclear, it is thought that these mutations play a role in altering pregenomic secondary structure that enhances viral replication and this has been demonstrated by increased HBV DNA levels in patients with core promoter mutations compared to those with no core promoter mutations.

Lastly, mutations in the PreS/S have been of interest. S mutations involving glycine to arginine substitution at position 145 (G145R) have been shown to play a role in immune escape by altering HBV envelope proteins. PreS deletions play a role in forming the hepatocyte binding site, transportation out of the hepatocyte and are essential for virion assembly (Llovet and Lok 2008; Nguyen, Law et al. 2009). These mutations are thought to occur during pathogenesis of HBV infection and transmitted vertically. Thus there is a potential for these mutations to serve as HCC screening markers.

In HCC screening, it is important to take into consideration the HBV genotypes as they have a role in the clinical outcome, treatment efficacy, prevalence patterns of HBV mutants and the geographic spread of HCC. There are known genotypes A through H with specific geographic distribution. HBV genotypes B and C are predominant in Southeast Asia. Genotype C has been found to be associated with more severe liver disease with higher frequency of HBeAg, higher serum HBV DNA levels, delayed HBeAg seroconversion, higher frequency of basal core promoter mutation, and lower response rate to interferon therapy compared to genotype B. However genotype B is associated with development of HCC in younger populations. Genotype A which is frequent in North America Europe, India, and parts of Africa holds a predominant nucleotide at position 1858 and as a result incur less frequent precore mutations. While genotypes B, C, and D which hold a predominant nucleotide T at position 1858 is more frequent in the Mediterranean and Asia have a much higher frequency of precore mutations. Genotypes F is found in South America while genotypes E (Africans), F (aboriginal populations of South America), H (Amerindian populations of Central America), and G (HBV carriers in France, Georgia, USA, and Germany) are less well studied (Kao 2003; Yuen, Tanaka et al. 2008). Furthermore, in Caucasian and Indian populations genotype D is associated with greater risk of HCC development compared to genotype A indicating host factors in combination with genotype can play a role in HCC risk.

Moreover, HCC, like other cancers, is extremely heterogeneous and has a complex etiology, even within the HBV-infected group (Buamah, Gibb et al. 1984; Bressac, Kew et al. 1991; Arbuthnot and Kew 2001; Block, Mehta et al. 2003; Boyault, Rickman et al. 2007; Aravalli, Steer et al. 2008; Hoshida, Nijman et al. 2009). Any single DNA marker is unlikely to have sufficient sensitivity and specificity to detect HCC such that it can be used as a stand-alone diagnostic test. Thus, a panel of multiple genetic and epigenetic markers, such as HCC-associated HBV mutations, as discussed above, mutations in p53 and CTNNB1 genes (Bressac, Kew et al. 1991; de La Coste, Romagnolo et al. 1998; Miyoshi, Iwao et al. 1998; Huang, Fujii et al. 1999; Legoix, Bluteau et al. 1999; Terris, Pineau et al. 1999; Wong, Fan et al. 2001; Taniguchi, Roberts et al. 2002; Edamoto, Hara et al. 2003; Kirk, Lesi et al. 2005; Zhang, Rossner et al. 2006; Boyault, Rickman et al. 2007; Hussain, Schwank et al. 2007; Cieply, Zeng et al. 2009; Jain, Singhal et al. 2010) and aberrant methylation of p16, APC, and GSTP-1 genes (Lee, Lee et al. 2003; Jicai, Zongtao et al. 2006; Katoh, Shibata et al. 2006; Su, Lee et al. 2007; Chang, Yi et al. 2008; Gao, Kondo et al. 2008; Harder, Opitz et al. 2008; Su, Zhao et al. 2008; Feng, Stern et al. 2010; Hernandez-Vargas, Lambert et al. 2010; Jain, Singhal et al. 2010) could be assembled that cumulatively result in a level of sensitivity and specificity for HCC screening that is superior or complimentary to alpha fetoprotein and its L3 glycoform or to ultrasound imaging, the methods currently used for HCC screening.

5. Conclusion

With the current technology in assay development, it is feasible to design assays targeting clinically relevant mutations in HBV for HCC screening. Given the heterogeneity of HCC and the genotypes of HBV, the challenge lies in developing a panel of assays which can then give a better performance than current screening tests. Also, given the long window period between HBV infection and HCC development, it is important that the test be as noninvasive and cost-effective as possible. The urine based tests can meet both of these demands and are also suitable for developing nations with fewer resources. The next step should be to test-drive the performance of the assays for HBV mutations in a larger study population. This will allow evaluation of these mutations as diagnostic biomarkers and investigate their association with HCC development, prognosis, treatment efficacy and overall survival.

6. Acknowledgment

This work is supported by NIH R01 CA125642 (YHS), The Prevent Cancer Foundation (Postdoctoral fellowship to SJ), and a translational research grant award from the Wallace Coulter Foundation (YHS).

7. References

Aravalli, R. N., C. J. Steer, et al. (2008). "Molecular mechanisms of hepatocellular carcinoma." Hepatology 48(6): 2047-2063.

Arbuthnot, P. and M. Kew (2001). "Hepatitis B virus and hepatocellular carcinoma." International Journal of Experimental Pathology 82(2): 77-100.

Baptista, M., A. Kramvis, et al. (1999). "High prevalence of 1762T 1764A mutations in the basic core promoter of hepatitis B virus isolated from black Africans with hepatocellular carcinoma compared with asymptomatic carriers." Hepatology 29(3): 946-953.

Block, T. M., A. S. Mehta, et al. (2003). "Molecular viral oncology of hepatocellular carcinoma." Oncogene 22: 5093-5107.

Botezatu, I., O. Serdyuk, et al. (2000). "Genetic analysis of DNA excreted in urine: a new approach for detecting specific genomic DNA sequences from cells dying in an organism." Clinical chemistry 46(8): 1078.

Boyault, S., D. S. Rickman, et al. (2007). "Transcriptome classification of HCC is related to gene alterations and to new therapeutic targets." Hepatology 45 42-45.

Bressac, B., M. Kew, et al. (1991). "Selective G to T mutations of p53 gene in hepatocellular carcinoma from southern Africa." Nature 350: 429-431.

Buamah, P. K., I. Gibb, et al. (1984). "Serum alpha fetoprotein heterogeneity as a means of differentiating between primary hepatocellular carcinoma and hepatic secondaries." Clinica Chimica Acta 139: 313-316.

Chan, K. C., S. F. Leung, et al. (2008). "Quantitative analysis of the transrenal excretion of circulating EBV DNA in nasopharyngeal carcinoma patients." Clinical Cancer Research 14(15): 4809.

Chang, H., B. Yi, et al. (2008). "Methylation of tumor associated genes in tissue and plasma samples from liver disease patients." Experimental and Molecular Pathology 85(2): 96-100.

Chen, C. J., U. H. Iloeje, et al. (2007). "Long-term outcomes in hepatitis B: the REVEAL-HBV study." Clinics in liver disease 11(4): 797-816.

Cieply, B., G. Zeng, et al. (2009). "Unique phenotype of hepatocellular cancers with exon-3 mutations in beta-catenin gene." Hepatology 49(3): 821,831.

de La Coste, A., B. Romagnolo, et al. (1998). "Somatic mutations of the beta-catenin gene are frequent in mouse and human hepatocellular carcinomas." Proc Natl Acad Sci U S A 95(15): 8847,8851.

Edamoto, Y., A. Hara, et al. (2003). "Alternations of RB1, p53 and Wnt pathways in hepatocellular carcinomas associated with hepatitis C, hepatitis B and alcoholic liver cirrhosis." International Journal of Cancer 106: 334-341.

Feng, Q., J. E. Stern, et al. (2010). "DNA methylation changes in normal liver tissues and hepatocellular carcinoma with different viral infection." Experimental and Molecular Pathology 88(2): 287-292.

Gao, W., Y. Kondo, et al. (2008). "Variable DNA methylation patterns associated with progression of disease in hepatocellular carcinomas." Carcinogenesis 29(10): 1901-1910.

Garcia, M., A. Jemal, et al. (2007). "Global cancer facts & figures 2007." Atlanta, GA: American Cancer Society 1(3).

Hannoun, C., P. Horal, et al. (2002). "Mutations in the X region and core promoter are rare and have little impact on response to interferon therapy for chronic hepatitis B." Journal of medical virology 66(2): 171-178.

Harder, J., O. G. Opitz, et al. (2008). "Quantitative promoter methylation analysis of hepatocellular carcinoma, cirrhotic and normal liver." International Journal of Cancer 122(12): 2800-2804.

Hernandez-Vargas, H., M.-P. Lambert, et al. (2010). "Hepatocellular Carcinoma Displays Distinct DNA Methylation Signatures with Potential as Clinical Predictors." PLoS One 5(3): e9749.

Hoshida, Y., S. M. B. Nijman, et al. (2009). "Integrative Transcriptome Analysis Reveals Common Molecular Subclasses of Human Hepatocellular Carcinoma." Cancer Res 69(18): 7385-7392.

Hou, J., G. K. K. Lau, et al. (1999). "T1762/A1764 variants of the basal core promoter of hepatitis B virus; serological and clinical correlations in Chinese patients." Liver 19(5): 411-417.

Hsia, C. C., H. Yuwen, et al. (1996). "Hot-spot mutations in hepatitis B virus X gene in hepatocellular carcinoma." Lancet 348(9027): 625.

Huang, H., H. Fujii, et al. (1999). "Beta-catenin mutations are frequent in human hepatocellular carcinomas associated with hepatitis C virus infection." Am J Pathol 155(6): 1795,1801.

Hussain, S. P., J. Schwank, et al. (2007). "TP53 mutations and hepatocellular carcinoma: insights into the etiology and pathogenesis of liver cancer." Oncogene 26(15): 2166,2176.

Jain, S., S. Singhal, et al. (2010). "Molecular genetics of hepatocellular neoplasia " Am J Transl Res 2(1): 105-118.

Javitt, N. B. (1990). "Hep G2 cells as a resource for metabolic studies: lipoprotein, cholesterol, and bile acids." The FASEB Journal 4(2): 161.

Jicai, Z., Y. Zongtao, et al. (2006). "Persistent infection of hepatitis B virus is involved in high rate of p16 methylation in hepatocellular carcinoma." Molecular Carcinogenesis 45(7): 530-536.

Kao, J. H. (2003). "Hepatitis B virus genotypes and hepatocellular carcinoma in Taiwan." Intervirology 46(6): 400-407.

Katoh, H., T. Shibata, et al. (2006). "Epigenetic Instability and Chromosomal Instability in Hepatocellular Carcinoma." American Journal of Pathology 168(4): 1375-1384.

Kim, H., M. J. Lee, et al. (2000). "Expression of cyclin D1, cyclin E, cdk4 and loss of heterozygosity of 8p, 13q, 17p in hepatocellular carcinoma: comparison study of childhood and adult hepatocellular carcinoma." Liver 20(2): 173-178.

Kirk, G. D., O. A. Lesi, et al. (2005). "249ser TP53 mutation in plasma DNA, hepatitis B viral infection, and risk of hepatocellular carcinoma." Oncogene 24(38): 5858-5867.

Kuang, S. Y., P. E. Jackson, et al. (2004). "Specific mutations of hepatitis B virus in plasma predict liver cancer development." Proceedings of the National Academy of Sciences of the United States of America 101(10): 3575.

Kuang, S. Y., S. Lekawanvijit, et al. (2005). "Hepatitis B 1762T/1764A mutations, hepatitis C infection, and codon 249 p53 mutations in hepatocellular carcinomas from Thailand." Cancer Epidemiology Biomarkers & Prevention 14(2): 380.

Laskus, T., J. Rakela, et al. (1995). "Hepatitis B virus core promoter sequence analysis in fulminant and chronic hepatitis B." Gastroenterology 109(5): 1618-1623.

Lee, S., H. J. Lee, et al. (2003). "Aberrant CpG Island Hypermethylation Along Multistep Hepatocarcinogenesis." American Journal of Pathology 163(4): 1371-1378.

Legoix, P., O. Bluteau, et al. (1999). "Beta-catenin mutations in hepatocellular carcinoma correlate with a low rate of loss of heterozygosity." Oncogene 18(27): 4044,4046.

Llovet, J. M. and A. Lok (2008). "Hepatitis B virus genotype and mutants: risk factors for hepatocellular carcinoma." Journal of the National Cancer Institute 100(16): 1121.

Melkonyan, H. S., W. J. Feaver, et al. (2008). "Transrenal nucleic acids: from proof of principle to clinical tests." Annals of the New York Academy of Sciences 1137(1): 73-81.

Miyoshi, Y., K. Iwao, et al. (1998). "Activation of the beta-catenin gene in primary hepatocellular carcinomas by somatic alterations involving exon 3." Cancer Res 58(12): 2524,2527.

Nguyen, V., M. Law, et al. (2009). "Hepatitis B-related hepatocellular carcinoma: epidemiological characteristics and disease burden." Journal of viral hepatitis 16(7): 453-463.

Pang, A., M. F. Yuen, et al. (2004). "Real-time quantification of hepatitis B virus core-promoter and pre-core mutants during hepatitis E antigen seroconversion." Journal of Hepatology 40(6): 1008-1017.

Ren, X. D., S. Y. Lin, et al. (2009). "Rapid and sensitive detection of hepatitis B virus 1762T/1764A double mutation from hepatocellular carcinomas using LNA-mediated PCR clamping and hybridization probes." Journal of virological methods 158(1-2): 24-29.

Serdyuk, O., I. Botezatu, et al. (2001). "Detection of mutant k-ras sequences in the urine of cancer patients." Bulletin of Experimental Biology and Medicine 131(3): 283-284.

Shekhtman, E. M., K. Anne, et al. (2009). "Optimization of transrenal DNA analysis: detection of fetal DNA in maternal urine." Clinical chemistry 55(4): 723.

Sikora, A., B. G. Zimmermann, et al. (2010). "Detection of increased amounts of cell-free fetal DNA with short PCR amplicons." Clinical chemistry 56(1): 136.

Su, H., J. Zhao, et al. (2008). "Large-scale analysis of the genetic and epigenetic alterations in hepatocellular carcinoma from Southeast China." Mutation Research/Fundamental and Molecular Mechanisms of Mutagenesis 641(1-2): 27-35.

Su, P. F., T. C. Lee, et al. (2007). "Differential DNA methylation associated with hepatitis B virus infection in hepatocellular carcinoma." International Journal of Cancer 121(6): 1257-1264.

Su, Y.-H., M. Wang, et al. (2005). "Detection of a K-ras mutation in urine of patients with colorectal cancer." Cancer Biomarkers 1.

Su, Y. H., J. Song, et al. (2008). "Removal of High Molecular Weight DNA by Carboxylated Magnetic Beads Enhances the Detection of Mutated K ras DNA in Urine." Annals of the New York Academy of Sciences 1137(1): 82-91.

Su, Y. H., M. Wang, et al. (2004). "Human urine contains small, 150 to 250 nucleotide-sized, soluble DNA derived from the circulation and may be useful in the detection of colorectal cancer." Journal of Molecular Diagnostics 6(2): 101.

Su, Y. H., M. Wang, et al. (2008). "Detection of Mutated K ras DNA in Urine, Plasma, and Serum of Patients with Colorectal Carcinoma or Adenomatous Polyps." Annals of the New York Academy of Sciences 1137(1): 197-206.

Takahashi, K., K. Aoyama, et al. (1995). "The precore/core promoter mutant (T1762A1764) of hepatitis B virus: clinical significance and an easy method for detection." Journal of general virology 76(12): 3159.

Taniguchi, K., L. R. Roberts, et al. (2002). "Mutational spectrum of beta-catenin, AXIN1, and AXIN2 in hepatocellular carcinomas and hepatoblastomas." Oncogene 21(31): 4863,4871.

Terris, B., P. Pineau, et al. (1999). "Close correlation between beta-catenin gene alterations and nuclear accumulation of the protein in human hepatocellular carcinomas." Oncogene 18(47): 6583,6588.

Wong, C. M., S. T. Fan, et al. (2001). "Beta-catenin mutation and overexpression in hepatocellular carcinoma: clinicopathologic and prognostic significance." Cancer 92(1): 136,145.

Yang, H. I., S. H. Yeh, et al. (2008). "Associations between hepatitis B virus genotype and mutants and the risk of hepatocellular carcinoma." Journal of the National Cancer Institute 100(16): 1134.

Yang, J. D. and L. R. Roberts (2010). "Hepatocellular carcinoma: a global view." Nature Reviews Gastroenterology and Hepatology 7(8): 448-458.

Yuan, J. M., A. Ambinder, et al. (2009). "Prospective evaluation of hepatitis B 1762T/1764A mutations on hepatocellular carcinoma development in Shanghai, China." Cancer Epidemiology Biomarkers & Prevention 18(2): 590.

Yuen, M. F., Y. Tanaka, et al. (2008). "Risk for hepatocellular carcinoma with respect to hepatitis B virus genotypes B/C, specific mutations of enhancer II/core promoter/precore regions and HBV DNA levels." Gut 57(1): 98.

Zhang, M., Y. Gong, et al. (2002). "Rapid detection of hepatitis B virus mutations using real time PCR and melting curve analysis." Hepatology 36(3): 723-728.

Zhang, Y. J., P. Rossner, Jr., et al. (2006). "Aflatoxin B 1 and polycyclic aromatic hydrocarbon adducts, p53 mutations and p16 methylation in liver tissue and plasma of hepatocellular carcinoma patients " International Journal of Cancer 119(5): 985-991.

8

Usual and Unusual Gross Appearance of Hepatocellular Carcinomas

Keita Kai[1], Atsushi Miyoshi[2], Kenji Kitahara[2],
Kohji Miyazaki[2], Hirokazu Noshiro[2] and Osamu Tokunaga[1]
[1]Department of Pathology & Microbiology
[2]Department of Surgery
Saga University Faculty of Medicine
Japan

1. Introduction

Hepatocellular carcinoma (HCC) usually shows a typical gross appearance and the gross classification and gross diagnosis of resected specimens is performed as routine clinical work. In the authors' institution, many surgical cases of HCC are encountered, including rare and unusual cases. This chapter documents the gross classification, features and diagnosis of usual and unusual HCCs with representative gross photographs and a review of the literature.

2. Gross findings

The gross appearances of HCCs are affected by various factors such as tumor size, tumor thrombus in the portal and hepatic veins, intrahepatic metastasis, necrosis and hemorrhage. Well-differentiated HCC often produces bilirubin and the tumor color will be greenish after formalin fixation. On the other hand, poorly differentiated HCC usually shows a whitish coloration on gross appearance. If the tumor is accompanied by steatosis, the tumor will be yellowish in color. HCC frequently presents with a nodular appearance showing fibrous capsules and septa. The occurrence of capsule and septum formation is closely related to tumor size. Both capsule and septum are unusual in small HCCs less than 2.0 cm in diameter. In the majority of HCCs over 2.0 cm in diameter, the tumor grows expansively and a capsule and septum are formed.

3. Gross classification of usual types of HCC

3.1 Eggel's classification

Eggel's classification [Eggel, 1901] was proposed more than 100 years ago, and has been widely used for the classification of autopsy cases, rather than surgical cases. This system classifies HCC into three major types according to gross appearance: nodular; massive; and diffuse. Nodular type consists of a single or multiple discrete nodular tumors with clear demarcation. Massive type is a large mass replacing almost the entire right or left lobe. Diffuse type is characterized by diffuse proliferation of numerous minute cirrhosis-like tumor nodules throughout the entire lobe or liver.

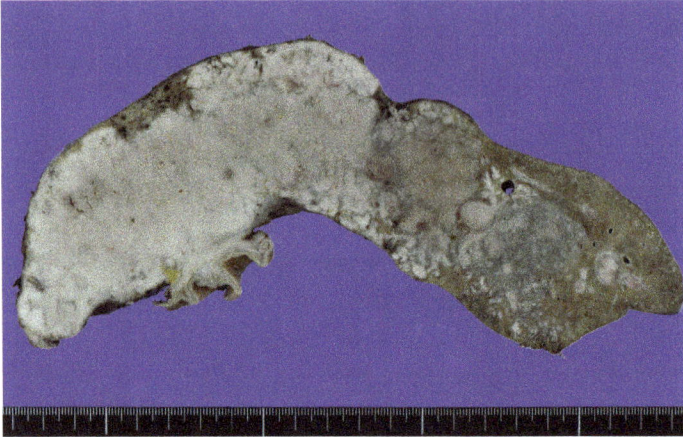

Fig. 1. Gross appearance of massive-type HCC in Eggel's classification.

3.2 Subclassification of nodular HCC

Eggel's classification is not applicable to many surgically resected HCCs. In order to cope with surgically resected HCCs, the Liver Cancer Study Group of Japan (LCSGJ) divided nodular HCC into three subtypes: simple nodular type; simple nodular type with extranodular growth; and confluent multinodular type [Kanai et al., 1987; LCSGJ, 1987]. The category of small nodular type with indistinct margin, as the typical gross appearance of early HCC, has recently been added to this subclassification [LCSGJ, 2000]. Several investigators have reported the predictive value of this subclassification, with favorable outcomes for simple nodular type compared to the other two subtypes in terms of recurrence and survival after hepatectomy [Hui et al., 2000; Shimada et al., 2001; Inayoshi et al., 2003].

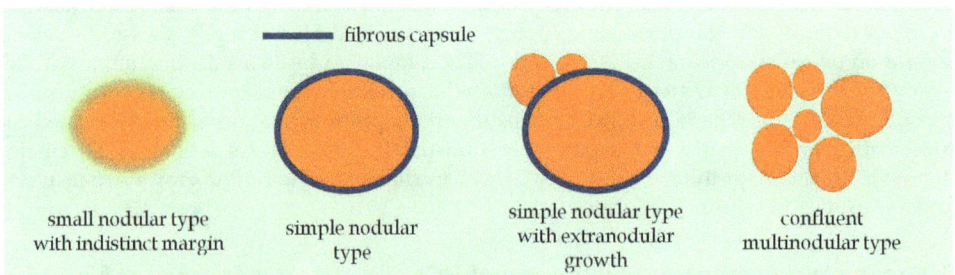

fibrous capsule

small nodular type with indistinct margin

simple nodular type

simple nodular type with extranodular growth

confluent multinodular type

Fig. 2. Schema for subclassification of nodular HCC on gross appearance

3.2.1 Small nodular type with indistinct margins

Grossly, small HCC less than about 2 cm in diameter can be classified into two major types: a small nodular type with indistinct margins (vaguely nodular type); and a distinctly nodular type [Kojiro & Nakashima, 1999]. The distinctly nodular type can be classified into one of the three subtypes: simple nodular type; simple nodular type with extranodular growth; and confluent multinodular type. On gross observation of the small nodular type with indistinct margins, distinguishing an obscure tumor nodule from surrounding cirrhotic liver is sometimes difficult. Histologically, most tumors of small nodular type with indistinct margins consist of uniformly distributed well-differentiated cancerous tissue showing a characteristic replacing growth at the tumor boundary. Although portal tracts are retained within the nodule, the number is markedly reduced [Nakashima et al., 1999]. Many of the retained portal tracts are deformed due to varying degrees of tumor cell invasion, designated as "stromal invasion", and this stromal invasion is regarded as the most helpful clue to distinguish small well-differentiated HCC from high-grade dysplastic nodules [Kondo et al., 1994, Tomizawa et al., 1995, Nakano et al, 1997]. Vascular invasion and intrahepatic micrometastasis are not usually observed in small nodular-type HCC with indistinct margins. Well-differentiated HCC of the small nodular type with indistinct margins has thus been designated as "early hepatocellular carcinoma", to separate this particular type of HCC from the classical form of HCC [Kojiro, 2006, 2007].

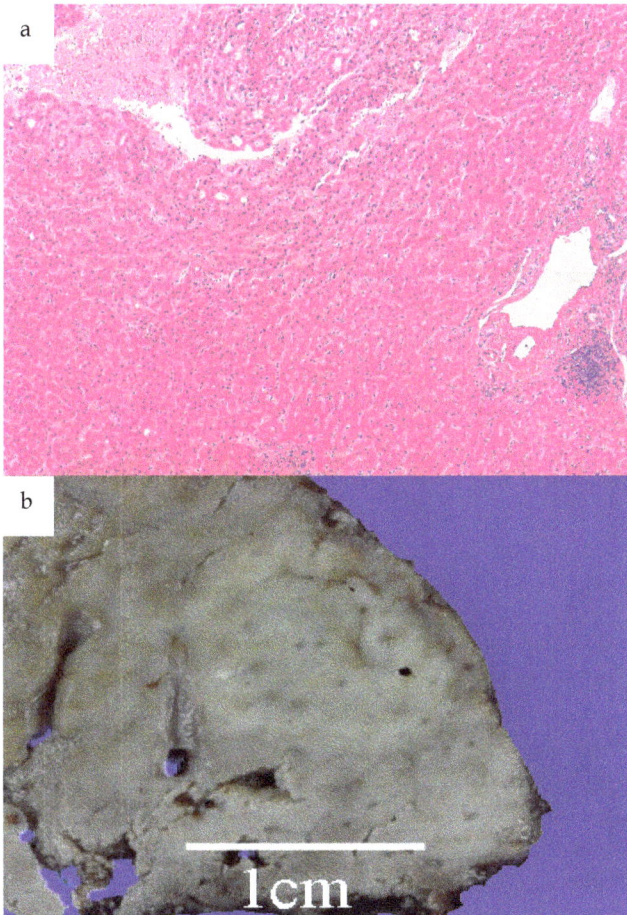

Fig. 3. a) Gross appearance of small nodular type with indistinct margins. b) Characteristic replacing growth at the tumor boundary (hematoxylin and eosin (HE), ×20).

3.2.2 Simple nodular type

This is a well-demarcated nodule, frequently surrounded by a fibrous capsule. Grossly, extranodular tumor growth, intrahepatic metastasis, and/or vascular invasion are not observed. The inside of the tumor often shows a mosaic appearance due to fibrous septa. Small HCC of the distinctly nodular type is also included in this category.

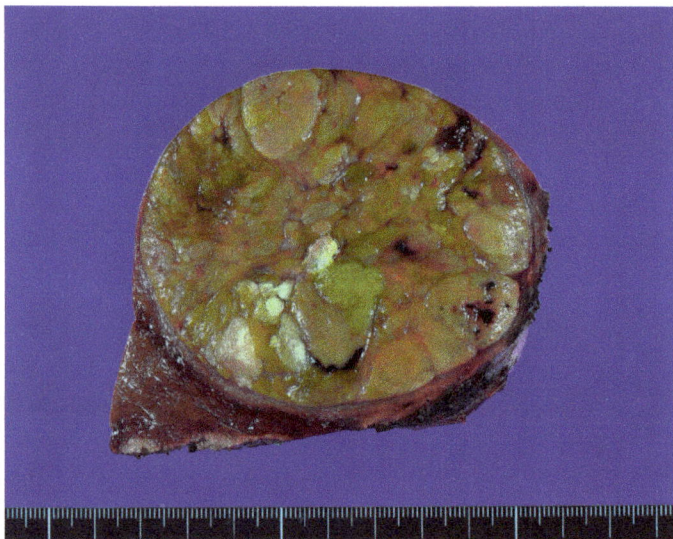

Fig. 4. Gross appearance of simple nodular type. A fibrous capsule and mosaic appearance due to fibrous septa are apparent.

3.2.3 Simple nodular type with extranodular growth

When a tumor of simple nodular type shows varying degrees of extranodular growth beyond the capsule, vascular invasion, and/or small metastases near the nodule, the tumor should be categorized as simple nodular type with extranodular growth. This criterion is not concerned with tumor size. Small tumors showing simple nodular type with extranodular growth sometimes need discrimination from confluent multinodular type and large tumors showing simple nodular type with extranodular growth sometimes need discrimination from massive-type HCC.

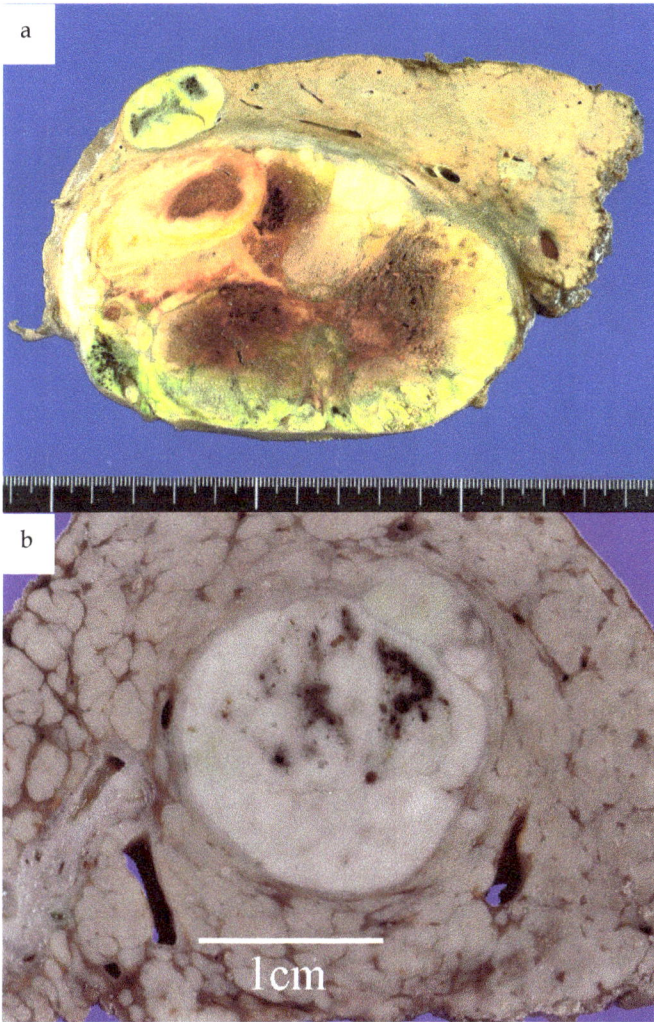

Fig. 5. Gross appearance of simple nodular type with extranodular growth. a) Small tumor of simple nodular type with extranodular growth. b) Large tumor of simple nodular type with extranodular growth. This type of tumor sometimes needs discrimination from massive-type and/or confluent multinodular-type HCC.

3.2.4 Confluent multinodular type

This is a tumor resulting from the joining together of a few to numerous small tumor nodules. No fibrous capsule is seen covering the entire tumor in this type and portal tracts are frequently entrapped between agglomerated small tumor nodules. The incidence of vascular invasion and/or intrahepatic metastasis is higher than in simple nodular types. Large confluent multinodular-type tumors sometimes need discrimination from massive-type HCC.

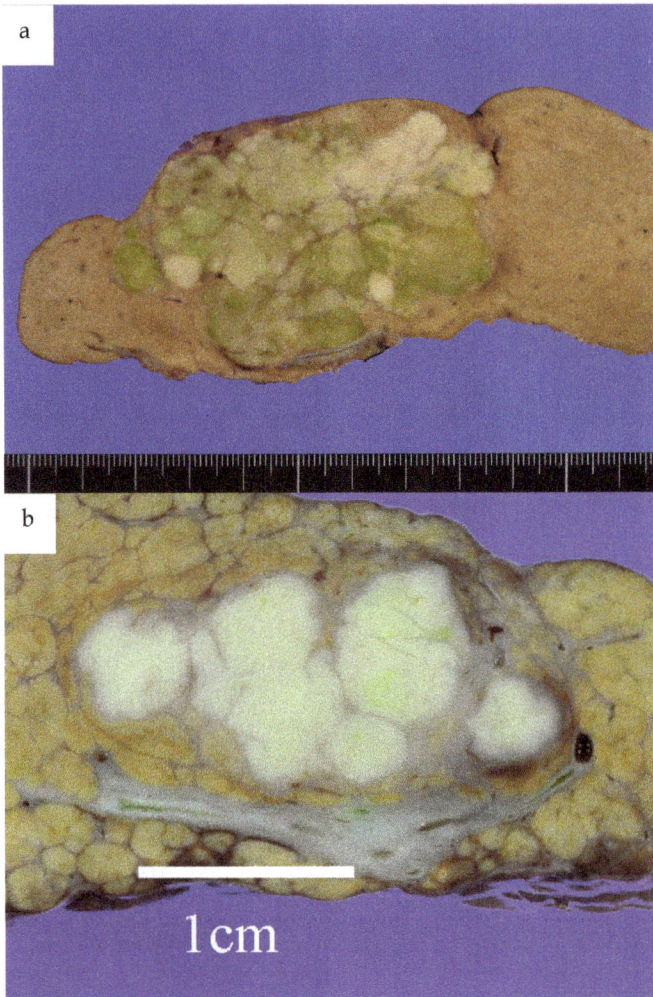

Fig. 6. Gross appearance of confluent multinodular-type HCC. a) Small tumor of confluent multinodular type. b) Large tumor of simple confluent multinodular type. No fibrous capsule covering the entire tumor is present.

4. Unusual gross types of HCC

4.1 Scirrhous HCC

About 5% of HCCs show a scirrhous growth pattern characterized by marked fibrosis along the sinusoid-like blood spaces with varying degrees of atrophy of the tumor trabeculae [Kurogi et al., 2006]. These tumors are subclassified as scirrhous HCC according to the WHO classification [Bosman et al., 2010]. Macroscopically, scirrhous HCCs are greyish-white, solid, lobulated, and unencapsulated, but well demarcated, stellate-shaped fibrosis is common. The gross appearance of scirrhous HCC mimics intrahepatic cholangiocarcinoma, combined hepatocellular and cholangiocarcinoma, and fibrolamellar carcinoma. Scirrhous HCC is histologically distinguishable from fibrolamellar carcinoma, because the cancer cells do not differ from those of ordinary HCC. Scirrhous HCC should also not be confused with diffuse fibrosis (scirrhous change) in HCC, a well-known feature of cases treated by various anticancer therapies such as chemotherapy, irradiation and chemoembolization. Preoperatively, scirrhous HCC is often misdiagnosed as intrahepatic cholangiocarcinoma or metastatic carcinoma on diagnostic imaging, because of atypical imaging findings due to the diffuse fibrosis [Kojiro, 2006; Bosman et al., 2010].

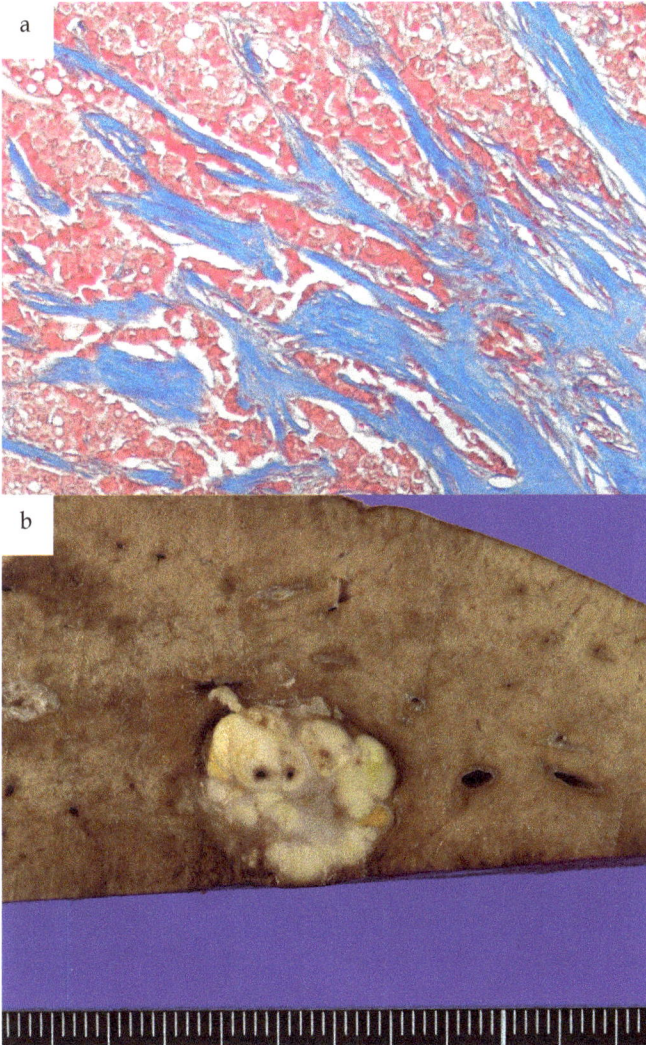

Fig. 7. a) Gross appearance of scirrhous HCC. Stellate-shaped fibrosis is present. b) Histology of the scirrhous HCC. Marked fibrosis (blue) is apparent along the sinusoid-like blood spaces. Cancer cells are no different from ordinary HCC (Azan staining, ×100).

4.2 Fibrolamellar HCC

The clinical and pathological features of fibrolamellar HCC (FLC) were first described by Edmondson [Edmondson, 1958]. The term "fibrolamellar carcinoma" was proposed by Craig et al. [Craig et al., 1980], and has been adopted worldwide. FLC shows marked geographic variations in incidence, and is extremely rare in Asian countries, including Japan [Magata et al., 2001]. Soreide et al. [Soreide et al., 1986] reviewed 80 cases of FLC (including their own 9 cases) reported between 1980 and 1986. This entity most frequently occurs in noncirrhotic livers of adolescents or young adults with a mean age of 23 years; only 6% are over 50 years old. Two thirds of the cases of FLC involve the left lobe and prognosis is more

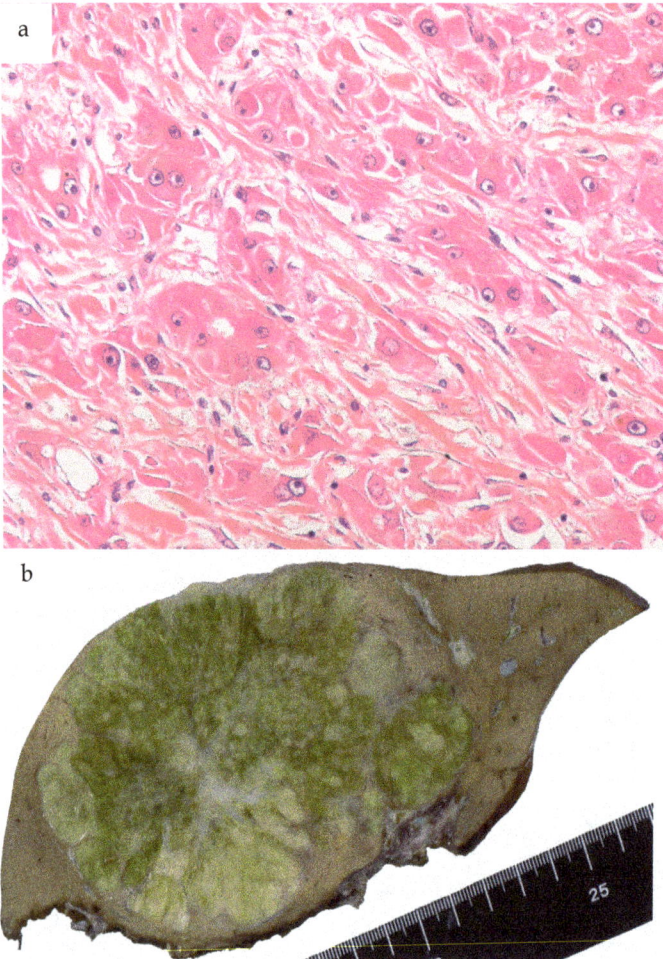

Fig. 8. a) Gross appearance of fibrolamellar hepatocellular carcinoma. White fibrous septa forming a central scar, lobulated appearance, and greenish coloration due to bile production can be observed. b) Tumor cells display abundant polygonal and deeply eosinophilic cytoplasm and characteristic lamellar fibrosis is observed (HE, ×200).

favorable than that of classical HCC. Grossly, the tumor is well demarcated but nonencapsulated and is light brown, tan or gray. The tumor is occasionally partially greenish due to bile production. Glistening white fibrous septa, sometimes forming a central scar, give the tumor a lobulated appearance. This gross appearance mimics focal nodular hyperplasia. Histologically, this particular type of HCC consists of tumor cells growing in sheets or small trabeculae, which are separated by fibrous collagen with a characteristic lamellar pattern of variable thickness and frequent hyalinization. Tumor cells display abundant polygonal and deeply eosinophilic cytoplasm and a distinct nucleolus. Intracytoplasmic inclusions, such as "pale bodies" that show immunohistochemically positive results for antifibrinogen and PAS-positive globules, are frequently observed [Ishak et al., 1999].

4.3 Green HCC

Nodular-type HCC accompanied by prominent bile production shows a yellowish coloration on a fresh specimen and deep greenish coloration after formalin fixation. Such tumors are generally called "green HCC".

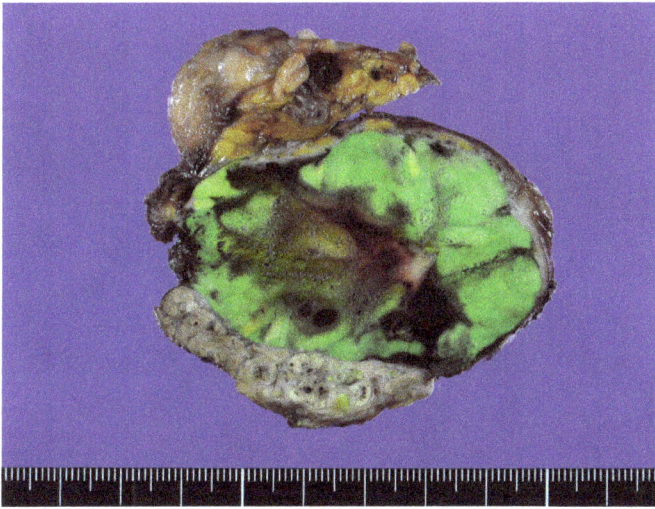

Fig. 9. Gross appearance of green HCC.

4.4 Pelioid type of HCC

Peliosis hepatis-like blood-filled cavities are frequently observed in HCC. HCC with this finding is generally called "HCC with peliotic change" or "pelioid-type HCC" [Ishak et al., 1999]. Another characteristic of HCC with peliotic change is that all tumors are completely or incompletely encapsulated. Several cases of extensive pelioid-type HCC have been reported [Kim, 2007, Hoshimoto, 2009, Kai, 2011]. Grossly, extensive pelioid-type HCC mostly consists of well-defined black-nodular components. Histologically, peliotic change is distinguished from hemorrhage by the presence or absence of degenerative changes and/or necrosis. In general, degenerative changes and/or necrosis are observed around hemorrhage in HCC tumors. On the other hand, the tumorous tissue around peliotic change is not at all degenerative or necrotic, and blood is localized within the spaces with clear margins. However, when peliotic change becomes extensive, rupture may occur and hemorrhage may develop [Kojiro, 2006].

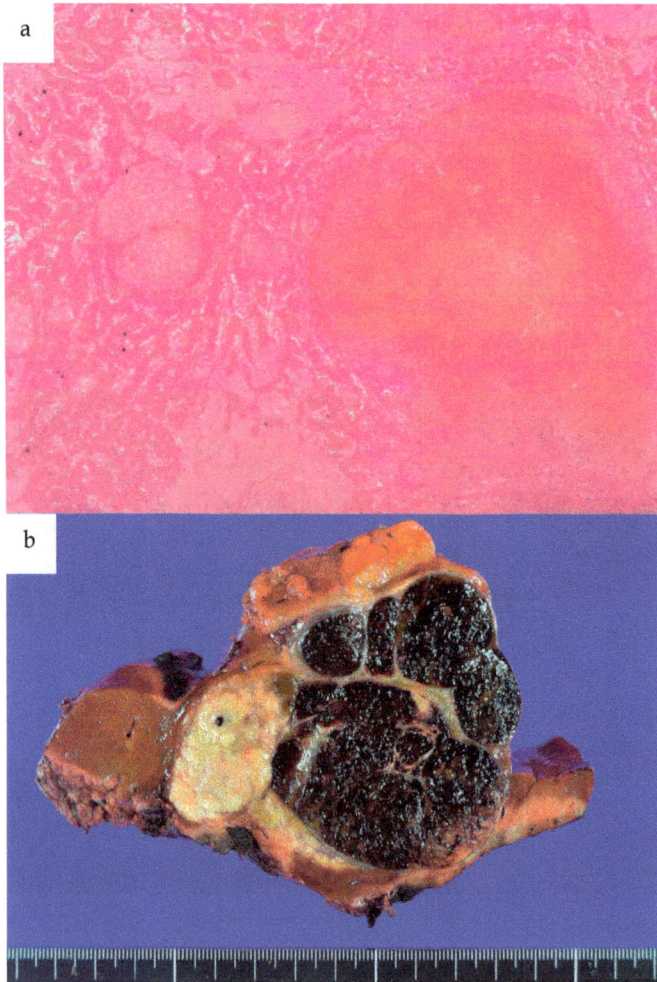

Fig. 10. a) The gross appearance of pelioid-type HCC. The tumor comprises well-defined black nodular components and white nodular components. b) Histologically, extensive pelioid change is apparent in the tumor tissue (HE, ×25).

4.5 Intraductal growth type of HCC

Rarely, HCC shows growth into the hepatic bile duct and/or common bile duct, causing progressive obstructive jaundice. In 1972, Lin [Lin, 1972] designated such cases as "icteric HCC". The reported incidence of icteric HCC varies from 0.2% to 5.4% in patients with HCC

[Kojiro et al., 1982; Huang et al., 1998]. Although intraductal tumor growth of HCC was once considered rare, advances in diagnostic imaging have revealed many cases of HCC presenting with intra-bile-duct growth [Kirk et al., 1994; Soyer et al., 1995; Wang et al., 2002]. Patients with the intraductal growth type of HCC rarely show no obvious intrahepatic tumor. Postoperative pathological examinations confirm the bile duct nodules causing obstructive jaundice as HCC. This type of HCC is difficult to diagnose, and only a few cases have been reported [Long et al., 2010]. In some cases, massive hemorrhage in the bile duct (hemobilia) forms due to tumor growth and can cause rapid death on rare occasions [Kojiro, 2006]. Huang et al. [Huang et al., 1998] stated that the prognosis might be improved if surgical resection of the tumor cast is performed at an earlier stage. In fact, many cases have been reported with good prognosis after tumor cast resection [Chen et al., 1994; Lau et al., 1997; Hu et al., 1999].

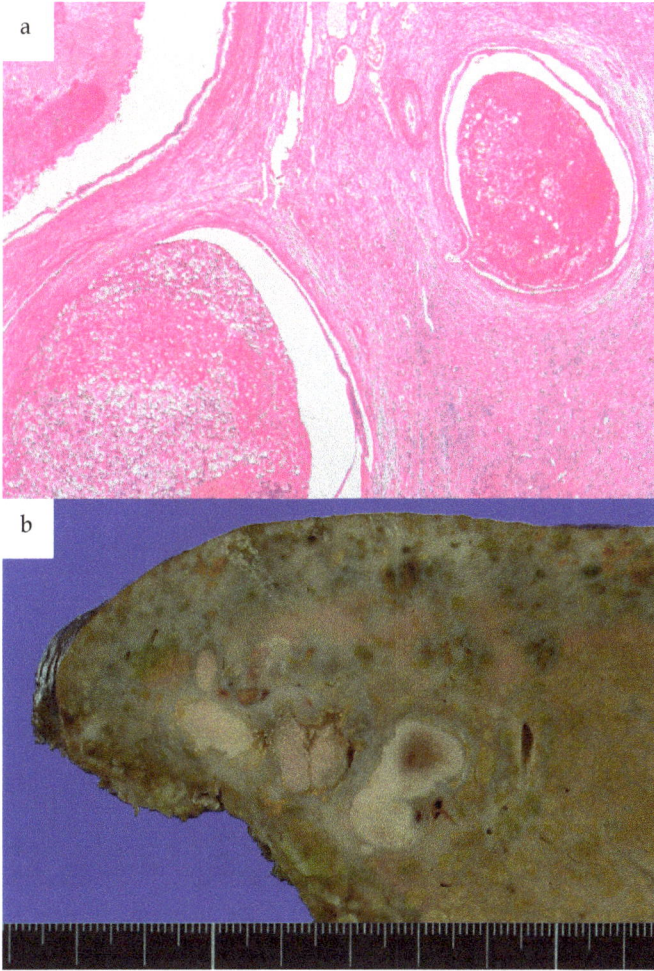

Fig. 11. a) Gross appearance for the intraductal growth type of HCC. This case shows no obvious intrahepatic mass lesion. b) Tumor cells with blood clot in dilated bile ducts (HE, ×20).

4.6 Spontaneous regression of HCC

Spontaneous massive necrosis or regression of HCC is a very rare event. The precise mechanisms underlying spontaneous regression of HCC remain unclear, but various factors

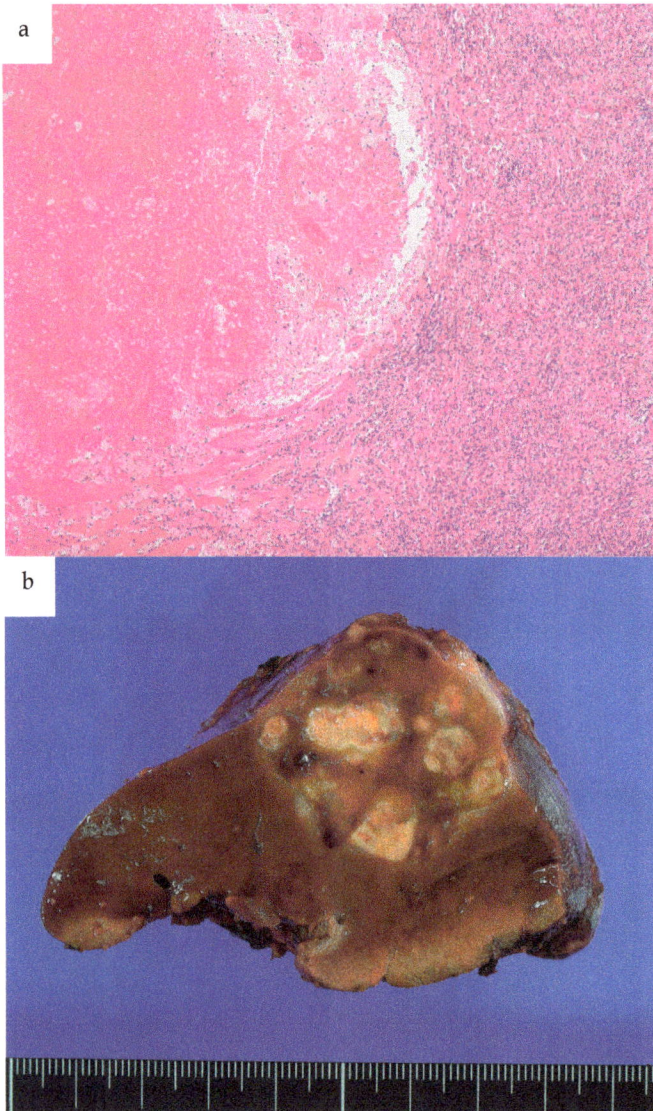

Fig. 12. a) Cut surface of the resected liver in a case of spontaneous regression. Yellow-white nodular lesions and brownish lesions coexist. The HCC measuring 11 cm in diameter showed a significant reduction to 3.7 cm after angiography. b) Coagulative necrosis and inflammatory granulation tissue are apparent in the nodule and small foci of viable HCC cells are observed in another specimen (HE, ×40).

have been speculated to play a role, such as alcohol withdrawal, androgen withdrawal, and intake of herbal medicines [Gottfried et al., 1982; Lam et al., 1982; McCaughan et al., 1985]. Secondary stimulation of cytokine production by tumor necrosis or bacterial infection has also been suggested to contribute to spontaneous regression [Watanabe et al., 1994; Markovic et al., 1996]. Another important factor might be insufficient blood supply to the tumor, possibly due to rapid natural tumor growth, spontaneous arterial thrombosis, thickened fibrous capsule or gastrointestinal bleeding [Suzuki et al., 1989; Gaffey et al., 1990; Tocci et al., 1990; Imaoka et al., 1994; Nakajima et al., 2004]. A few cases of spontaneous regression of HCC after angiography have been reported [Takayasu et al., 1986; Kai et al., 2010]. The characteristic histology in these cases is coagulative necrosis of tumor cells and inflammatory granulation tissue surrounding the coagulative necrosis. Grossly, yellow-white nodular lesions reflecting coagulative necrosis and brownish lesions reflecting inflammatory granulation tissue coexist.

5. Differential diagnosis by gross appearance

Various tumors and tumor-like lesions can arise in the liver. Some of these tumors show a similar gross appearance to HCC, but some are easily discriminated from HCC on gross appearance.

5.1 Intrahepatic cholangiocellular carcinoma

Intrahepatic cholangiocellular carcinoma (ICC) is also grossly classified into three types: mass-forming type; periductal infiltrating type; and intraductal growth type. Within these three types, the mass-forming type is grossly nominated as a differential diagnosis of classical HCC. This differential diagnosis is usually easily achieved based on the characteristic gross appearance of mass-forming ICC, such as a lobulated, firm and solid

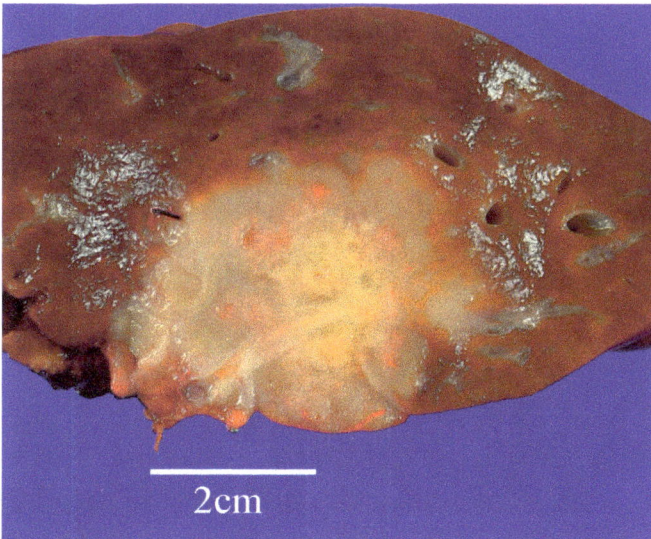

Fig. 13. Cut surface of the mass-forming type of ICC.

gray to gray-white mass without a fibrous capsule and often with central necrosis or scarring. Scirrhous-type HCC sometimes mimics mass-forming ICC. Intraductal growth-type HCC often mimics intraductal growth-type ICC and discrimination based on gross appearance is difficult.

5.2 Cholangiolocellular carcinoma

Cholangiolocarcinoma is a rare neoplasm with a reported incidence of 0.8-1.0% among primary liver cancers [Steiner & Higginson, 1959; Shiota et al., 2001]. Cholangiolocarcinoma

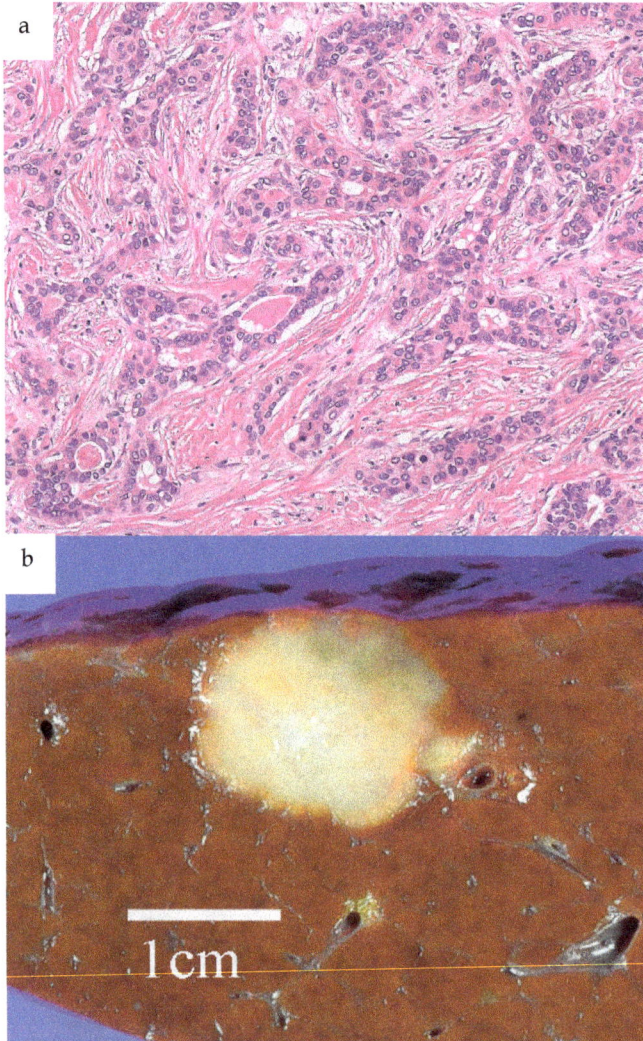

Fig. 14. a) Gross appearance of cholangiolocellular carcinoma. b) A tubular cordlike anastomosing pattern (as the so-called "antler pattern") of tumor cells (HE, ×100).

is now considered to be derived from Hering's canal or stem cells, which have intermediate features between hepatocytes and bile duct epithelium [Shiota et al., 2001; Kojiro, 2006]. Grossly, cholangiolocarcinoma is whitish in color and solid, not encapsulated, and resembles cholangiocellular carcinoma. Histologically, tumor cells display eosinophilic cytoplasm with ovoid nuclei, and mild atypia, and adopt a tubular cordlike anastomosing pattern (so-called antler pattern). These cell cords are continuous with liver cell cords at the tumor boundaries, showing a replacing pattern.

5.3 Hepatocellular adenoma (HCA)

HCA is a benign liver neoplasm comprising hepatocyte-like tumor cells. The incidence of HCA is about 3-4 per 100 000 population in Western countries [Rooks et al., 1979], but is

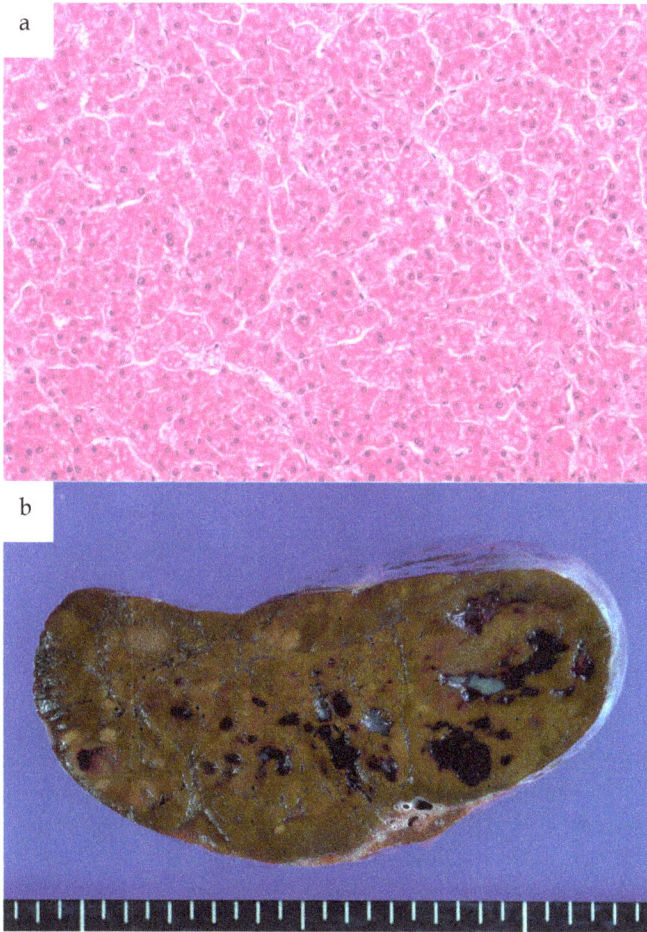

Fig. 15. a) Gross appearance of hepatocellular adenoma. Focal peliotic change is present. b) The nodule consists of tumor cells with abundant hydropic cytoplasm and little atypia arranged in a trabecular pattern.

lower in Japan and Asian countries. HCA predominantly occurs in females in the third and fourth decades of life, and a close etiological relationship between HCA and oral contraceptives has been described [Ishak & Rabin, 1975]. Patients taking androgens for Fanconi anemia or acquired anaplastic anemia are also at risk [Velazquez & Alter, 2004]. Nonhormonal risk factors include glycogenosis type 1 (von Gierke disease) or 3 (Forbes disease), galactosemia, tyrosinemia, familial polyposis coli, and hepatic iron overload with β-thalassemia [Shuangshoti & Thaicharoen, 1994]. Obesity has recently been shown to be a risk factor for a particular HCA subtype [Bosman et al., 2010]. Grossly, HCA is found in the normal liver as a well-demarcated, single or multiple solid tumor. Many HCAs are not encapsulated, but some are partly or entirely encapsulated. The tumor is yellowish and solid, sometimes associated with necrosis and hemorrhage and/or peliosis hepatis-like (pelioid) change and the tumor may be divided by fibrous septa. HCA developing close to the liver surface can protrude outside the liver, and is thus susceptible to rupture. Histologically, HCA consists of tumor cells with abundant hydropic cytoplasm and little atypia arranged in a trabecular pattern of one- or two-cell-thick plates, or round eosinophilic tumor cells in a thin trabecular pattern. However, because the sinusoid-like blood spaces of the tumor stroma are compressed by the swollen, hydropic tumor cells, the trabecular pattern is often obscured and the tumor takes on a solid appearance. The tumor contains many arterial and venous tumor vessels, and pelioid change is frequently observed.

5.4 Focal nodular hyperplasia (FNH)

FNH is not a true neoplasm, but rather a regenerative hyperplastic response of hepatocytes, secondary to localized vascular abnormalities with a marked female preponderance [Wanless et al., 1985; Fukukura et al., 1998]. This lesion was reported as liver cell adenoma for many years before the disease concept of FNH was defined by Edmondson in 1958 [Edmondson, 1958]. In two-thirds of cases, FNH is solitary [Wanless et al., 1989]. Most lesions are asymptomatic and discovered incidentally during laparotomy, autopsy or imaging studies for unrelated symptoms. Although it can now be precisely diagnosed by various imaging modalities, FNH is still considered one of the common lesions in the differential diagnosis of HCC. The size of FNH varies from a few millimeters to over 10 cm in diameter. Grossly, FNH is usually well demarcated, but not encapsulated. Most tumors are located close to the liver capsule, and 4.6-20% are reportedly pedunculated [Ishak, 1975; Klatskin, 1977; Luciani et al., 2002]. One of the characteristic gross features of FNH is the presence of a central fibrous scar with radiating fibrous bands dividing the tumor into lobules. The reported incidence of a central scar in FNH is 49-62.8% [Nguyen et al., 1999; Kojiro, 2006]. Histologically, classical FNH lesions are composed of benign hepatocytes arranged in a trabecular pattern of one- or two-cell-thick plates. The central scar consists of dense fibrous tissue with many artery-like or vein-like anomalous blood vessels and ductal proliferations. Hyperplastic features of hepatocytes in FNH comprise increased cellularity with an increased nuclear cytoplasmic ratio, an irregular thin trabecular pattern, and a pseudoglandular pattern. Areas showing prominent hyperplastic features mimic well-differentiated HCC.

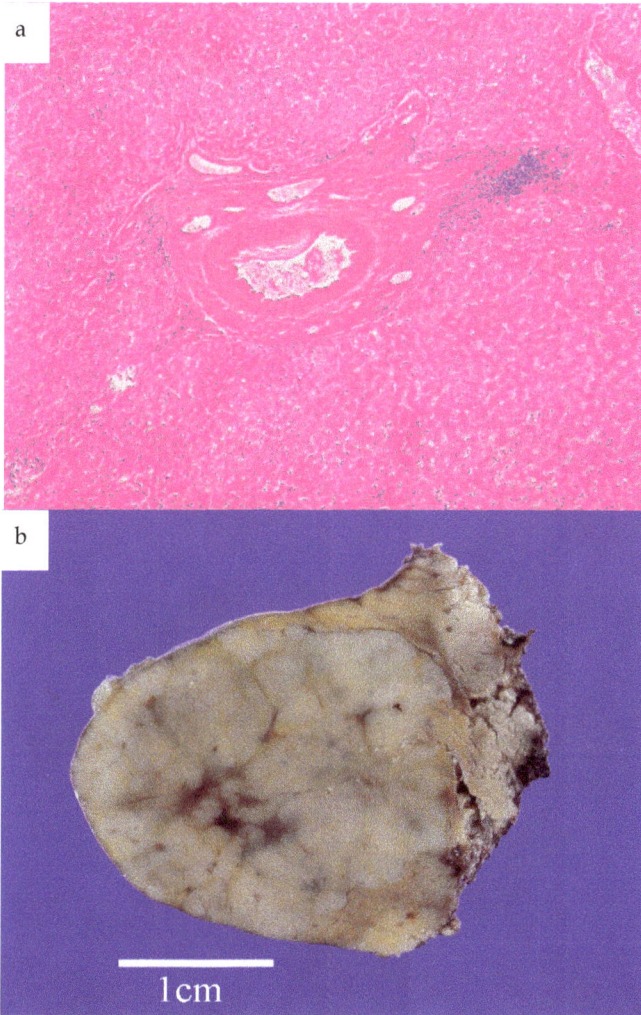

Fig. 16. a) Gross appearance of FNH. A faint central fibrous scar is apparent in this case. b) Artery-like anomalous blood vessels are observed in benign hepatocytes (HE, ×40).

5.5 Hepatocellular neoplasm with massive histiocyte infiltration

HCC usually contains various degrees of histiocyte infiltration. In the authors' institution, a case of unique hepatocellular nodule with infiltration of abundant histiocytes not previously described has been encountered [Kai, 2010]. This case involved a 73-year-old Japanese man with diabetes mellitus and mild obesity without viral hepatitis. Histologically, the nodule consisted of hepatocyte-like tumor cells and abundant foam cell-type histiocytes that filled up a sinusoid-like space and formed central loose fibrosis. The tumor showed characteristics of hepatocellular adenoma, but contained a focal HCC-like lesion. Similar hepatic nodules have not been reported and most of the clinicopathological features and pathology remain unknown.

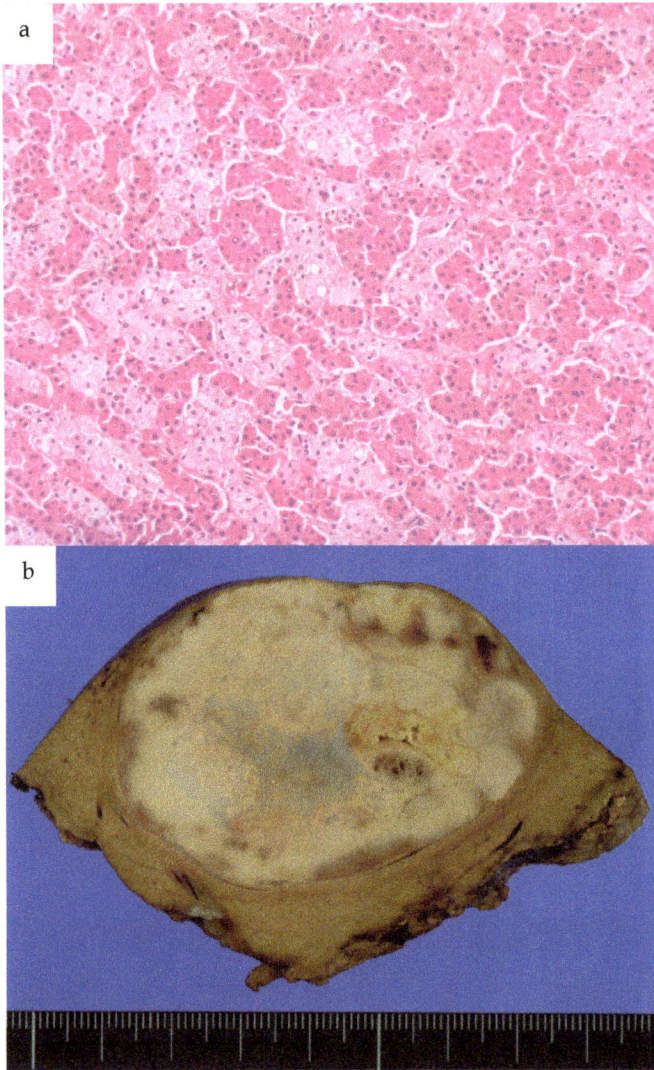

Fig. 17. a) Gross appearance of hepatocellular neoplasm with massive histiocyte infiltration. The nodule was solitary, and the cut surface was whitish with a partly necrotic yellowish area. A white myxoid fibrotic area was found at the center of the nodule. b) The nodule showed a two-cell pattern: hepatocyte-like cells with rich eosinophilic cytoplasm and little nuclear atypia; and light-pink cells considered to be foam cell-type histiocytes (HE, ×100).

5.6 Primary squamous cell carcinoma (SCC) of the liver

Primary SCC of the liver is very rare. Adenosquamous carcinoma of the liver is also rare and reported only sporadically. Various theories have been advanced concerning the pathogenesis of SCC of the liver. Chronic inflammation of the bile duct and various

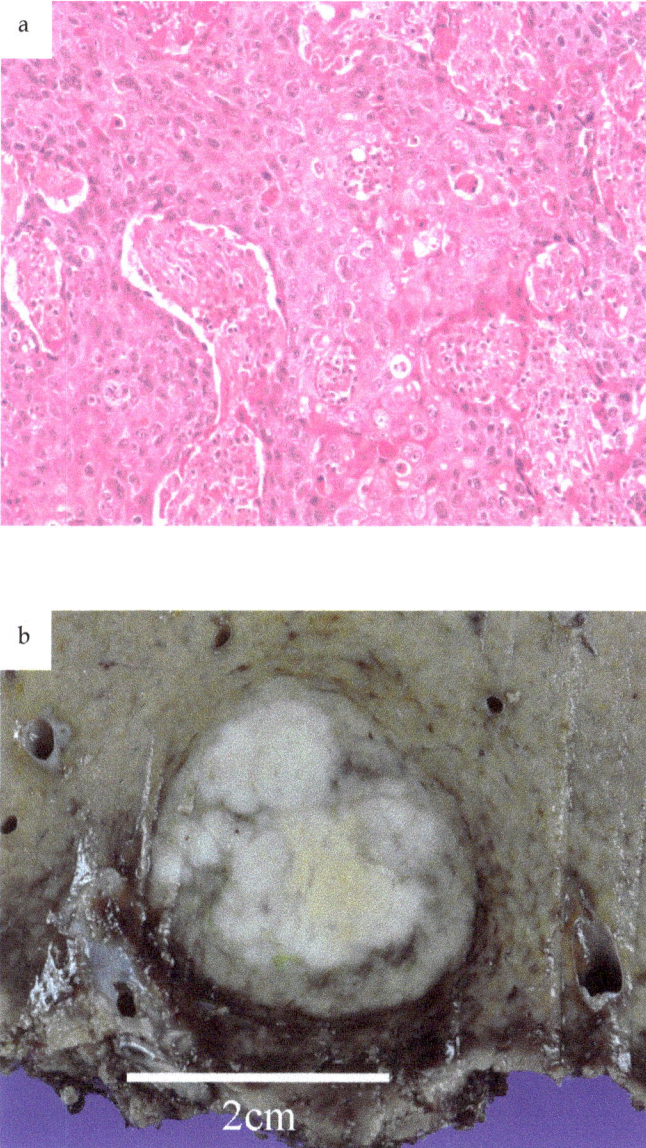

Fig. 18. a) Gross appearance of primary pure SCC of the liver in a patient with no history of prior liver insult. b) The nodule consists entirely of SCC tissue with or without keratinization.

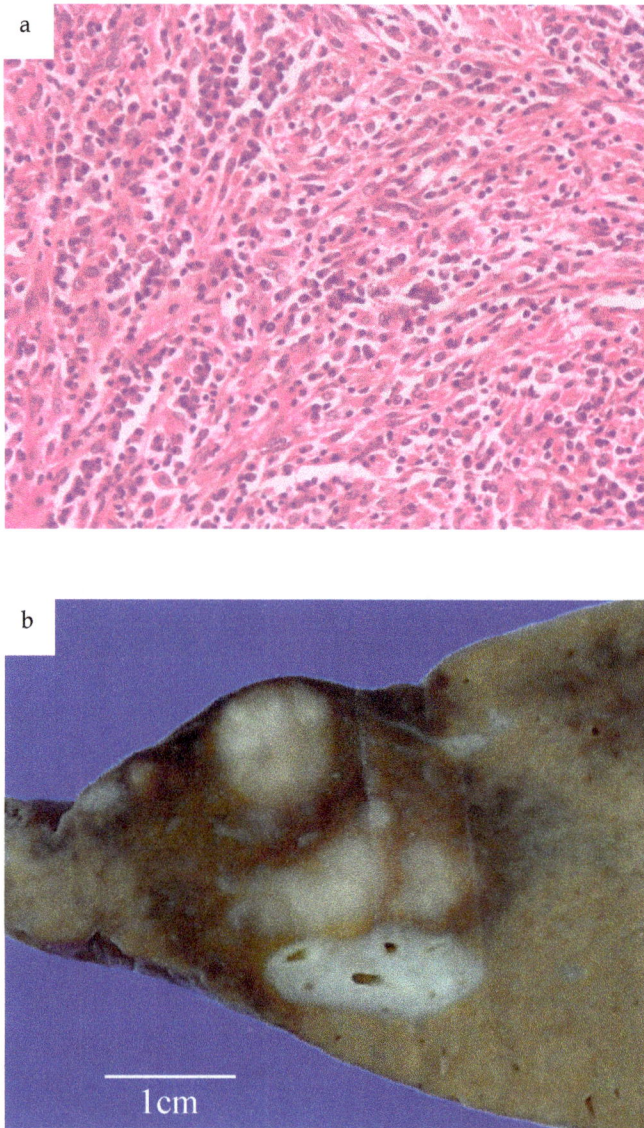

Fig. 19. a) A cross-section of inflammatory pseudotumor. Small, white nodules without fibrous capsules are observed. b) The tumor comprises chronic inflammatory cells, predominantly representing plasma cells (HE, ×200).

congenital cysts of the biliary tract have been proposed as etiological factors and continuous irritation due to chronic infection, followed by metaplastic changes in the biliary epithelium, has been thought to lead to neoplasia [Clements et al., 1990; Nieweg et al., 1992; Banbury et al., 1994]. On the other hand, some investigators have suggested that adenosquamous carcinoma could arise from squamous metaplasia of adenocarcinoma cells [Barr and Hancock, 1975; Tomioka et al., 1987]. Primary SCC of the liver without history of prior liver insult suggesting development from squamous metaplasia of adenocarcinoma cells has recently been reported [Naik et al., 2009]. Gross appearance depends on the presence or absence of congenital cysts. The mass lesion in that case appeared as a solid, whitish firm mass without fibrous capsule and with a necrotic area of keratin deposits observed inside the nodule.

5.7 Inflammatory pseudotumor / inflammatory myofibroblastic tumor

Inflammatory pseudotumor is defined as a benign, non-neoplastic mass consisting of fibrous tissue and proliferated myofibroblasts and fibroblasts, with marked infiltration of chronic inflammatory cells, predominantly comprising polyclonal plasma cells, histiocytes, and macrophages [Coffin et al., 1995]. Lesions of known cause, such as healing abscess, tuberculosis, and parasitic infestations, and post-traumatic granulation tissue, are excluded from this category. Patients with hepatic lesions generally complain of recurrent fever, malaise, abdominal pain, vomiting, and/or diarrhea, but those clinical symptoms are not specific. The morphology of inflammatory pseudotumor apparently differs according to the stage of inflammation when the lesion is detected. Grossly, the lesion appears as a yellowish or whitish nodule with relatively clear margins and a widely varying diameter, usually within the range of 1-3 cm. Histological appearance also varies considerably, sometimes consisting of nonspecific inflammatory granulation tissue with prominent plasma cell infiltration, sometimes associated with necrotic foci, and sometimes appearing as a scar-like fibrous nodule with mild inflammatory cell infiltration [Kojiro, 2006]. Phlebitis involving peripheral portal or hepatic veins is often seen. Rarely, major hepatic and/or portal veins or the vena cava are involved by phlebitis mimicking malignant tumor [Broughan et al., 1993; Kai et al., 2007]. Lately, IgG4-related disease has been identified as an important subgroup of inflammatory pseudotumor [Zen et al., 2004, 2007]. Inflammatory myofibroblastic tumor has recently been considered as a possible neoplastic counterpart of inflammatory pseudotumor [Coffin et al., 1998], based on the finding that approximately half of inflammatory myofibroblastic tumors show an ALK gene translocation [Lawrence et al., 2000; Bridge et al., 2001; Chan et al., 2001].

6. Conclusion

This chapter documented the gross appearance and pathology of various types of tumor, along with a review of the literature. We believe that the observation of gross features with contrasting pathological and clinical findings is helpful in clarifying the nature of tumors. In rare cases, a picture of the gross specimen is necessary for case reports. Careful storage of good-quality images of gross specimens is thus important in daily clinical work.

7. References

Banbury J, Conlon KC, Ghossein R, et al. (1994). Primary squamous cell carcinoma within a solitary nonparasitic hepatic cyst. *J Surg Oncol*, 57, pp.210-212.

Barr RJ, Hancock DE (1975). Adenosquamous carcinoma of the liver. *Gastroenterology*, 69, pp.1326-1330

Bosman FT, Carnerio F, Hruban RH, Theise ND, Eds. (2010) *WHO classification of Tumors of the Digestive System*. IARC, Lyon.

Bridge JA, Kanamori M, Ma Z, et al. (2001). Fusion of the ALK gene to the clathrin heavy chain gene, CLTC, in inflammatory myofibroblastic tumor. *Am J Pathol.*, 159, pp.411-415.

Broughan TA, Fischer WL, Tuthill RJ. (1993). Vascular invasion by hepatic infl ammatory pseudotumor. A clinicopathologic study. *Cancer*, 71, pp.2934-2940.

Chan JK, Cheuk W, Shimizu M. (2001), Anaplastic lymphoma kinase in inflammatory pseudotumors. *Am J Surg Pathol.*, 25, pp.761-768.

Chen MF, Jan YY, Jeng LB, et al. (1994). Obstructive jaundice secondary to ruptured hepatocellular carcinoma into the common bile duct. Surgical experiences of 20 cases. *Cancer*, 73, pp.1335-1340.

Clements D, Newman P, Etherington R,et al. (1990). Squamous carcinoma in the liver. *Gut*, 31, pp.1333-1334.

Coffin CM, Dehner LP, Meis-Kindblom JM. (1998). Inflammatory myofibroblastic tumor, inflammatory fibrosarcoma, and related lesions: an historical review with differential diagnostic considerations. *Semin Diagn Pathol.*, 15, pp.102-110.

Coffin CM, Watterson J, Priest JR, et al. (1995). Extrapulmonary inflammatory myofi broblastic tumor (inflammatory pseudotumor). A clinicopathologic and immunohistochemical study of 84 cases. *Am J Surg Pathol.*,19(8), pp.859-872.

Craig JR, Peters RL, Edmondson HA, et al. (1980). Fibrolamellar carcinoma of the liver: a tumor of adolescents and young adults with distinctive clinico-pathologic features. *Cancer*, 15, 46(2), pp.372-379.

Edmondson HA. (1958). Focal nodular hyperplasia. In: *Atlas of Tumor Pathology: Tumors of the Liver and Intrahepatic Bile Ducts*, 1st Series, Fascicle 25. Armed Forces Institute of Pathology, Washington DC, pp. 193-195.

Edmondson HA. (1958). Hepatocelllar carcinoma. In: *Atlas of Tumor Pathology: Tumors of the Liver and Intrahepatic Bile Ducts*, 1st Series, Fascicle 25. Armed Forces Institute of Pathology, Washington DC, pp. 32.

Eggel, H. (1901). Uber das prime Carcinoma der Leber. *Beitr Pathol Anat Allg Pathol*, 30, pp.506-604.

Fukukura Y, Nakashima O, Kusaba A, et al. (1998). Angioarchitecture and blood circulation in focal nodular hyperplasia of the liver. *J Hepatol.*, 29(3), 470-475.

Gaffey MJ, Joyce JP, Carlson GS, et al. (1990). Spontaneous regression of hepatocellular carcinoma. *Cancer*, 65, pp.2779-2783.

Gottfried EB, Steller R, Paronetto F, et al. (1982). Spontaneous regression of hepatocellular carcinoma. *Gastroenterology*, 82, pp.770-774

Hoshimoto S, Morise Z, Suzuki K, et al. (2009). Hepatocellular carcinoma with extensive peliotic change. *J Hepatobiliary Pancreat Surg.*,16, pp.566-570.

Hu J, Pi Z, Yu MY, et al. (1999). Obstructive jaundice caused by tumor emboli from hepatocellular carcinoma. Am Surg., 65(5), pp.406-410.

Huang GT, Sheu JC, Lee HS, rt al. (1998). Icteric type hepatocellular carcinoma: revisited 20 years later. *J Gastroenterol.*, 33(1), pp. 53-56.

Hui AM, Takayama T, Sano K, et al. (2000). Predictive value of gross classification of hepatocellular carcinoma on recurrence and survival after hepatectomy. *J Hepatol.*, 33(6), pp.975-979.

Imaoka S, Sasaki Y, Masutani S, et al. (1994). Necrosis of hepatocellular carcinoma caused by spontaneously arising arterial thrombus. *Hepatogastroenterology*, 41, pp.359-362.

Inayoshi J, Ichida T, Sugitani S, et al. (2003) Gross appearance of hepatocellular carcinoma reflects E-cadherin expression and risk of early recurrence after surgical treatment. *J Gastroenterol Hepatol.*, 18(6), pp.673-677.

Ishak KG, Goodman ZD, StockerJT. (1999). Hepatocelllar carcinoma. In: *Atlas of Tumor Pathology: Tumors of the Liver and Intrahepatic Bile Ducts*, 3rd Series, Fascicle 31. Armed Forces Institute of Pathology, Washington DC.

Ishak KG, Rabin L. (1975). Benign tumors of the liver. *Med Clin North Am.*, 59(4), pp.995-1013.

Kai K, Matsuyama S, Ohtsuka T, et al. (2007). Multiple inflammatory pseudotumor of the liver, mimicking cholangiocarcinoma with tumor embolus in the hepatic vein: report of a case. *Surg Today.*, 37(6), pp.530-533.

Kai K, Miyoshi A, Ario K, et al. (2010). The two cases of massive spontaneous necrosis of hepatocellular carcinoma after angiography. *Kanzo* , 51, pp.312-318.

Kai K, Miyoshi A, Egashira Y, et al. (2011). A case of Pelioid type of Hepatocellular carcinoma composed of the two different nodules. *Kanzo*, 52(2), pp.112-119.

Kai K, Miyoshi A, Tokunaga O, et al. (2010) A hepatocellular neoplasm accompanied with massive histiocyte infiltration. *Clin J Gastroenterol*, 3, pp.40–44.

Kanai T, Hirohashi S, Upton MP, et al. (1987) Pathology of small hepatocellular carcinoma. A proposal for a new gross classification. *Cancer*, 15, 60(4), pp.810-819.

Kim YK, Jang KY, Cho BH, et al. (2007). Three-phase dynamic CT of pelioid hepatocellular carcinoma. *Am J Roentgenol.*, 189, pp.160-162.

Kirk JM, Skipper D, Joseph AE, et al. (1994). Intraluminal bile duct hepatocellular carcinoma. *Clin Radiol*, 49, pp. 886-888.

Klatskin G. (1977). Hepatic tumors: possible relationship to use of oral contraceptives. *Gastroenterology.*, 73(2), 386-394.

Kojiro M, Kawabata K, Kawano Y, et al. (1982). Hepatocellular carcinoma presenting as intrabile duct tumor growth: a clinicopathologic study of 24 cases. *Cancer.*, 15, 49(10), pp.2144-2147.

Kojiro M, Nakashima O. (1999). Histopathologic evaluation of hepatocellular carcinoma with special reference to small early stage tumors. *Semin Liver Dis,* 19(3), pp.287-296.

Kojiro M. (2006). *Pathology of Hepatocellular Carcinoma*, Blackwell publishing inc., Massachusetts.

Kojiro M. (2007) Diagnostic discrepancy of early hepatocellular carcinoma between Japan and West. *Hepatology Research*, 37 (Suppl. 2), pp.S121–S124.

Kondo F, Kondo Y, Nagato Y, et al. (1994). Interstitial tumour cell invasion in small hepatocellular carcinoma. Evaluation in microscopic and low magnification views. *J Gastroenterol Hepatol*, 9(6), pp. 604-612.

Kurogi M, Nakashima O, Miyaaki H, et al. (2006) Clinicopathological study of scirrhous hepatocellular carcinoma. *J Gastroenterol Hepatol.*, 21(9), pp.1470-1477.

Lam KC, Ho JC, Yeung RT. (1982). Spontaneous regression of hepatocellular carcinoma: a case study. *Cancer*, 50, pp.332-336

Lau W, Leung K, Leung TW, et al. (1997). A logical approach to hepatocellular carcinoma presenting with jaundice. *Ann Surg.*, 225(3), pp.281-285.

Lawrence B, Perez-Atayde A, Hibbard MK, et al. (2000). TPM3-ALK and TPM4-ALK oncogenes in inflammatory myofibroblastic tumors. *Am J Pathol.*, 157, pp.377-384.

Lin TY. (1972). Tumors of the liver, part 1: primary malignant tumors. In : Bockus HL, Berk JE, Haubrich WS, et al. (eds). *Gastroenterology*, 3rd edn. WB Saunders, Philadelphia, pp.527.

Liver Cancer Study Group of Japan. (1987). *General Rules for the Clinical and Pathological Study of Primary liver cancer*, 2nd edn. Kanehara, Tokyo.

Liver Cancer Study Group of Japan. (2000). *General Rules for the Clinical and Pathological Study of Primary liver cancer*, 4th edn. Kanehara, Tokyo.

Long XY, Li YX, Wu W,et al. (2010). Diagnosis of bile duct hepatocellular carcinoma thrombus without obvious intrahepatic mass. *World J Gastroenterol.*, 21, 16(39), pp. 4998-5004.

Luciani A, Kobeiter H, Maison P, et al. (2002). Focal nodular hyperplasia of the liver in men: is presentation the same in men and women? *Gut*, 50(6), 877-880.

Magata S, Kitahara K, Watanabe K, et al. (2001). Fibrolamellar hepatocellular carcinoma-a case report. *Kanzo*, 42(8), pp.414-419.

Markovic S, Ferlan-Marolt V, Hlebanja Z. (1996). Spontaneous regression of hepatocellular carcinoma. *Am J Gastroenterol*; 91, pp.392-393.

McCaughan GW, Bilous MJ, Gallagher ND. (1985) Long-term survival with tumor regression in androgen-induced liver tumors. *Cancer*, 56, pp.2622-2626.

Naik S, Waris W, Carmosino L, et al. (2009). Primary squamous cell carcinoma of the liver. *J Gastrointestin Liver Dis.*, 18(4), 487-489.

Nakajima T, Moriguchi M, Watanabe T, et al. (2004). Recurrence of hepatocellular carcinoma with rapid growth after spontaneous regression. *World J Gastroenterol.*, 15, 10(22), pp.3385-3387.

Nakano M, Saito A, Yamamoto M, et al. (1997). Stromal and blood vessel wall invasion in well-differentiated hepatocellular carcinoma. *Liver*, 17(1), pp.41-46.

Nakashima Y, Nakashima O, Hsia CC, et al. (1999). Vascularization of small hepatocellular carcinomas: correlation with differentiation. *Liver*, 19(1), pp.12-18.

Nguyen BN, Fléjou JF, Terris B, et al. (1999). Focal nodular hyperplasia of the liver: a comprehensive pathologic study of 305 lesions and recognition of new histologic forms. *Am J Surg Pathol.*, 23(12), 1441-1454.

Nieweg O, Slooff MJ, Grond J. (1992). A case of primary squamous cell carcinoma of the liver arising in a solitary cyst. *HPB Surg*, 5, pp.203-208.

Rooks JB, Ory HW, Ishak KG, et al. (1979). Epidemiology of hepatocellular adenoma. The role of oral contraceptive use. *JAMA.*, 17, 242(7), pp.644-648.

Shimada M, Rikimaru T, Hamatsu T, et al. (2001). The role of macroscopic classification in nodular-type hepatocellular carcinoma. *Am J Surg.*, 182(2), pp.177-182.

Shiota K, Taguchi J, Nakashima O, et al. (2001) Clinicopathologic study on cholangiolocellular carcinoma. *Oncol Rep.*, 8(2), pp.263-268.

Shuangshoti S, Thaicharoen A. (1994). Hepatocellular adenoma in a beta-thalassemic woman having secondary iron overload. *J Med Assoc Thai.*, 77(2), pp.108-112.

Soreide O, Czerniak A, Bradpiece H, et al. (1986). Characteristics of fibrolamellar hepatocellular carcinoma. A study of nine cases and a review of the literature. *Am J Surg.*, 151(4), pp.518-523.

Soyer P, Laissy JP, Bluemke DA, et al. (1995). Bile duct involvement in hepatocellular carcinoma: MR demonstration. *Abdom Imaging.*, 20(2), pp.118-121.

Steiner PE, Higginson J. (1959) Cholangiolocellular carcinoma of the liver. Cancer., 12(4), pp.753-759.

Suzuki M, Okazaki N, Yoshino M. (1989). Spontaneous regression of a hepatocellular carcinoma: a case report. *Hepatogastroenterology*, 36, pp.160-163.

Takayasu K, Muramatsu Y, Shima Y, et al. (1986). Necrosis of hepatocellular carcinoma as a result of subintimal injury incurred by hepatic angiography: report of two cases. *Am J Gastroenterol.*, 81, pp.979-983.

Tocci G, Conte A, Guarascio P, et al. (1990). Spontaneous remission of hepatocellular carcinoma after massive gastrointestinal haemorrhage. *BMJ.*, 300, pp.641-642.

Tomioka T, Tsunoda T, Harada N, et al. (1987). Adenosquamous carcinoma of the liver. *Am J Gastroenterol.*, 82, pp.1203-1206.

Tomizawa M, Kondo F, Kondo Y. (1995). Growth patterns and interstitial invasion of small hepatocellular carcinoma. *Pathol Int.*, 45(5), pp.352-358.

Velazquez I, Alter BP. (2004). Androgens and liver tumors: Fanconi's anemia and non-Fanconi's conditions. *Am J Hematol.*, 77(3), pp.257-267.

Wang JH, Chen TM, Tung HD, et al. (2002). Color Doppler sonography of bile duct tumor thrombi in hepatocellular carcinoma. *J Ultrasound Med.*, 21(7), pp.767-772.

Wanless IR, Albrecht S, Bilbao J, et al. (1989). Multiple focal nodular hyperplasia of the liver associated with vascular malformations of various organs and neoplasia of the brain: a new syndrome. *Mod Pathol.*, 2(5), 456-462.

Wanless IR, Mawdsley C, Adams R. (1985). On the pathogenesis of focal nodular hyperplasia of the liver. *Hepatology.*, 5(6), pp.1194-1200.

Watanabe N, Yamauchi N, Maeda M, et al. (1994). Recombinant human tumor necrosis factor causes regression in patients with advanced malignancies. *Oncology*, 51, pp.360-365

Zen Y, Fujii T, Sato Y, et al. (2007). Pathological classification of hepatic inflammatory pseudotumor with respect to IgG4-related disease. *Mod Pathol.*, pp.884-894.

Zen Y, Harada K, Sasaki M, et al. (2004). IgG4-related sclerosing cholangitis with and without hepatic inflammatory pseudotumor, and sclerosing pancreatitis-associated sclerosing cholangitis: do they belong to a spectrum of sclerosing pancreatitis? *Am J Surg Pathol.*, 28(9), pp.1193-1203.

Part 2

Surgical Treatment

9

Major Hepatectomy without Allogeneic Blood Transfusion for Hepatocellular Carcinoma

Jing An Rui
Peking Union Medical College Hospital
Chinese Academy of Medical Sciences
China

1. Introduction

Hepatocellular carcinoma (HCC) is the fifth most common cancer in the world and the third leading cause of cancer-related deaths. More than 80% of HCC cases are from the Asian and African continents, and more than 50% of cases are from mainland China. It is estimated that more than 50% of liver cancers worldwide are attributable to HBV and up to 89% of HBV-related HCC are from developing countries. Recently, increasing trends in HCC incidence have been reported from several Western countries, including France, Australia, and the United States, mainly because of the rising incidence of HCV (McClune & Tong, 2010). At least one million new cases of HCC occur annually and mortality from this disease remains high (Munoz et al., 1988; Rustgi, 1987; Simonnetti et al., 1991). Surgery, including hepatectomy and transplantation, remains the main curative strategy for hepatocellular carcinoma. The history of hepatic surgery is strongly involved with the history of use of bleeding-control during hepatic operations. In the early 1900s a small but significant step forward was made in liver surgery by J. Hogarth Pringle, who in 1908 described a method for digital compression of the hilar vessels to control hepatic bleeding from traumatic injuries. Credit for the first anatomic liver resection is usually given to Lortat- Jacob, who performed a right hepatectomy in 1952 in France. Wang Chen En in 1961 was first to report a successful hepatic resection for liver cancer in China.

Blood loss during liver resection is one of the most important factors affecting the perioperative outcomes of patients undergoing liver resection. It has been accepted that intraoperative blood transfusion is a risk factor for tumor recurrence, and that infiltrative tumor type, surgical margin <10 mm and intraoperative blood transfusion are independent prognostic factors for overall survival.

1.1 Background

Blood transfusion has been found to be a highly significant factor which influences outcome of hepatectomy, and major bleeding and major blood transfusion during major hepatectomy are of especial importance.

The long-term survival of patients with hepatocellular carcinoma after hepatectomy depends on tumor staging, hepatic functional reserve before operation and history of blood transfusion. Preventing major intraoperative bleeding and avoiding allogeneic blood transfusion can significantly improve the disease free and overall survival rates in HCC patients. Rui et al., reported (Rui et al.; 2004) that major hepatectomy without allogeneic blood transfusion can reduce postoperative morbidity and recurrence rate of patients with HCC.

1.2 Selection of patients for right-trisectionectomy of huge liver tumor

Up to now, treatment of huge liver cancers is still very difficulty due to poor outcomes and higher mortality and mobidity (Hanazaki et al, 2001; Regimbeau et al, 1999). Since the middle of last century the right trisetionectomy (previous trisegmentectomy) has been used for huge hepatic neoplasms which involve the right and left medial sections of the liver (Quattlebaum 1953). Starzl described and clearly defined in detail a safe technique for right trisectionectomy (Starzl et al 1975). Most reports have indicated that right trisectionectomy is effective for extensive hepatic malignancy, based on patients who have had long-term survival after this operation (Sugiura et al., 1994; Yamamoto et al 1995). Rui reported on a retrospective series of patients in which thirty three cases of right trisectionectomy were all performed under normothermic interruption of the porta hepatis at single time for huge primary liver cancer. The 1-, 3- and 5- year survival rates after right trisectionectomy were 71.9%, 40.6% and 34.4%, respectively. Among the 33 cases of right trisectionectomy, 2 cases did not utilize allogeneic blood transfusion and had good recoveries (Rui et al., 2003). Up to now, the longest cancer free survival in our series is 23 years. This patient is still alive in Beijing.

The feasibility of right trisectionectomy for a given patient must be carefully evaluated according to the following criteria: (1). Tumor(s) (including less than 2 satellite nodules) limited to the right lobe and left medial portion of the liver. There must be no evidence of cancer invasion in the left lateral segment; (2). Tumor mass must have clear borders or a pseudocapsule, and there must be no tumor thrombus in the trunk of the portal vein and hepatic vein, but liver resection remains the only therapeutic option that may offer a chance of cure for HCC with PVTT (Lau WY et al 2008). There were 17 cases (51.5%) with tumor thrombi in the right branch of the portal vein in our right trisectionectomy patients (Rui JA et al 2003). (3). There must be no evidence of distant metastasis; (4). Compensatory enlargement of the left lateral section should be obvious; (5). The Child-Pugh classification of liver function must be "A" and the indocyanine green retention rate (ICGR 15) at 15 minutes should be lower than 15 % before surgery; (6). During the Child-Pugh classification of liver function is "A" and ICGR is less than 15%, the remnant liver volume can be at least 25% of whole liver. The CT volumetry can be utilized to determine the liver and tumor volume before surgery (Mandli et al 2008).

2. Surgical technology for major hepatectomy without allogenic blood transfusion

Major hepatectomy has recently been defined as a resection of four or more liver segments (Reddy et al., 2011) which differs from the former definition of "resection of three liver segment". Based on the evaluations of CT volumetry and liver functions (including Child-Pugh classification and ICGR test) the major hepatectomy under single time interruption of porta hepatis (continuous Pringle) can be done safely.

Control of hemorrhage is the key factor in liver resection for HCC. Blood loss of more than 1000 ml is defined as major bleeding. In patients with risk factors for bleeding, it is necessary to take effective steps in order to minimize intraoperative blood loss in hepatectomy for patients with HCC, so that allogeneic blood transfusion can be avoided. Surgeons play an important role in avoiding allogeneic blood transfusion and thus improving the prognosis of these patients. Rui performs major hepatectomy without allogeneic blood transfusion via a number of surgical techniques, including normothermic interruption of the porta hepatis at a single time and application of supplementary instruments. Moreover, the surgical procedures characterized by single time interruption of the porta hepatis for major hepatectomy, including right trisectionectomy have been used in more than thirty county and town hospitals located in thirteen provinces in China and have been demonstrated to be feasible and successful.

2.1 Surgical procedures characterized by single time interruption of the porta hepatis is requisite for major hepatectomy without allogeneic blood transfusion

Foster said: "Surgical technique is an art form. It can be very personal, based mostly on experience, or it can take a cookbook approach. For many standard operations, we follow in the ruts created by our teachers, perhaps adding a nuance or two called forth by an unusual situation or by a creative mind. Unfortunately, many years ago when I needed help, there was no available to teach me to operate on the liver." (Foster, 1989).

179 cases of hepatectomy for huge HCC were performed in our hospital from January 1995 to December 2002. Among these patients, 155 (86.6%) cases were males and 24 (13.4%) females, with ages ranging from 15 to 77 years (mean ± SD, 56.3 ± 13.7 years). 138 (77.1%) were hepatitis B surface antigen (HBsAg) positive and 144 (80.4%) had liver cirrhosis. 165 patients (92.2%) were evaluated as grade A and 14 (7.8%) were grade B in the Child-Pugh's classification prior to surgery. Tumor sizes ranged from 5 to 30 cm (mean ± SD, 7.9 ± 4.6 cm). Serum alpha-fetoprotein (AFP) in 63 patients (35.2%) was higher than 400 ng/ml and 75 patients were TNM stage II, 60 were stage III, 37 were stage IVa, and 7 were stage IVb. These hepatectomies were all performed under single time normothermic interruption of the porta hepatis. Interruption of flow through the porta hepatis lasted 15 to 40 minutes (mean ± SD, 25.3 ± 6.8 minutes). The ultrasonic dissector (CUSA System 200) was applied for dissecting hepatic parenchyma. These hepatectomy procedures included right trisectionectomy in 23 patients, left trisectionctomy in 4 patients, extended right hepatectomy in 11 patients, extended left hepatectomy in 3 patients, central hepatectomy in 4, right hepatectomy in 30, and left hepatectomy in 14 patients. The postoperative complication rate was 10.6% (19/179), and operative mortality was 1.1%. Postoperatively, overall and cancer-free survival rates at 1, 2, 3, 4 and 5 years were 82.0%, 56.7%, 51.1%, 46.2% and 40.2%; and 73.1%, 53.2%, 46.0%, 44.5% and 38.1%, respectively (Zhou et al., 2007). These results demonstrate that hepatectomy applying normothermic continuous single interruption of the porta hepatis, but not intermittent multiple occlusions of hepatic inflow is safe and tolerable for selected patients with HCC including many who also have cirrhosis.

At the same time, no damage to the liver has been found by either the electron microscopic examination of liver tissue biopsies or by liver function tests within 20 minutes of single time normothermic interruption of the porta hepatis. Our clinical practice has shown that a single time 20-42 minute normothermic interruption of the porta hepatis is safe with use of skilled surgical technique. Since 1984 we have applied single time normothermic interruption of the porta hepatis for all surgical hepatectomy procedures. We have carried out one hundred cases of hepatic resection without mortality under single time normothermic interruption of the porta hepatic in a period of 4 years (1984-1988), and our subsequent surgical mortality has been shown to be less than 1.3%.

Diminished bleeding by applying single time interruption of porta hepatis serves to avoid allogeneic blood transfusion during liver resection. We have conducted a retrospectively study of 51 patients who received hepatectomy without allogeneic blood transfusion. Of these patients whose ages ranged from 24 to 77 years (mean 46.5 years), 40 were men and 11 were women. Clinical diagnosis showed primary liver cancer in 29 patients, metastatic liver cancer in 6, hepatic hemangioma in 10, and benign hyperplasia in 6. TNM staging of the primary liver cancer showed 15 patients were stage II (51.8%), 10 patients were stage III (34.5%), and 4 were stage IVa. The mean tumor diameter was 8.7 cm (range 6.5 to 18 cm). Preoperative Child-Pugh classification for liver function was grade A in 34 patients (66.7%) and grade B in 17 (33.3%). Surgical procedures included right trisectionectomy in 2 patients (3.9%), right lobectomy in 6 (11.8%), left lobectomy in 7 (13.7%), medial hepatectomy in 3 (5.9%), and trisegmentectomy in 33 (64.7%). The mean operative time was 181 minutes (range 90 to 300 minutes). Single time normothermic interruption of the porta hepatis was applied in all procedures, with a mean interruption time of 16 minutes (range 8 to 35 minutes). The ultrasound dissector (CUSA System 200) was used for dissecting parenchyma of the liver, and intraoperative ultrasonography was used for localization of tumors. The mean blood loss was 755ml (range 400 to 2000 ml). Thirty-two patients (63.0%) accepted autologous blood transfusion (mean volume, 326 ml; range 200 to 600 ml). Pathologic examination showed hepatocellular carcinoma in 27 patients, mixed hepatocellular-cholangiocarcinoma in 2, liver metastasis of malignancies from colorectal cancer in 6 patients, hepatic cavernous hemangioma in 10 patients, and hepatic focal nodular hyperplasia in 6. At the same time there were 60 patients in the control group who received hepatectomy with allogeneic blood transfusion, including 48 cases of primary liver cancer. Blood was transfused routinely if the haemoglobin level fell to < 8g/dl. Fresh frozen plasma was transfused if the prothrombin time rose to >30s. As a result the operative mortality and morbidity rates in the study group (without allogeneic blood transfusion) were o%, and 9.8% respectively, while in the control group (allogeneic blood transfusion) mortality and morbidity were 3.3% and 28.3%, respectively. Cancer recurrence within three years was discovered in 9 of 51 pateints in the study group. The 1, 2 and 3 year cancer recurrence rates in the study group were 24.1%, 27.6%, and 31.0%, respectively; while in the control group 27 of 46 patients had tumor recurrence in the same period, and the 1, 2 and 3 year recurrence rates were 43.5%, 54.3% and 58.7%, respectively. Significant differences ($p < 0.05$) were present between these two groups (Rui et al., 2004) demonstrating the advantages of major hepatectomy applying single interruption of porta hepatis without allogeneic blood transfusion.

2.2 Application of supplementary instruments

2.2.1 Intraoperative ultrasound

Intraoperative ultrasonography (US) of the liver provides the surgeon with useful real-time diagnostic and staging information that may result in an alteration of the planned surgical approach. Current applications for intraoperative US of the liver include evaluation of tumor staging and metastatic survey, guidance for metastasectomy and various tumor ablation procedures, documentation of vessel patency, evaluation of intrahepatic biliary disease, and guidance for whole-organ or split-liver transplantation. To obtain the most useful information with intraoperative US, the sonographer must use a dedicated transducer and a scanning method appropriate for the purpose of the examination. Motohide applied 3D-US in 24 patients undergoing hepatic resection, and found that this technique allowed easy visualization of the tumors and vascular anatomy. It is thus considered to be an efficient and safe navigation system in liver surgery (Motohide et al., 1998). In addition, application of intraoperative US of the liver with current transducer resolution permits the identification of lesions larger than 2 mm. Sensitivity of more than 90% has been documented for detection of lesions in the liver, with positive and negative predictive values of 90% and 78%, respectively (Guimaraes et al., 2004). Since 1983, we have utilized intraoperative ultrasonography of the liver for patients with liver tumors. The sensitivity is more than 90% in our series which is consistent with what reported by Zacherl (2002).

2.2.2 Ultrasound dissector for dissecting parenchyma of the liver

Since November 1992 we have applied the ultrasonic dissector (CUSA system 200) for dissecting hepatic parenchyma, instead of using the previous finger fracture technique. Combined application of single time interruption of the porta hepatis and ultrasonic dissector can reduce intraoperative bleeding in liver resection. The advantages of applying this technique are: (1) It can reveal small vessels and segments of the biliary tree which are less than 2mm; (2) It allows damage to the portal vein and hepatic vein to be diminished resulting in less blood loss; (3) It promotes quick portal hepatic dissection and tumor resection. However, the disadvantage may be prolongation of operating time.

Fan reported that they performed major hepatectomy in 69 patients with the assistent of the ultrasonic dissector, and found that it is better than the crushing clamp and finger fracture technique in hepatectomy for hepatocellular carcinoma (Fan et al., 1996).

2.2.3 RF (radiofrequency) assisted liver resection technique

Milicevic et al reported that the sequential coagulate-cut, RF–assisted liver resection technique is a safe liver transection technique associated with minimal blood loss and it has facilitated tissue-sparing liver resection (Milicevic et al., 2007). Navarra reported RF-assisted liver resection (Navarra et al., 2004), in which the median resection time was 47.5 minutes (range 30-110) with median blood loss of 30 mls (range 15-992) and mean pre-operative and post-operative hemaglobin values of 13.5 g/dL (SD ± 1.7) and 11.6 g/dL (SD ± 1.4) respectively. No blood transfusion was registered, nor was any mortality observed. There was one post-operative complication which was a sub-phrenic abscess. The median postoperative stay was 8 days (range 5-86). Long reported: Over the past few years, a new technique for liver resection assisted with radiofrequency has been developed at the author's hospital, expanding the role of radiofrequency in liver surgery from mere tumor ablation to routine hepatic resection (Long R Jiao et al 2008). Ayav concluded that major hepatectomy using RF can decrease the rates of blood transfusion, postoperative liver failure, ICU admission, and postoperative stay. Moreover the price is significantly lower as compared to total vascular exclusion (Ayav et al., 2007).

3. Advantages from single time interruption of the portal hepatis without allogeneic blood transfusion in hepatectomy

3.1 Advantages from single time interruption of the porta hepatis

Since there is a lack of donors for liver trasplantation, liver resection continues to be the first choice for patients with resectable hepatocellular carcinoma with liver cirrhosis but compensated liver function. Univariate analysis has shown that the presence of portal vein tumor thrombosis and satellite nodules, high TNM stage, high Edmondson-Steiner grading, and blood transfusion are all associated with worsened prognosis (Zhou et al., 2007).

In a period of 8 years (from January 1995 to 2002) we successfully performed major hepatectomy in 81 patients with HCC combined with cirrhosis applying normothermic continuously single interruption of the porta hepatis. The mortality and morbidity rates were 1.2% and 24.7% respectively, indicating that the procedure can be carried out safely. Less blood loss and shorter operating time have been achieved in our cohort.

The significance of intermittent hepatic inflow occlusion for safe hepatectomy has been generally recognized (Man et al., 2003). Some surgeons have argued that intermittent interruption of flow through the porta hepatis leads to less liver injury during hepatic resection than with continuous flow interruption (Belghiti et al., 1999). Belghiti and Pol reported that the mean ischemic time under intermittent interruption of flow through the porta hepatis for hepatectomy was approximately 40 min (Belghiti et al., 1999; Pol et al., 1999), which is far longer than the mean ischemic time of 20.6 min that we reported with a single interruption of the porta hepatic for major hepatectomy. Our experience is similar to results of a recent prospective, randomized clinical trial from Italy (Capussotti et al., 2003). It is established that major hepatectomy under normothermic continuous interruption of flow through the porta hepatis is well tolerated by HCC patients, including those with liver cirrhosis, when the interruption time was well controlled. Thus, intermittent interruption of the porta hepatis may not be necessary (Zhou et al., 2007). It is easily understood that compared with intermittent multi hepatic inflow occlusions, continuous single interruption can simplify procedures, shorten operating time, and reduce blood loss, especially during transaction of liver parenchyma.

It is well known that reperfusion injury following ischemia is a clinically important process that contributes significantly to tissue damage (Mitchell & Cotran, 2003). Single time interruption of the porta hepatis during liver resection not only diminishes blood loss, but also attenuates reperfusion injury following ischemia as compared with multi-interruption of the porta hepatis.

3.2 Advantages of avoiding allogeneic blood transfusion

We have successfully performed major hepatectomy applying single time normothermic interruption of the porta hepatis in 51 patients without allogeneic blood transfusion, and have effectively limited intraopertive bleeding. It is evident that postoperative complications of major hepatectomy can be markedly reduced, recurrence rate can be decreased, and mortality can be decreased by avoiding allogeneic blood transfusion. Our results confirmed the conclusion that perioperative allogeneic blood transfusion is responsible for a relatively poor prognosis.

Poon reported that in a prospective study of 377 patients over 10 years, absence of perioperative transfusion is an independent favorable prognostic factor for disease-free survival, and improves survival results after resection for HCC (Poon et al., 2001).

3.3 Immunomodulation and blood transfusion

It is known that allogeneic blood transfusion-associated immunomodulation has been associated with alterations in immune function in transfusion recipients, including decreased ratio of helper T-lymphocytes to suppressor T-lymphocytes, attenuated function of natural killer cells, defective antigen presentation, and reduction in cell-mediated immunity (Blajchman, 2002). Perioperative allogeneic blood transfusion may play an important role in suppressing the host immune system, for example by decreasing natural killer cell activity (Hanna et al., 1980; Herberman, 1984) and/or increasing suppressor T-cell activity and inhibition of lymphocyte transformation, thereby diminishing specific and non-specific immune responses. These effects are possibly due to the cytological and immunological factors for tumor recurrence after blood transfusion allowing for progression of residual cancer and leading to a poor prognosis (Kaplan et al., 1984). Therefore, it is suggested that avoiding intraoperative and perioperative allogeneic blood transfusion is beneficial to patients with resectable HCC, particularly to those with large tumors (Rui et al., 2004; Sugita et al., 2007). For a better prognosis including prevention of recurrence and metastasis, and prolongation of survival time, the surgeon must master skilled surgical techniques, and apply suitable surgical procedures and supplementary instruments for hepatectomy, especially for major hepatectomies. In summary, hepatectomy without allogeneic blood transfusion is advantageous to diminishing surgical complications and improving the prognosis of HCC patients (Kaplan et al., 1984; Rui et al., 2004).

4. Case report

Case 1: A 15 years old boy was diagnosed with hepatocellular carcinoma, and a right trisectionectomy was performed with single time interruption of the porta hepatis. The resected tumor weighted 2000 gm (Figure1). The postoperative cancer free survival time was 6 years and the patient died of non-neoplastic disease.

Case 2: A 57 years old woman was diagnosed with hepatocellular carcinoma, and a right trisectionectomy was performed with single time interruption of the porta hepatic in 1988. The resected tumor weighted 2200gm (Figure2). She is still alive in Beijing 23 years after right trisectionectomy without recurrence.

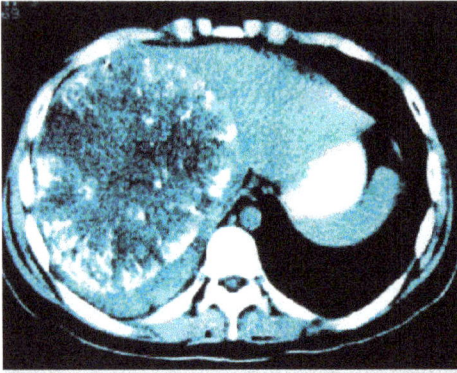
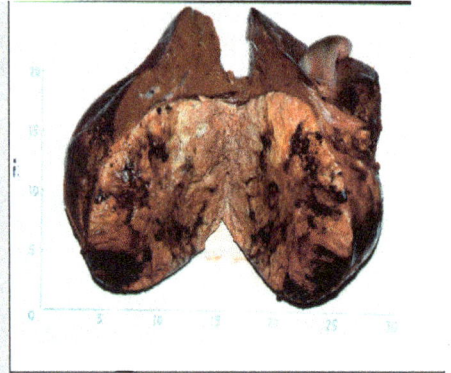

CT   Specimen

Fig. 1. The resected tumor tumor weighted 2000 gm from a 15 years old boy. This patient was operated for right trisectionectomy under single time interruption of the porta hepatis, and postoperative cancer free survival for 6 years, died of noncancerous disease.

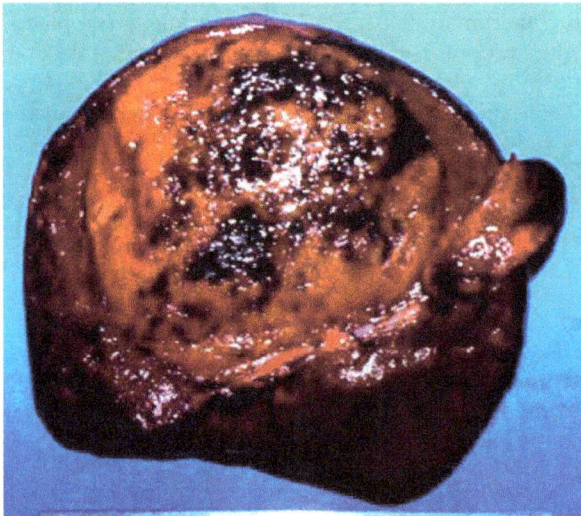

Fig. 2. The resected tumor weighted 2200gm with a diameter of 15X18cm from a 57 years old woman. This patient was operated for right trisectionectomy under single time interruption of the porta hepatis in 1988 and is still alive in Beijing 23 years after right trisectionectomy.

Case 3: A 24 years old man was diagnosed with hepatocellular carcinoma. A right trisectionectomy was performed under single time interruption of the porta hepatis, loss blood of intraoperation 1500ml, accepted autologous blood transfusion 600ml, without allogeneic blood transfution. The resected tumor weighted 2500 gm (Figure3). The patient was discharged from hospital after recovery at 32 days after operation.

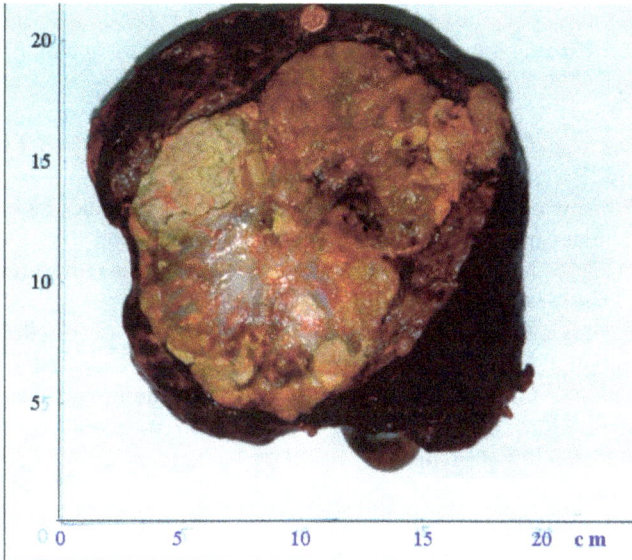

Fig. 3. The resected tumor weighted 2500gm with a diameter of 17.5X13.7cm from a 24 years old man. This patient was operated for right trisectionectomy under single time interruption of the porta hepatis without allogeneic blood transfusion and discharged from hospital after recovery at 32 days after operation. The pathologic disnosis was hepatocellular carcinoma.

5. References

Ayav, A., Navarra, G., Basaglia, E., Tierris, J., Healey, A., Spalding, D., Canelo, R ., Habib, NA. & Jiao, LR. (2007). Results of major hepatectomy without vascular clamping using radiofrequency-assisted technique compared with total vascular exclusion. *Hepatogastroenterology.*Vol. 54 , No.75, pp.806-809.

Belghiti, J., Noun, R., Malafosse,R., et al. (1999). Continuous versus intermittent portal triad clamping for liver resection : a controlled study . *Ann Surg,*Vol. 229, pp. 369- 375.

Blajchman, MA. (2002). Immunomodulation and blood transfusion. *American Journal of Therapeutics.* Vol.9, No.5, pp.389-395.

Capussotti, L., Muratore, A., Massucco, P, et al. (2004). Major liver resections for hepatocellular carcinoma on cirrhosis : early and long-term outcomes. *Liver Transpl.* *Vol.10 (Suppl 1),* pp. 64-68 。

Capussotti, L., Nuzzo, G., Polastri, R., et al. (2003) Continuous versus intermittent portal triad clamping during hepatectomy in clinical trial. *Hepatogastroenterology.* Vol. 50, pp.1073-1077.

Foster, JH. (1989). Liver Resection Techniques .*Surgical C linics of North America.* Vol. 69, No. 2, pp. 235-249.

Fan, ST., Lai, EC., Lo, CM., Chu, KM., Liu, CL.,& Wong, J. (1996). Hepatectomy with an ultrasonic dissector for hepatocellular carcinoma. *Br J Surg*, Vol. 83, No.1, pp.117-120.

Guimaraes ,CM., Correia, MM.,& Baldisserotto, M.(2004). Intraoperative ultrasonography of the liver in patients with abdominal tumors : a new approach. *J Ultrasound Med*, Vol.23, pp.1549-1555.

Hanazaki, K., Kajikawas, S. & Shimozawa, N. (2001). Hepatic resection for large hepatocellular carcinoma. *Am J Surg*, .Vol. 181, pp. 347-353.

Herberman, RB., (1984). Natural killer cells and their possible roles in host resistance against tumors. *Transplant Proc*, Vol.16, pp.476–478.

Hanna, N., Fidler, IJ. (1980). Role of natural killer cells in the destruction of circulating tumor emboli. *J Natl Cancer Inst*, Vol.65, pp.801–809.

Kaplan, J., Sarnaik, S., Gitlin, J. & Lusher, J. (1984). Diminished helper/suppressor lymphocyte ratios and natural killer activity in recipients of repeated blood transfusion. *Blood*, Vol.64, pp.308–310.

Li, CH., Chau, GY., Lui ,WY., Tsay, SH., King, KL., Hsia, CY. & Wu, CW. (2003). Risk factors associated with intra-operative major blood loss in patients with hepatocellular carcinoma who underwent hepatic resection. *Journal of the Chinese medicine Assocication : JMCA*.Vol. 66, No.1, pp. 669- 675.

Lau, WY., Lai, Eric CH. & Yu, Simon CH. (2008). Management of Portal Vein Tumor Thrombus, In: *Hepatocellular carcinoma*, Lau WY, pp.739-760, World Scientific, Singapore.

Long, R.Jiao. & Habib, NA. (2008). Radiofrequency-Assisted Liver Resection, In: *Hepatocellular carcinoma*, W.Y. Lau, pp.551-567, World Scientific, Singapore.

Munoz, N. & Bosch, X.. (1988). Epidemiology of hepatocellular carcinoma. In: Okuda, K., Ishak, KG. eds. *Neoplasms of the liver*. Springer-Yerlag, Berlin, Germany, pp.3-19.

Man, K., Lo, CM., Liu, CL, et al . (2003) Effects of the intermittent Pringle manoeuvre on hepatic gene expression and ultrastructure in a randomized clinical study. *Br J Surg*.Vol. 90, pp.183-198.

Mandli T, Fazakas J, Ther G. et al. (2008). Evaluation of liver function before living donor liver transplantation and liver resection. *Orv Hetil*. Vol.149, No.17, pp.779-786.

McClune, AC. & Tong M J. (2010). Chronic Hepatitis B and Hepatocellular Carcinoma, *Clinics in Liver Disease*, Vol.14, No. 3, pp. 461-476

Mitchell, RN. & Cotran, RS. (2003). Cell injury, adaptation and death, In: *Basic Pathology* (7th edition), Kuman Vinay, Cotran Ramzi S. and Robbins Stanley L., pp.9, Elsevier, ISBN: 0-7216-9274-5, Singapore

Milicevic, M., Bulajic, P., Zuvela, M., Dervenis, C., Basaric ,D. & Galun, D. (2007). A radiofrequency-assisted minimal blood loss liver parenchyma dissection technique. *Digestive Surgery*, Vol.24, No.4, pp.306-313.

Morris A Blajchman. (2002). Immunomodulation and Blood Transfusion. *America Journal of Therapeutics*, Vol.9, No. 5, pp. 389-395.

Motohide, S., Go, W., Masahiro, O., Hiroshi, H. & Masaki, K. (1998)Clinical application of three-dimensional ultrasound imaging as intraoperative navigation for liver surgery. Nihon Geka Gakkai Zasshi. Vol.99, No.4, pp.3-7.

Navarra, G., Lorenzini, C., Currò, G., Sampiero, G., & Habib, NH., (2004). Radiofrequency-assisted hepatic resection--first experience. *Ann Ital Chir,* Vol.75, No.1, pp.53-67.

Pringle, JH. (1908). Notes on arrest of hepatic hemorrhage due to trauma. *Ann Surg* ,Vol.48, pp.541-549.

Pol, B., Campan, P., Hardwigsen, J., et al. (1999). Morbidity of major hepatic resections: a 100-case prospective study. *Eur J Surg,* Vol.165, pp. 446-453.

Poon, RT., Fan, ST., Lo, CM., Ng, IO., Liu, CL., Lam ,CM. & Wong,J. (2001). Improving survival results after resection of hepatocellular carcinoma: a prospective study of 377 patients over 10 years. *Ann Surg,* Vol. 234, No.1, pp. 63-70.

Quattlebaum ,JK. (1953) .Massive resection of the liver. *Ann Surg,* Vol. 137. pp.787-796.

Reddy, SK., Barbas, AS., Turley, RS., Steel, JL., Tsung, A., Marsh, JW., Geller, DA. & Clary,BM. (2011). A standard definition of major hepatectomy: resection of four or more liver segments. *HPB,* Vol.13, N0. 7, pp. 494-502.

Rustgi, VK. (1987). Epidemiology of hepatocellular carcinoma. *Gastroenrol, Clin North Am* . Vol.16, pp. 545-551

Rui, JA., Wang, SB., Chen, SG., & Zhou, L . (2003). Right trisectionectomy for primary liver cancer. *World J Gastroenterol,* Vol. 9, No. 4, pp. 706-709.

Regimbeau, JM., Farges, O. & Shen, BY. (1999). Is surgery for large hepatocellular carcinoma justified ? *J Hepatol* , Vol. 31, pp.1062-1068.

Rui, JA., Zhou, L,, Liu, FD., Chu, QF, Wang, SB., Chen, SG., Qu, Q., Wei, X., Han, K., Zhang, N. & Zhao, HT. (2004). Major hepatectomy without blood transfusion : report of 51 cases.*Chinese Medical Journal.* Vol.117, No.5, pp.673-676.

Simonnetti, RG., Camma, C., Fiorello, F.et al. (1991). Hepatocellular carcinoma. A worldwide probelem and the major risk factors. *Dig Dis Sci.* Vol.36, pp.962-972.

Starzl, TE., Bell, RH., & Beart ,RW .(1975). Hepatic trisegmentectomya and other liver resections. *Surg Gynecol Obstet.* Vol.141, pp. 429-437.

Sugiura,Y., Nakamura, S. & Lida S. (1994). Extensive resection of the bile ducts combined with liver resection for cancer of the main hepatic duct junction: a cooperative study of the keio Bile Duct Cancer Study Group . *Surgery,* Vol.155, pp. 445-451.

Sugita,S., Sasaki, A, Iwaki,K, Uchida, H., Kai, S., Shibata, K. & Ohtab, S. (2008). Prognosis and postoperative lymphocyte count in patients with hepatocellular carcinoma who received intraoperative allogenic blood transfusion: A retrospective study. *EJSO,* Vol. 34, pp. 339-345

Thompson, HH., Tompkins, RK. & Longmire, WP Jr .(1983). Major hepatic resection. A 25-year experience. *Ann Surg.* Vol.197, pp.375-388.

Tjandra, J J., Fan, ST., & Wong, J. (1991). Peri-operative mortality in hepatic resection. *Aust. NZJ* , *Surg.* Vol.61, pp.201-206.

Yamamoto, M., Miura, K. &Yoshioka, M. (1995). Disease-free survival for 9 years after liver resection for stage IV gallbladder cancer: report of a case. *Surg Today* , Vol.25, pp.750-753.

Zhou,Li., Rui, JA.& Wang, SB. (2007). Outcomes and prognostic factors of cirrhotic patients with hepatocellular carcinoma after radical major hepatectomy. *World J Surg* ,Vol. 31, pp. 1782-1787.

Zacherl, J., Scheuba, C., Imhof, M., et al. (2002). Curret value of intraoperative sonography during surgery for hepatic neoplasms. *World J Surg,* Vol. 26, No.5, pp. 550-554.

10

Pure Laparoscopic Hepatectomy for HCC Patients

Zenichi Morise
Department of Surgery, Fujita Health University School of Medicine
Banbuntane Houtokukai Hospital, Otobashi Nakagawa-ku, Nagoya Aichi
Japan

1. Introduction

Pure laparoscopic hepatectomy is thought to be a less invasive procedure than conventional open hepatectomy for the resection of hepatic lesions (1). Recent development of devices facilitates expansion of the indication of the procedure (2, 3). At the present moment, common advantages of laparoscopic surgery, such as early recovery and discharge with smaller postoperative pain and earlier intake, have been reported (4). However, specific advantages and/or disadvantages of pure laparoscopic hepatectomy for the settlement of the indication have yet to be sufficiently discussed.

On the other hand, at the treatment of hepatocellular carcinoma (HCC) with liver cirrhosis, considerations for the control of invasive surgical stress, especially to impaired liver, should be placed besides oncological therapeutic effects. Patients with severe liver cirrhosis have various (overt and preliminary) symptoms, such as 1) deteriorations of protein synthesis and metabolism, 2) congestion of GI tract, ascites, pancytopenia due to portal hypertension and hypersplenism, 3) susceptibility to infectious diseases and hepatopulmonary syndrome (hypoxaemia) due to increased shunt vessels (5). Cirrhotic patients have high morbidity and mortality at undergoing anesthesia and surgery (6) and the risk of abdominal operations increases according to the preoperative Child's class of the patients (7). Hepatic resection for severe cirrhotic patients, even minimum, often develops refractory ascites which leads to fatal complications (8, 9). In Japan, the criteria based on 3 parameters (the presence or absence of ascites, total serum billirubin level, and indocyanine green retension rate at 15 minutes (ICG R15)) have been widely used for patient selection of hepatectomy (10). Nowadays, surgical resection, local ablation therapy or transarterial chemoembolization is adapted to each HCC patient with liver cirrhosis depending on the tumor condition and the liver function.

However, not small number of HCC patients with severe liver dysfunction exists who is not able to undergo those treatment modalities due to liver function, tumor size and/or localization, especially after repeat treatments for the disease. Furthermore, not small portion of patients need the repeat treatments for multicentric metachronous lesions occurred in chronic impaired liver. For thosee patients, "less invasive" pure laparoscopic hepatectomy may provide a good option.

2. Pure laparoscopic hepatectomy for HCC patients with liver cirrhosis- our experiences

From May 2005, 21 patients with hepatocellular carcinoma and chronic liver disease underwent pure laparoscopic hepatectomy. There were 6 out of 21 patients had severe liver cirrhosis (Child-Pugh B/C and ICG R15 of 40% or above) (Table 1). These 6 patients and the other 14 patients (Child A and ICG R15: 10.1- 27.4 (median: 13.4) %, excluded the patient with HCC and rectal carcinoma) were compared in operating time, intraoperative blood loss, day of oral ingestion started, day of drain removal, total dose of drain discharge from the operation day to post operative day 3, complication, and postoperative hospital stay.

Age, Sex	Background liver disease	Child-Pugh (ICGR15 (%))	TB/DB (mg/dl)	PT (%)	Alb (g/dl)	Tumor location, Tumor size (mm)	Postoperative Complication
64, M	B,C	B (42.8%)	1.3/0.3	79	3.2	S4 and 2-3, 44	Cholecyctitis
53, M	B	B (41.2%)	1.5/0.4	75	3.4	S5-6, 28	no
68, F	C	C (58.2%)	2.2/0.5	58	2.6	S8, 13	no
40, M	Alc	B (52.5%)	1.7/0.4	74	2.8	S6-7, 20	no
50, M	C	C (48.9%)	2.1/1.0	66	2.7	S5, 18	no
75, F	C	B (42.5%)	1.3/0.8	63	3.2	S3, 30	no

Table 1. Patients with severe liver cirrhosis who underwent pure laparoscopic hepatectomy
B: type-B viral hepatitis, C: type-C viral hepatitis, Alc: alcoholic hepatitis

For 6 patients with HCC and severe liver cirrhosis who underwent pure laparoscopic hepatectomy, the operating time was 140-341 (median: 232) minutes (for other patients with mild/moderate liver cirrhosis: 216-528 (295) minutes), the intraoperative blood loss was uncountable-213 (median: 58) ml (for other patients with mild/moderate liver cirrhosis: uncountable -696 (43) ml), the day of oral ingestion started was postoperative day 1-3 (median: 2) (for other patients with mild/moderate liver cirrhosis: day 2-3 (2)), the day of drain removal was postoperative day 3-6 (median: 4) (for other patients with mild/moderate liver cirrhosis: day 4-6 (5)), the total dose of drain discharge from the operation day to post operative day 3 was 279-1990 (median: 820) ml (for other patients with mild/moderate liver cirrhosis: 141-1275 (416) ml), and the postoperative hospital stay was 11-21 (median: 17) days (for other patients with mild/moderate liver cirrhosis: 9-254 (20) days). One patient developed postoperative complication of cholecystitis among 6 patients with severe liver cirrhosis, and 2 patients developed postoperative complication of ileus and refractory ascites among other 14 patients. There was no post-operative mortality in both groups. These results of perioperative course were comparable without statistically significant difference in the two groups. Perioperative course of HCC patients with severe liver cirrhosis who underwent pure laparoscopic hepatectomy was favorable and comparable to that of the other HCC patients with mild/moderate liver cirrhosis. (A case is shown in figures 1-5)

Also, repeat pure laparoscopic hepatectomy (and combined treatments) for patients with liver cirrhosis and multicentric/metachronous HCCs was feasible and safe with advantage of less post-operative adhesion. (A case is shown in figures 6-10)

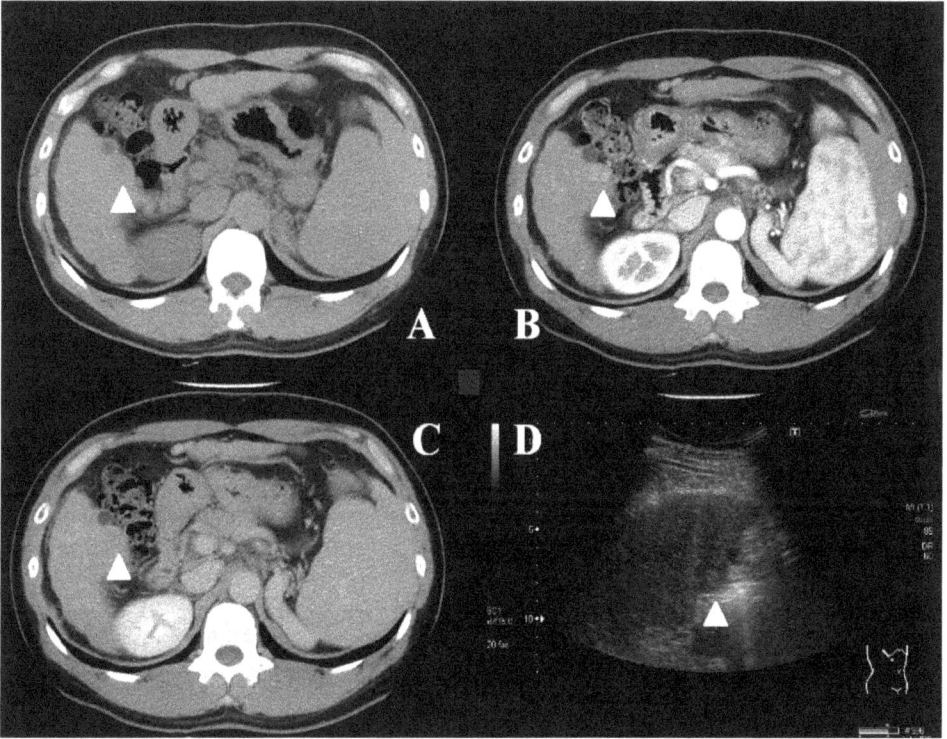

Fig. 1. A case with hepatocellular carcinoma and severe liver cirrhosis treated with pure laparoscopic hepatectomy
50 years old man with type-C severe liver cirrhosis (Table 1, patient 5) developed 2 cm hepatocellular carcinoma (HCC) at the undersurface area of the segments 5, revealed in computed tomography (plain (A), arterial phase with contrast (B), venous phase (C)) and ultrasonography (D).

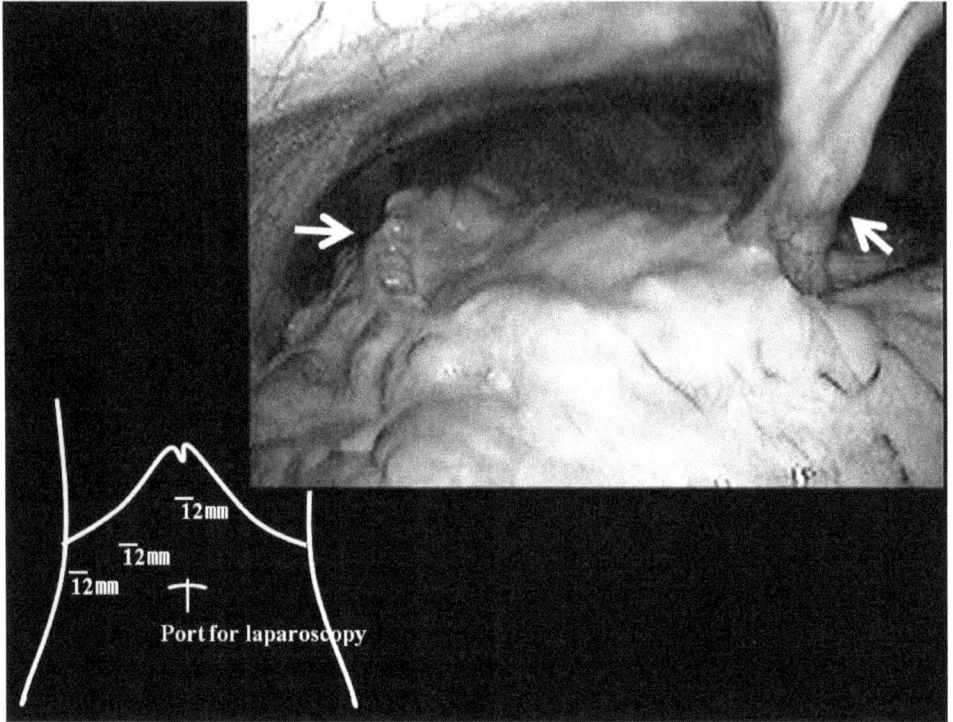

Fig. 2. Intraoperative findings of the case in figure 1 (1)
The liver was highly atrophic with large shunt vessels in the round ligament and the hepatic flexure of the colon was migrating into the subphrenic space.

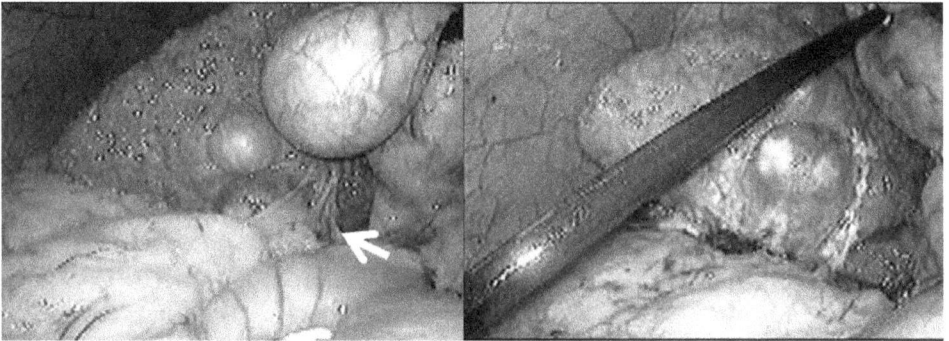

Fig. 3. Intraoperative findings of the case in figure 1 (2)
There were mild adhesions around the tumor. Dissection of the adhesion was performed, but not the mobilization of the liver. Since the liver was highly atrophic and the tumor was located deeply in the subphrenic space, mobilization of the liver was necessary for safe resection of the tumor under laparotomy. However, with laparoscopy, good direct vision and safe resection was obtained without mobilization.

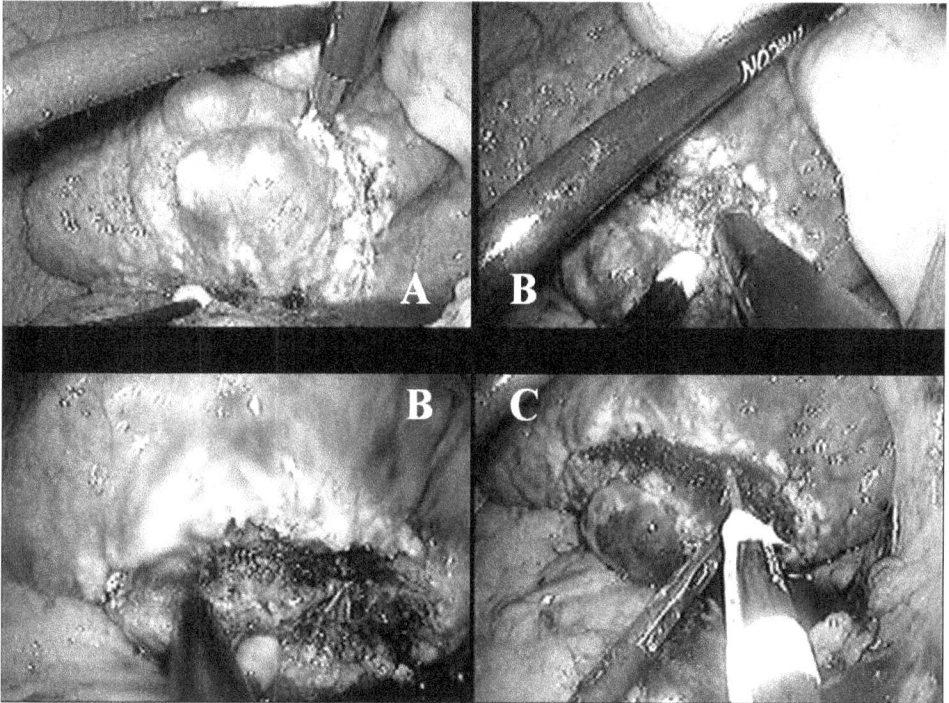

Fig. 4. Intraoperative findings of the case in figure 1 (3)

(A) After intraoperative ultrasonography, shallow cut in the surface area of the liver was made with harmonic scalpel.

(B) In the deeper area of the liver, dissection was performed with CUSA, monopolar and bipolar electric cautery. Thicker vessels were clipped or ligated and divided.

(C) The tissue with good coagulation with bipolar and monopolar was cut with scissors.

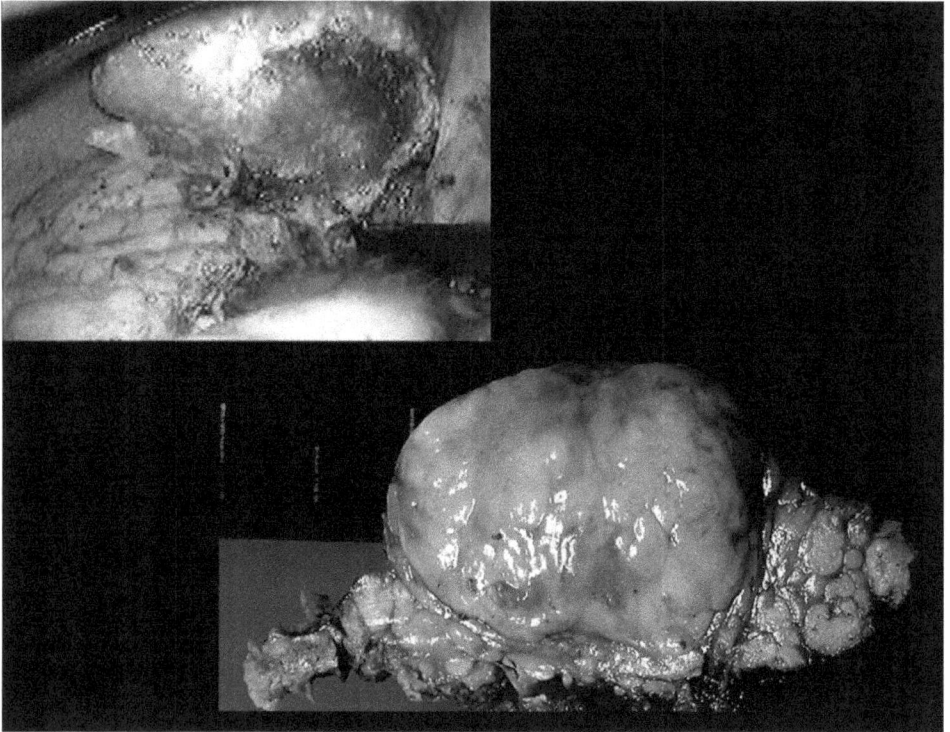

Fig. 5. Intraoperative findings (4) and resected specimen of the case in figure 1
The operation time was 140 minutes and intraoperative blood loss was 100ml. His post-operative hospital stay was uneventfull and 11 days. Pathologically, the tumor was moderately differentiated HCC in well differentiated HCC. He is alive without recurrence at 16 months after surgery

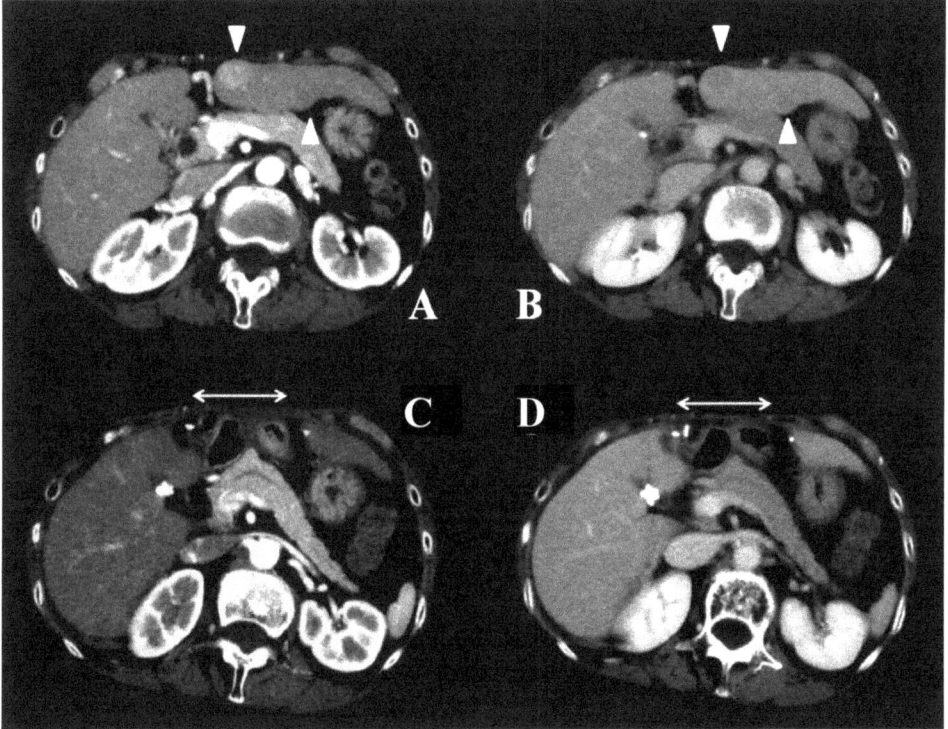

Fig. 6. A case with multicentric metachronous hepatocellular carcinomas and liver cirrhosis treated repeatedly with pure laparoscopic hepatectomy
69 years old woman with type-C liver cirrhosis developed 2 cm HCC in the segments 3 and 1.5cm in the border of segments 2 and 3, revealed in computed tomography (upper, arterial phase with contrast (A), venous phase (B)) and underwent pure laparoscopic hepatectomy (lower, arterial phase with contrast (C), venous phase (D)) in 2008. Pathological findings of the tumors were moderately (S3) and well (S2-3) differentiated hepatocellular carcinomas.

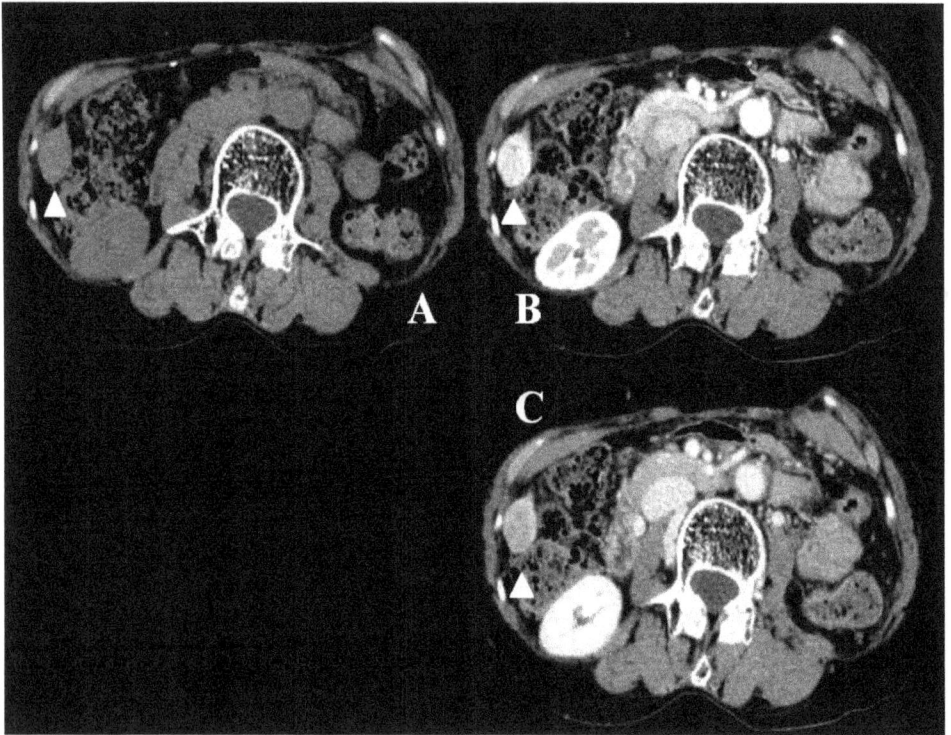

Fig. 7. A case with multicentric metachronous hepatocellular carcinomas and liver cirrhosis treated repeatedly with pure laparoscopic hepatectomy (2)

In 2010, she developed 2.5 cm HCC at the undersurface area of the segments 6, revealed in computed tomography (plain (A), arterial phase with contrast (B), venous phase (C)) and ultrasonography. She also had two small hypovascular lesions in the borders of segments 3 and 4, and of segments 4 and 8.

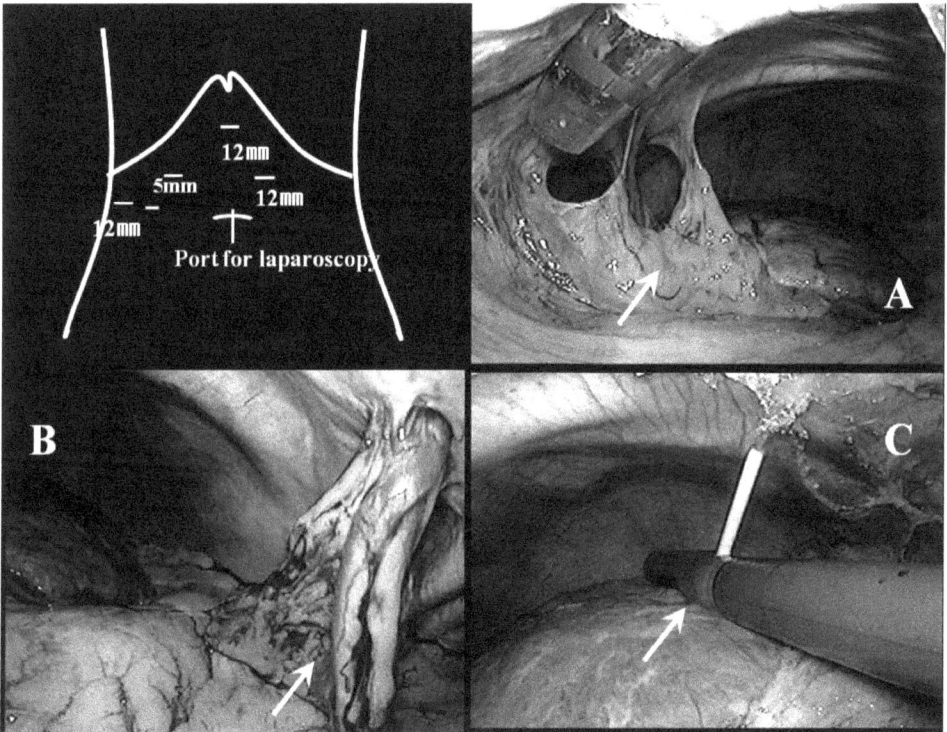

Fig. 8. Intraoperative findings of the case in figure 7 (1)
Adhesions were observed at the resected area of the liver (A) and the port site (B). There was shunt vessel formation in the port site adhesion. Two small hypovascular lesions in the borders of segments 3 and 4, and of segments 4 and 8 were ablated with US-guided intraoperative MCT (C).

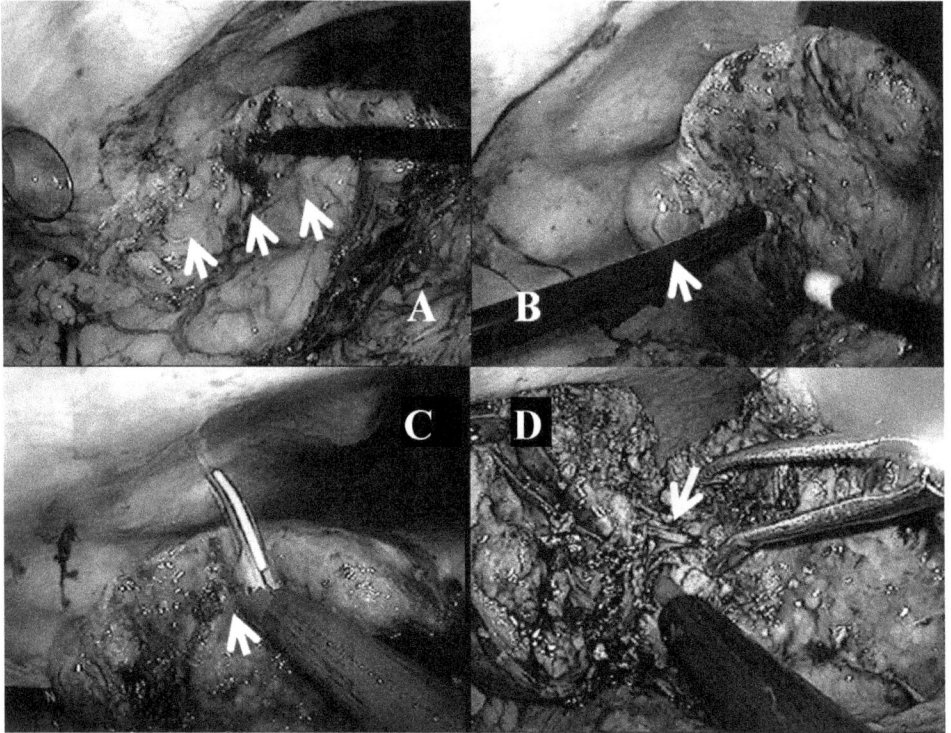

Fig. 9. Intraoperative findings of the case in figure 7 (2)
There were also adhesions at the undersurface area of the right lobe of the liver after
laparoscopic cholecystectomy performed 8 years ago (A). Dissection of the adhesion, but not
the mobilization of the liver, exposed the tumor (B). After intraoperative ultrasonography,
shallow cut in the surface area of the liver was made with harmonic scalpel (C). In the
deeper area of the liver, dissection was performed with CUSA, monopolar and bipolar
electric cautery. Thicker vessels were clipped or ligated and divided (D).

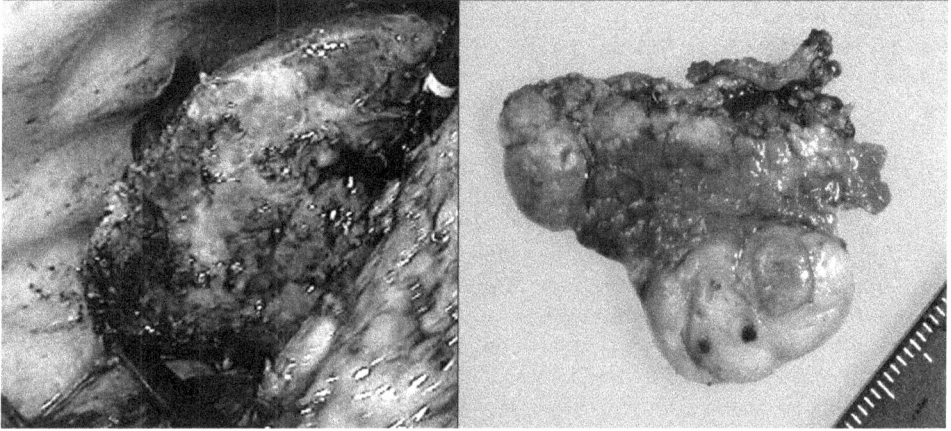

Fig. 10. Intraoperative findings of the case in figure 7 (3) and resected specimen of the case in figure

The operation time was 168 minutes and intraoperative blood loss was 30ml. Her post-operative hospital stay was uneventfull 9 days. Pathologically, the tumor was moderately differentiated HCC. She is alive without recurrence at 6 months after surgery

3. Discussion

Mirnezami et al recently reported systematic review and meta-analysis for short- and long-term outcomes after laparoscopic and open hepatic resection, with twenty-six studies met the inclusion criteria with a population of 1678 patients (60% of the patients had malignant liver tumor) (11). In their study, laparoscopic hepatectomy resulted in longer operating time, but reduced blood loss, portal clamp time, overall and liver-specific complications, and length of post-operative hospital stay. No difference was found between two groups for oncological outcomes. The benefits of laparoscopy may be particularly great for cirrhotic patients, given the potential for lower levels of parietal and hepatic injury and the preservation of venous and lymphatic collateral circulation. The safety and feasibility of the laparoscopic approach and its short-term benefits for HCC have been demonstrated by a few series to date (12-19). Tranchart et al recently reported laparoscopic resection of HCC for selected patients gave a better postoperative outcome without long- and short-term oncologic consequences from their series (42 each laparoscopic- and open-hepatectomy patients, with more than 96% Child A patients and mostly anatomical resection) (20). In our experience, perioperative course of 6 HCC patients with severe liver cirrhosis (Child B/C and ICG R15 of 40% or above) who underwent pure laparoscopic hepatectomy was favorable and comparable to that of the other HCC patients with mild/moderate liver cirrhosis.

Early postoperative recovery and discharge with smaller postoperative pain and earlier intake are advantages in pure laparoscopic hepatectomy for severe cirrhotic patients as the other laparoscopic surgery. On top of that, we consider that relatively small amount (median 230 ml/day) of drain discharge of severe liver cirrhosis patients, some (case 3, 5, 6 in table 1) of whom had mild or controllable ascites before surgery, was the other benefit of pure laparoscopic hepatectomy for these patients in our series. Pure laparoscopic hepatectomy might have possible advantage of minimal postoperative drain discharge (ascites) which leads to lower risk of disturbance in water/electrolyte balance and hypoproteinemia. These disorders could trigger fatal liver failure. There are also reports which described little development of postoperative ascites on laparoscopic hepatectomy (14, 17). In case of pure laparoscopic hepatectomy for severe cirrhotic patients, this feature could be the most remarkable specific advantage for postoperative course. Patients who undergo hepatectomy are exposed three different types of stresses, 1) general surgical stress for whole body depends on operating time, amount of bleeding etc, 2) reduced liver function due to resected liver volume, 3) injury for liver parenchyma and environment around the liver by surgical procedure (destruction of the collateral blood and lymphatic flow caused by laparotomy and mobilization of the liver and, also, mesenchymal injury caused by compression of the liver). We consider that the reduction of the third type of stress mentioned above with pure laparoscopic hepatectomy leads to lowering the risk of refractory ascites, resulting in reduced risk of successive complications and smooth recovery for HCC patients with severe liver cirrhosis.

Liver surface HCC with severe liver cirrhosis is not the good candidate of percutaneous ablation therapy due to the concern about hemorrhage, tumor dissemination, and injury of adjacent organs. There are reports of microwave or radiofrequency ablation therapy under mini-laparotomy or laparoscopy for those tumors as safe and less invasive procedure (21). However, surgery should obtain better control for the tumor located in the surface area with minimum reduction of liver function, as Buell et al described (22). We think pure laparoscopic hepatectomy for those tumors with minimum invasiveness could be established as a feasible and more effective treatment modality. The tumor located deep in the liver with severe cirrhosis should be good candidate of percutaneous ablation therapy. The resection of the tumor located in the surface but bare area of the liver should need dissection of the attachments and mobilization of the liver. For these tumors, transpleural or retroperitoneal approach may need to be considered for reducing invasiveness. For the extension of the indication, hand-assisted laparoscopic hepatectomy with the incision for hand port in the lower abdomen (2), robotic hepatectomy (23), and single-incision laparoscopic hepatectomy (24) might be a good option as conventional pure laparoscopic hepatectomy, although further investigation is needed.

In conclusion, our experiences suggest that pure laparoscopic hepatectomy for HCC patients with severe liver cirrhosis has specific advantage of minimal postoperative ascite production which leads to lower risk of disturbance in water/electrolyte balance and hypoproteinemia. The procedure minimize destruction of the collateral blood and lymphatic flow caused by laparotomy and mobilization of the liver and, also, mesenchymal injury caused by compression of the liver. It restrains the complications, which lead to the postoperative serious liver failure, such as massive ascites. Severe cirrhotic patients with tumors on the surface of the liver, in case of difficult adaptation of percutaneous ablation therapy and/or local recurrence after repeat treatments, are the good candidates for this procesure. Furthermore, repeat pure laparoscopic hepatectomy (and combined treatments) for patients with liver cirrhosis and multicentric/metachronous HCCs was feasible and safe with advantage of less post-operative adhesion and the procedure could be good option of bridging therapy to liver transplantation for the patients with severe liver cirrhosis and small HCC.

4. References

[1] Kaneko H, Tsuchiya M, Otsuka Y, Yajima S, Minagawa T, Watanabe M, Tamura A. Laparoscopic hepatectomy for hepatocellular carcinoma in cirrhotic patients. J Hepatobiliary Pancreat Surg. 2009;16(4):433-8.

[2] World Consensus Conference on Laparoscopic Surgery. The international position on laparoscopic liver surgery: The Louisville Statement, 2008. Ann Surg. 2009;250(5):825-30.

[3] Tsuchiya M, Otsuka Y, Tamura A, Nitta H, Sasaki A, Wakabayashi G, Kaneko H. Status of endoscopic liver surgery in Japan: a questionnaire survey conducted by the Japanese Endoscopic Liver Surgery Study Group. J Hepatobiliary Pancreat Surg. 2009;16(4):405-9.

[4] Viganò L, Tayar C, Laurent A, Cherqui D. Laparoscopic liver resection: a systematic review. J Hepatobiliary Pancreat Surg. 2009;16(4):410-21.

[5] Hoeper MM, Krowka MJ, Strassburg CP. Portopulmonary hypertension and hepatopulmonary syndrome. Lancet. 2004;363(9419):1461-8.

[6] Ziser A, Plevak DJ, Wiesner RH, Rakela J, Offord KP, Brown DL. Morbidity and mortality in cirrhotic patients undergoing anesthesia and surgery. Anesthesiology. 1999;90(1):42-53.

[7] Mansour A, Watson W, Shayani V, Pickleman J. Abdominal operations in patients with cirrhosis: still a major surgical challenge. Surgery. 1997;122(4):730-5.

[8] Belghiti J, Hiramatsu K, Benoist S, Massault P, Sauvanet A, Farges O. Seven hundred forty-seven hepatectomies in the 1990s: an update to evaluate the actual risk of liver resection. J Am Coll Surg. 2000;191(1):38.

[9] Lai EC, Fan ST, Lo CM, Chu KM, Liu CL, Wong J. Hepatic resection for hepatocellular carcinoma. An audit of 343 patients. Ann Surg. 1995;221(3):291–8.

[10] Torzilli G, Makuuchi M, Inoue K, Takayama T, Sakamoto Y, Sugawara Y, Kubota K, Zucchi A. No-mortality liver resection for hepatocellular carcinoma in cirrhotic and noncirrhotic patients: is there a way? A prospective analysis of our approach. Arch Surg. 1999;134(9):984-92.

[11] Mirnezami R, Mirnezami AH, Chandrakumaran K, Abu Hilal M, Pearce NW, Primrose JN, Sutcliffe RP. Short- and long-term outcomes after laparoscopic and open hepatic resection: systematic review and meta-analysis. HPB 2011;13(5):295–308.

[12] Chen HY, Juan CC, Ker CG. Laparoscopic liver surgery for patients with hepatocellular carcinoma. Ann Surg Oncol 2008;15(3):800–806

[13] Dagher I, Lainas P, Carloni A, Caillard C, Champault A, Smadja C, Franco D. Laparoscopic liver resection for hepatocellular carcinoma. Surg Endosc 2008;22(2):372–378

[14] Laurent A, Cherqui D, Lesurtel M, Brunetti F, Tayar C, Fagniez PL. Laparoscopic liver resection for subcapsular hepatocellular carcinoma complicating chronic liver disease. Arch Surg. 2003;138(7):763–9.

[15] Kaneko H, Takagi S, Otsuka Y, Tsuchiya M, Tamura A, Katagiri T, Maeda T, Shiba T. Laparoscopic liver resection of hepatocellular carcinoma. Am J Surg 2005;189(2):190–194

[16] Cherqui D, Laurent A, Tayar C, Chang S, Van Nhieu JT, Loriau J, Karoui M, Duvoux C, Dhumeaux D, Fagniez PL. Laparoscopic liver resection for peripheral

hepatocellular carcinoma in patients with chronic liver disease: midterm results and perspectives. Ann Surg 2006;243(4):499–506

[17] Belli G, Fantini C, D'Agostino A, et al. Laparoscopic versus open liver resection for hepatocellular carcinoma in patients with histologically proven cirrhosis: short- and middle-term results. Surg Endosc. 2007;21(11):2004–11.

[18] Shimada M, Hashizume M, Maehara S, Tsujita E, Rikimaru T, Yamashita Y, Tanaka S, Adachi E, Sugimachi K. Laparoscopic hepatectomy for hepatocellular carcinoma. Surg Endosc 2001;15(6):541–544

[19] Lai EC, Tang CN, Ha JP, Li MK. Laparoscopic liver resection for hepatocellular carcinoma: 10-year experience in a single center. Arch Surg 2009;144(2):143–147

[20] Tranchart H, Di Giuro G, Lainas P, Roudie J, Agostini H, Franco D, Dagher I. Laparoscopic resection for hepatocellular carcinoma: a matched-pair comparative study. Surg Endosc. 2010;24(5):1170-6.

[21] Santambrogio R, Podda M, Zuin M, Bertolini E, Bruno S, Cornalba GP, Costa M, Montorsi M. Safety and efficacy of laparoscopic radiofrequency ablation of hepatocellular carcinoma in patients with liver cirrhosis. Surg Endosc. 2003;17(11):1826-32.

[22] Buell JF, Thomas MT, Rudich S, Marvin M, Nagubandi R, Ravindra KV, Brock G, McMasters KM. Experience with more than 500 minimally invasive hepatic procedures. Ann Surg. 2008;248(3):475-86.

[23] Giulianotti PC, Coratti A, Sbrana F, Addeo P, Bianco FM, Buchs NC, Annechiarico M, Benedetti E. Robotic liver surgery: results for 70 resections. Surgery. 2011 Jan;149(1):29-39.

[24] Barbaros U, Sümer A, Tunca F, Gözkün O, Demirel T, Bilge O, Randazzo V, Dinççağ A, Seven R, Mercan S, Budak D. Our early experiences with single-incision laparoscopic surgery: the first 32 patients. Surg Laparosc Endosc Percutan Tech. 2010 Oct;20(5):306-11.

Part 3

Non-Surgical Treatment

11

Medical Management Options for Hepatocellular Carcinoma

Mehmet Sitki Copur[1] and Angela Mae Obermiller[2]
[1]Medical Director, Saint Francis Cancer Center, Grand Island, Nebraska
University of Nebraska Medical Center,
Omaha, Nebraska
[2]Pharmacy Supervisor, Saint Francis Medical Center, Grand Island, Nebraska
University of Nebraska Medical Center,
Omaha, Nebraska
USA

1. Introduction

Hepatocellular carcinoma (HCC) is typically diagnosed late in the course of patients with chronic liver disease and cirrhosis. Hepatic reserve of the patient, as indicated by the Barcelona Clinic or Child-Pugh staging system, can be helpful in determining therapeutic options. Because of rapidly evolving new treatment options and varying availability of therapeutic approaches to individual patients attempts in generating algorithmic approaches for the treatment of patients with hepatocellular carcinoma may not be applicable to all situations. General treatment options can be divided into surgical or non-surgical approaches. Non-surgical approaches may be liver directed (such as transarterial chemoembolozation, percutaneous ethanol injection, radiofrequency ablation) or sysytemic therapy. Systemic palliative therapy of HCC has not been used routinely for a number of reasons; First, due to high rate of expression of drug resistance genes, including p-glycoprotein, glutathione-S-transferase, heat shock proteins, and mutations in p53, HCC has been considered a relatively chemotherapy-refractory tumor. Second, systemic chemotherapy has been difficult to be tolerated by patients with significant underlying hepatic dysfunction and may have less efficacy in patients with significant cirrhosis. Third, clinical investigations of chemotherapy in advanced HCC have been undertaken in diverse patient populations (Asian versus North American/European) making the interpretation of the results difficult for the overall population. Recently there has been a resurgence of interest and enthusiasm for systemic therapy of HCC with the emergence of data showing benefit from several targeted therapies.

This chapter will focus on the non-surgical systemic treatment of HCC which includes chemotherapy, immunotherapy, molecularly targeted therapy, hormonal therapy, Immunomodulatory/antiangiogenic therapy and ongoing clinical trials of new targeted agents.

2. Chemotherapy/immunotherapy

2.1 Single agent regimens

2.1.1 Antracyclines

Although there is no approved treatment for HCC in the United States, the European Union, or elsewhere in the world, doxorubicin has been commonly used as a first-line chemotherapy treatment for this disease. First approved by the US Food and Drug Administration in 1974 for breast cancer, doxorubicin has been the subject of multiple clinical trials in HCC. Early encouraging response rates as high as 79% of doxorubicin single agent (Olweny et al.,1975) has not been supported by later studies. Most studies have reported an objective response rate around 20 percent with doxorubicin doses of 75 mg/m². Despite the modest objective response rate one clinical trial involving 106 patients has shown that doxorubicin had a small survival advantage compared to best supportive care alone (median survival 10.6 versus 7.5 weeks)(Lai et al.,1988) While the clinical trials that occurred from 1977 to 1990 performed in HCC with doxorubicin as a single agent at doses ranging from 40 to 75 mg/m2 demonstrated a survival range from 3.0 to 4.1 months, (Ihde et al., 1977; Johnson et al.,1978; Falkson et al., 1984a; Falkson et al., 1984b; Colombo et al.,1985; Melia et al.,1987; Kalayci C et al., 1990) a more recent trial comparing single agent doxorubicin to nolatrexed showed a median survival of 32 versus 22 weeks in favor of doxorubicin (Gish et al.,2007). The higher than expected survival in both treatment groups might be due to advances in the management of patients with HCC including better supportive therapies, such as growth factors and greater expertise in the treatment of patients with cirrhosis. A limited number of phase III studies note higher response rates but no survival benefit with doxorubicin monotherapy compared to non-oxaliplatin 5-FU-based regimens and single agent etoposide (Choi et al.,1984; Falkson et al., 1978; Melia et al.,1983).

Both epirubicin and mitoxantrone have an approximately similar level of antitumor efficacy as doxorubicin (response rates 10 to 25 percent) (Pohl et al.,2001; Dunk et al.,1985). In contrast, the single agent activity of pegylated liposomal doxorubicin (PLD) is limited (Lind et al., 2007).

2.1.2 Fluoropyrimidines

Although there is extensive hepatic metabolism, 5-Fluorouracil (5-FU) has been utilized in the treatment of HCC with acceptable low toxicity and efficacy. Adequate doses have been able to be administered in the setting of hepatic dysfunction or jaundice. Response rates with 5-FU monotherapy have been low. However, when given in combination with leucovorin, response rates as high as 28 percent have been reported (Porta et al., 1995).

While single agent treatment with the oral fluoropyrimidine capecitabine (Patt et al., 2004) has shown an encouraging 25% response rate in one small study, a lower objective response rate (three partial responses among 50 treated patients) was noted in a subsequent larger phase II study evaluating the same dose of capecitabine in combination with oxaliplatin (Bogie et al., 2007).

2.2 Interferon alfa immunotherapy

Although interferon alfa has shown activity in preclinical models against HCC, several clinical trials have shown inconclusive results. An early Chinese randomized trial of 75 patients suggested superior response rates and better tolerability of interferon alfa compared to single agent doxorubicin (Lai et al., 1989). In another randomized trial, 75 patients with inoperable HCC were randomly assigned to receive interferon alfa 50 mU/m^2 intramuscularly three times weekly or best supportive care. Reported median survival was significantly improved in the interferon group (14.5 versus 7.5 weeks) with an objective response rate of 31 percent. Treatment was well tolerated with fatigue being the most common side effect requiring a dose reduction in only 34 percent of patients (Lai et al., 1993). On the contrary in a second trial utilizing a much lower dose of interferon alfa 3 mU three times weekly for one year versus symptomatic treatment only 6.6 percent of patients achieved a partial response with no survival benefit (Llovet et al., 2000).

Other chemotherapy and immunotherapy single agents with reported modest activity (mostly partial response and/or disease stabilization in HCC include irinotecan, gemcitabine and thalidomide (O`Reilly et al., 2002; Yang et al. et al., 2000; Lin et al., 2005).

2.3 Combination chemotherapy and immunotherapy regimens

2.3.1 Folfox

In an Asian trial of 371 patients with advanced or metastatic HCC modified FOLFOX-4 was directly compared to single agent doxorubicin (50 mg/m^2 every three weeks) the median survival in the FOLFOX arm, was 6.5 versus 4.9 months, p = .00425. FOLFOX was associated with better median PFS, objective response rate, and disease control rate, 53 versus 33 percent. Although the FOLFOX group had higher sensory neuropathy, most cases were mild, and there were no significant differences in the rate of grade 3 or 4 toxicities(Qin et al., 2010).

2.3.2 Xelox

Bogie et al. evaluated capecitabine (1000 mg/m^2 twice daily for 14 of every 21 days) in combination with oxaliplatin (130 mg/m^2 every three weeks), there were only three partial responses among 50 treated patients (objective response rate 6 percent) Stable disease in 29 patients led to a disease control rate of 72 percent. Median overall and progression-free survival was 9.3 and 4.1 months, respectively (Bogie et al. 2007).

2.3.3 Gemox

In a phase II study involving 32 cirrhotic patients with previously untreated advanced HCC, gemcitabine (1000 mg/m^2 by fixed dose rate infusion) on day 1 was followed by oxaliplatin (100 mg/m^2) on day 2, with both drugs repeated every two weeks. The objective response rate was 18 percent, and an additional 58 percent had disease stabilization. Median survival was 11.5 months. Treatment seemed to be more effective in patients with nonalcoholic rather than alcoholic cirrhosis (Louafi et al., 2007).

2.4 Gemcitabine plus pegylated liposomal doxorubicin

In a phase II trial, 41 patients were treated with gemcitabine (1000 mg/m^2 days 1 and 8) plus pegylated liposomal doxorubicin (30 mg/m^2 on day 1) every 28 days. There were three complete and seven partial responses (overall response rate 24 percent), the median TTP was 5.8 months, and median overall survival was 22.5 months. Treatment was well tolerated, with grade 3 to 4 toxicity limited to neutropenia (17 percent) and thrombocytopenia (2 percent) (Lombardi et al. 2011).

2.5 Gemcitabine and cisplatin

Parikh et al. evaluated the combination of gemcitabine (1250 mg/m^2 on days 1 and 8) and cisplatin (70 mg/m^2 on day 1 of every 21-day cycle) was associated with an overall response rate of 20 percent (Parikh et al., 2005). Grade 3 to 4 toxicities included anemia (37 percent), neutropenia (13 percent), thrombocytopenia (7 percent), transaminitis and mucositis (3 percent each). A second trial using a slightly different dosing regimen (cisplatin 25 mg/m^2 on days 1 and 8, gemcitabine 1000 mg/m^2 on days 1 and 8) reported a more favorable toxicity profile but a lower response rate (one partial response among 15 patients (Chia et al., 2008).

Other combination regimens include cisplatin plus doxorubicin with response rates 18 to 49 percent (Lee et al., 2004; Czauderna et al., 2002), cisplatin, mitoxantrone, and continuous infusion 5-FU with objective response rates 24 to 27 percent in two different studies (Yang et al., 2004; Ikeda et al., 2005), cisplatin, epirubicin and infusional 5-FU with a response rate 15 percent (Boucher et al., 2002;) cisplatin, doxorubicin plus capecitabine with a response rate of 24 percent (Park et al., 2006).

2.6 Combination of chemotherapy with interferon-alfa

2.6.1 The PIAF regimen

The immunomodulatory cytokine interferon alfa has been utilized in combination with different chemotherapy drugs in the treatment of HCC. One of the most aggressive combinations of this drug involves cisplatin, interferon alfa and infusional 5-FU, the so called PIAF regimen. Leung et al. evaluated this combination in 50 advanced stage HCC patients and found an objective response rate of 26 percent. Overall median survival of the entire population was nine months and eight of the resected patients remained in complete remission from eight to 26 months. Toxicity was mainly myelosupression and mucositis with no treatment related deaths (Leung et al., 1999). In another trial 188 unselected patients with chemotherapy-naive unresectable HCC were randomly assigned to doxorubicin monotherapy (60 mg/m^2 every three weeks) versus PIAF (cisplatin 20 mg/m^2 on days 1 through 4, interferon alfa 5 MU/m^2 subcutaneously on days 1 through 4, doxorubicin 40 mg/m^2 on day 1, and 5-FU 400 mg/m^2 on days 1 through 4) (Yeo et al., 2005). Objective response rates and median survival favored the PIAF regimen but the difference did not reach statistical significance. Toxicity was more in the PIAF arm, with more pronounced myelosupression and hypokalemia (Yeo et al.,2005).

Although the role of PIAF regimen in the treatment of HCC remains unclear, it may be considered for patients with a good performance status and liver function.

2.6.2 5-FU plus interferon alfa

Patt et al. evaluated 43 patients with advanced HCC on a regimen of infusional 5-FU (200 mg/m2 daily for 21 of 28 days) plus interferon alfa (4 mU/m2 three times weekly and found an objective response rate of 33 percent(Patt et al.,2003 (Patt et al., 2003). Two of four patients with HCC who were subsequently resected had a complete histologic response.

Despite the presence of cirrhosis in 71 percent of the patients with HCC, toxicity was moderate, with grade 3 or 4 stomatitis, fatigue, and hematologic toxicity in 33, 5, and 9 percent of patients, respectively. A similar level of benefit (objective response rates between 33 and 50 percent, one-third to one-half complete) has been seen with combinations of systemic interferon alfa with intrahepatic arterial 5-FU in patients with advanced HCC and major portal vein thrombus (a contraindication to transhepatic arterial chemoembolization) (Sakon et al., 2002; Ota et al., 2005; Nagano et al. 2007). A weekly bolus regimen of 5-FU 750 mg/m2 plus interferon alfa 9 MU three times weekly however, was much more toxic and ineffective in a small series of 10 patients with no sustainable responses (Stuart et al., 1996).

3. Molecularly targeted therapy

Existing evidence points to the possible role of epidermal growth factor receptor (EGFR)/EGF (HER1) signaling pathway in the carcinogenesis of HCC (Huether et al.,2005; Hung et al., 1993; Yamaguchi et al., 1995; Myaki et al., 2000; Schiffer et al.., 2005; Hopfner et al., 2004; Wu et al., 2003; Ito et al., 2001; Thomas et al., 2005). These data have led to the clinical trials evaluating the role of biologics such as erlotinib and cetuximab in HCC patients. HCCs are highly vascular tumors with high levels of expression of vascular endothelial growth factor (VEGF), thus suggesting a possible therapeutic role for agents targeting VEGF and/or the VEGF receptor (VEGFR). Similarly the Raf/MAP kinase pathway has been implicated in HCC tumorigenesis (Huynh et al.,2003) with a potential therapeutic role for drugs that inhibit Raf kinase pathway. There is a constant research to find less toxic more active targeted treatments in this disease.

3.1 Sorafenib

Efficacy of sorafenib, an oral small molecule tyrosine kinase inhibitor, was first noted on a phase I trial (Liu I et al., 2006; Strumberg D. et al., 2005). Further studies did not suggest a high level of objective tumor shrinkage but provided stable disease (Abou-Alfa GK et al., 2006). Eventually SHARP trial confirmed a survival benefit compared to best supportive care alone. SHARP trial randomly assigned 602 patients with inoperable HCC and Child-Pugh A cirrhosis to sorafenib (400 mg twice daily) versus placebo (Llovet et al., 2008). Overall survival, the primary endpoint, was significantly longer in the sorafenib-treated patients (10.7 versus 7.9 months), as was time to radiologic progression (5.5versus2.8months). Treatment was well tolerated with manageable side effects. These results established sorafenib monotherapy as the new reference standard systemic treatment for advanced HCC. In another trial 226 Asian patients with Child-Pugh A cirrhosis and no prior systemic therapy for HCC received sorafenib 400 mg twice daily versus placebo (Cheng et al., 2009). Patients receiving sorafenib had significantly better median overall survival (6.5 versus 4.2 months) and TTP (2.8 versus 1.4 months). The treated group in the Asian trial had a shorter survival duration than the control group in the SHARP trial (6.5 versus 7.9 months), despite the fact that both trials used the same entry criteria. Patients accrued to the Asian study were more ill at the start of therapy than those in the SHARP trial, with a generally worse performance status and more advanced stage of disease (Raoul et al., 2008). Preliminary data suggest that patients with hepatitis C virus (HCV) infection as the etiology of their cirrhosis may have a better response to sorafenib as compared to those with other etiologies of the HCC (Huitzel-Melendez et al., 2007; Bolondi et al., 2008). However, the available data are scant, and further study is needed to establish the influence of underlying liver disease on sorafenib treatment responsiveness. With the advances in our understanding of the pathophysiology of this disease and the development of new biomarkers, we may be able to better identify patients who might benefit most from sorafenib treatment.

3.2 Sorafenib plus doxorubicin

The benefit of adding sorafenib to doxorubicin was studied in a phase II trial in which all patients received doxorubicin (60 mg/m^2 every 21 days), and they were randomly assigned to sorafenib 400 twice daily for a maximum of six cycles or placebo (Abou-Alfa et al., 2010). Combination therapy was associated with a similarly low objective response rate (4 versus 2 percent with doxorubicin alone), but a significantly longer time to tumor progression (6.4 versus 2.8 months) and median overall survival duration (13.7 versus 6.5 months). The side effect profile was not significantly worse with combined therapy.

The degree to which this improvement represents synergism between sorafenib and doxorubicin remains to be defined. Before this approach can be considered standard, this combination must be compared to sorafenib alone in a large-scale phase III trial, which is ongoing.

3.3 Sunitinib

Sunitinib is another orally active TKI that targets a variety of TKs in addition to VEGFR, including platelet-derived growth factor receptors (PDGFRs), KIT, RET, and FLT3. Antitumor activity is suggested by the following early observations:A phase II study included 37 patients with unresectable HCC who were treated with sunitinib (50 mg daily for four of every six weeks) and assessed by monthly CT scans (Faivre et al.,2009). There was one confirmed partial response, and 35 percent had stable disease for over three months.

3.4 Small molecule TK inhibitors

Small molecule TKI, erlotinib has shown some activity in phase II studies of advanced HCC patients with tumors expressing EGFR/HER1. Philip et al. treated 38 patients with advanced HCC, one half of whom had prior chemotherapy using 150 mg of erlotinib orally daily on 28-day cycles. Twelve patients out of 38 (32 percent) were progression free at six months while three had a radiographic response that lasted for two, 10 and 11 months respectively. (Philip et al., 2005). The median survival of the entire cohort was 13 months. A second trial included 40 patients with previously untreated unresectable HCC who received erlotinib 150 mg daily as monotherapy (Thomas et al., 2007). There were no objective responses, but 17 achieved stable disease with 16 weeks of continuous therapy. The median overall survival was 11 months. Additional studies with other receptor TKIs, both as monotherapy and in combination with cytotoxic chemotherapy are ongoing.

3.5 Bevacizumab

Bevacizumab, a monoclonal antibody against the VEGF, has been shown to be active in HCC. In one study involving 46 patients with locally advanced HCC single agent bevacizumab was given at 5 mg/kg or 10 mg/kg every two weeks.(Siegel et al.,2008) An objective response was documented in six (13 percent, one complete), and the median progression-free survival was 6.9 months. The most common grade 3 or 4 toxicities were hypertension (15 percent), thrombosis (6 percent) and major bleeding (11 percent). A similar level of efficacy was seen in a second trial, reported in abstract form only (Malka et al., 2007). Using bevacizumab 5 to 10 mg/kg every 14 days, there were three partial responses and 13 disease stabilizations among 30 patients, and six had to discontinue therapy because of variceal bleeding.

3.6 Erlotinib plus bevacizumab

In a study of bevacizumab (10 mg/kg every two weeks) plus erlotinib (150 mg orally daily, continuously), was associated with a response rate of 25 percent and a stable disease rate of 37 percent. The median progression-free and overall survival durations were 9 and 15.6 months, respectively (Thomas et al.,2009). These results appear favorable compared with those reported in phase II and III trials of sorafenib as a single agent (median survival 6.5 to 14 months). Randomized trials are needed to confirm the superiority of erlotinib and bevacizumab over other systemic regimens.

3.7 Bevacizumab plus gemcitabine plus oxaliplatin

In a small phase II trial 30 patients received gemcitabine (1000 mg/m^2) followed by oxaliplatin (85 mg/m^2) on days 2 and 16, plus bevacizumab (10 mg/m^2 on day 1 of the first cycle and thereafter, on days 1 and 15 of each cycle) (Zhu et al., 2006). The objective response rate was 20 percent, the six-month progression-free survival rate was 48 percent, and median overall survival was 9.6 months. Whether any combination regimens are better than bevacizumab alone will require a randomized trial.

3.8 Cetuximab

Early results suggest activity for cetuximab in combination with GEMOX (Louafi et al., 2007). In a preliminary report of 44 patients who received gemcitabine 1000 mg/m^2 on day 1 and oxaliplatin 100 mg/m^2 on day 2 every 14 days, in combination with cetuximab (400 mg/m^2 initially, then 250 mg/m^2 weekly), there were eight partial responses, and the total disease control rate (partial response plus stable disease) was 65 percent. Treatment was well tolerated with only one grade 4 toxicity (thrombocytopenia) and no grade 5 toxicities. Grade 2 and 3 neurotoxicity occurred in 16 and 5 percent of patients, respectively.

4. Hormone therapy

4.1 Tamoxifen

HCC known to express hormonal receptors and the striking gender disparity observed in the incidence of hepatocellular carcinoma has suggested an important role of sex hormones in HCC pathogenesis. Though the studies began as early as in 1980s, the precise role of sex hormones and the significance of their receptors in HCC still remain poorly understood and perhaps contribute to current controversies about the potential use of hormonal therapy in HCC(Kalra M et al., 2008). Several prospective randomized trials and a systematic review of tamoxifen in patients with advanced HCC have failed to show a survival benefit or improved functional status (Castells et al., 1995; Chow et al., 2002; Nowak et al., 2004; Barbare et al., 2005). One possible reason for the lack of efficacy may be the presence of variant ERs in some of these tumors (Villa et al., 1996; Villa et al., 2001). Tamoxifen may also function as a potential inhibitor of p-glycoprotein, the MDR (multidrug resistance) gene product, and this has led to trials of tamoxifen combined with various chemotherapeutic agents. Unfortunately, these studies have also failed to demonstrate any benefit for the addition of tamoxifen (Cheng et al.., 1996; Raderer et al., 1996).

4.2 Megestrol

Unlike tamoxifen there has been some modest benefit with the use of megestrol in some studies involving patients with HCC. In a study of 24 patients with advanced HCC who were randomly assigned to megestrol (160 mg daily) or supportive care only, median survival was significantly better with megestrol (18 versus 7 months) despite no objective responses(Farinati et al., 2001). In another study, one of 37 patients receiving megestrol (160 mg daily) for at least 60 days had a partial response, while two others had a significant decline in serum alpha-fetoprotein (AFP) levels (Chao et al., 1997).

4.3 Octreotide and lanreotide

In a review of four randomized controlled trials (three of which were high quality trials) published in 1998 or later with a total of 373 patients only one (126 patients) suggested that octreotide could improve survival and quality of life of HCC patients, whereas the other two(189 patients) suggested octreotide did not have survival benefit in HCC; moreover, none of the three trials indicated that octreotide has significant beneficial effect on tumor regression or decrease of tumor mass. Nonetheless, serious adverse effects were not reported in these included trials. In order to detect a realistic treatment advantage, further larger well-designed multicenter randomized trials will have to be conducted(Jia et al., 2010).

Lanreotide is a long acting somatostatin analog that is available in a depot formulation that has comparable efficacy to octreotide when injected intramuscularly two to three times per month. Although limited antitumor activity has been suggested in nonrandomized studies a randomized trial of lanreotide versus placebo in 272 patients with advanced HCC failed to show any advantage for drug treatment in terms of progression-free or overall survival, and treatment was associated with worse quality of life (Barbare et al., 2009).

5. Immunomodulatory/antiangiogenic therapy

5.1 Lenalidomide

Last but not he least, Lenalidomide, an immunomodulatory analog of thalidomide, an anti-angiogenic agent with inhibitiory effects on basic fibroblast growth factor (FGF) and vascular endothelial growth factor (VEGF) has shown promising and in some patients dramatic activity. FGF is an important growth factor in HCC. In a phase II study to determine the activity of lenalidomide in Second-line HCC therapy, patients with advanced HCC who progressed or were intolerant to sorafenib were treated with lenalidomide 25 mg orally days 1-21 of a 28 day cycle until disease progression or unacceptable toxicity. A preplanned interim analysis was undertaken when study enrollment reached 13 out of the total planned 40 patients. Of the first 13 patients, the median age was 66 years (44-86 years). Eight patients were Child-Pugh A, 3 patients were B, and 2 patients were C. Nine patients had extrahepatic disease. Five of 13 patients (38%) had a > 50% reduction in AFP including one patient with a reduction in AFP from 56,900 to 5 ng/mL. Two patients had radiographic partial responses including one patient with complete resolution of all areas of enhancement. Treatment was well tolerated with grade 3 neutropenia seen in 2 patients (Safran et al., 2010)

6. Active clinical trials in HCC

Clinical trials for patients with Advanced Hepatocellular Carcinoma (HCC) are listed below. The list of clinical trials includes treatment trials currently recruiting in the United States. Further information regarding each clinical trial can be reached at *www.canliv.org/Doctors--amp;-Researchers/Active-Clinical-Trials*

- Sorafenib and TRC105 in Hepatocellular Cancer
- A Study of LY2157299 in Patients With Hepatocellular Carcinoma
- Axitinib For The Treatment Of Advanced Hepatocellular Carcinoma
- A Study of Ramucirumab (IMC-1121B) Drug Product (DP) and Best Supportive Care (BSC) Versus Placebo and BSC as 2nd-Line Treatment in Patients With Hepatocellular Carcinoma After 1st-Line Therapy With Sorafenib
- A Study of the Effectiveness and Safety of AMG 386 and Sorafenib to Treat Advanced or Inoperable Hepatocellular Cancer
- Study of Bavituximab and Sorafenib In Patients With Advanced Liver Cancer
- Global Study Looking at the Combination of RAD001 Plus Best Supportive Care (BSC) and Placebo Plus BSC to Treat Patients With Advanced Hepatocellular Carcinoma.
- Efficacy and Tolerability of ABT-869 Versus Sorafenib in Advanced Hepatocellular Carcinoma (HCC)
- A Study of IMC-A12 in Combination With Sorafenib in Patients With Advanced Cancer of the Liver ABT-888 and Temozolomide for Liver Cancer
- A Randomized, Placebo-controlled, Double-blind Phase 2 Study With OSI-906 in Patients With Advanced HCC Bevacizumab and Erlotinib or Sorafenib as First-Line Therapy in Treating Patients With Advanced Liver Cancer

7. Conclusions

In this chapter we tried to summarize systemic therapy options for patients with advanced unresectable disease who are not candidates for locoregional therapy. This is a constantly evolving field. In general, efficacy with conventional cytotoxic chemotherapy has been modest at best, and the duration of benefit is limited. Although few randomized trials have been conducted, no single regimen seems to be superior and no drug or regimen has been unequivocally shown to improve survival. Newer data on the efficacy of molecularly targeted agents has been promising offering the potential for prolonged survival. Participation in ongoing clinical trials testing new therapeutic strategies is the best option for patients with advanced unresectable disease. For patients who are not eligible for a clinical trial or for whom protocol therapy is not available initial therapy with sorafenib 400 mg twice daily is the first line recommendation. To improve tolerability starting at 200 mg twice a day and increase the daily dose in 200 mg increments approximately every five days until the target dose is reached is a feasible option.

The efficacy of cytotoxic chemotherapy is at best modest in patients with HCC, and in general, the duration of benefit is limited. No single regimen has emerged as superior to any other, although few randomized trials have been conducted. Despite objective responses that are occasionally complete, median survival in all of these studies has been short (4.4 to 11.6 months), with the exception of those in which resection/transplantation is attempted after chemotherapy. There are insufficient data to routinely recommend any standard regimen. Systemic chemotherapy may still be considered for patients whose tumors progress while on sorafenib and whose performance status and baseline liver function are sufficient to tolerate it. The side effect profile of any chemotherapy regimen should be considered carefully in patients with advanced liver disease and a short life expectancy. Cytotoxic therapy should be reserved for medically appropriate patients with adequate hepatic function and preferably administered within the context of a clinical trial. Reactivation of viral hepatitis may occur in patients with HCC who are undergoing intensive systemic chemotherapy, so it is important to monitor and maintain antiviral medications during treatment.

8. References

Abou-Alfa GK, Johnson P, Knox JJ, et al. Doxorubicin plus sorafenib vs doxorubicin alone in patients with advanced hepatocellular carcinoma: a randomized trial. JAMA 2010; 304:2154.

Abou-Alfa GK, Schwartz L, Ricci S Phase II study of sorafenib in patients with advanced hepatocellular carcinoma. J Clin Oncol;2006 24(26):4293

Barbare JC, Bouché O, Bonnetain F, et al. Treatment of advanced hepatocellular carcinoma with long-acting octreotide: a phase III multicentre, randomised, double blind placebo-controlled study. Eur J Cancer 2009; 45:1788.

Barbare JC, Bouché O, Bonnetain F, et al. Randomized controlled trial of tamoxifen in advanced hepatocellular carcinoma. J Clin Oncol 2005; 23:4338.

Becker G, Allgaier HP, Olschewski M, et al. Long-acting octreotide versus placebo for treatment of advanced HCC: a randomized controlled double-blind study. Hepatology 2007; 45:9.

Bogie V, Raoul JL, Pignon JP et al. Multicnetre phase II trial of capecitabine plus oxaliplatin XELOX in patients with advanced hepatocellular carcinoma:Br J Cancer 2007;97:862.

Boige V, Raoul JL, Pignon JP, et al. Multicentre phase II trial of capecitabine plus oxaliplatin (XELOX) in patients with advanced hepatocellular carcinoma: FFCD 03-03 trial. Br J Cancer 2007; 97:862.

Bolondi L, Caspary W, Bennouna J, et al. Clinical benefit of sorafenib in hepatitis C patients with hepatocellular carcinoma (HCC): subgroup analysis of the SHARP trial (abstract). Data presented at the 2008 ASCO Gastrointestinal Cancers Symposium, Orlando, FL, January 25-27, 2008. (abstract 129).

Boucher E, Corbinais S, Brissot P, et al. Treatment of hepatocellular carcinoma (HCC) with systemic chemotherapy combining epirubicin, cisplatinum and infusional 5-fluorouracil (ECF regimen). Cancer Chemother Pharmacol 2002; 50:305.

Castells A, Bruix J, Brú C, et al. Treatment of hepatocellular carcinoma with tamoxifen: a double-blind placebo-controlled trial in 120 patients. Gastroenterology 1995; 109:917.

Chao Y, Chan WK, Wang SS, et al. Phase II study of megestrol acetate in the treatment of hepatocellular carcinoma. J Gastroenterol Hepatol 1997; 12:277.

Cheng AL, Kang YK, Chen Z, et al. Efficacy and safety of sorafenib in patients in the Asia-Pacific region with advanced hepatocellular carcinoma: a phase III randomised, double-blind, placebo-controlled trial. Lancet Oncol 2009; 10:25.

Cheng AL, Chen YC, Yeh KH, et al. Chronic oral etoposide and tamoxifen in the treatment of far-advanced hepatocellular carcinoma. Cancer 1996; 77:872.

Chia WK, Ong S, Toh HC, et al. Phase II trial of gemcitabine in combination with cisplatin in inoperable or advanced hepatocellular carcinoma. Ann Acad Med Singapore 2008; 37:554.

Choi TK, Lee NW, Wong J. Chemotherapy for advanced hepatocellular carcinoma. Adriamycin versus quadruple chemotherapy.Cancer. 1984;53(3):401.

Chow PK, Tai BC, Tan CK, et al. High-dose tamoxifen in the treatment of inoperable hepatocellular carcinoma: A multicenter randomized controlled trial. Hepatology 2002; 36:1221.

Colombo M, Tommasini MA, Del Ninno E, et al: Hepatocellular carcinoma in Italy: Report of a clinical trial with intravenous doxorubicin. Liver 5:336-341, 1985

Czauderna P, Mackinlay G, Perilongo G, et al. Hepatocellular carcinoma in children: results of the first prospective study of the International Society of Pediatric Oncology group. J Clin Oncol 2002; 20:2798.

Dunk AA, Scott SC, Johnson PJ et al. Mitoxantrone as single agent therapy in hepatocellular carcinoma. A phase II study J Hepatol 1985;1:395.

Faivre S, Raymond E, Boucher E, et al. Safety and efficacy of sunitinib in patients with advanced hepatocellular carcinoma: an open-label, multicentre, phase II study. Lancet Oncol 2009; 10:794.

Falkson G, MacIntyre JM, Schutt AJ, et al: Neocarzinostatin versus m-AMSA or doxorubicin in hepatocellular carcinoma. J Clin Oncol 2:581-584, 1984

Falkson G, MacIntyre JM, Moertel CG, et al: Primary liver cancer: An Eastern Cooperative Oncology Group trial. Cancer 54:970-977, 1984

Falkson G, Moertel CG, Lavin P et al. Chemotherapy studies in primary liver cancer:a prospective randomized clinincal trial. Cancer 1978;42:2149.

Farinati F, Gianni S, De Giorgio M, Fiorentini S. Megestrol treatment in patients with hepatocellular carcinoma. Br J Cancer 2001; 85:1606.

Gish RG, Porta C, Lazr L et al. Phase III randomized controlled trial comparing the survival of patients with unresectable hepatocellular carcinoma treated with nolatrexed or doxorubicin. J Clin Oncol 2007;25:3069.

Höpfner M, Sutter AP, Huether A, et al. Targeting the epidermal growth factor receptor by gefitinib for treatment of hepatocellular carcinoma. J Hepatol 2004; 41:1008.

Huether A, Höpfner M, Sutter AP, et al. Erlotinib induces cell cycle arrest and apoptosis in hepatocellular cancer cells and enhances chemosensitivity towards cytostatics. J Hepatol 2005; 43:661.

Huitzel-Melendez FD, Saltz LB, Song J, et al. Retrospective analysis of outcome in hepatocellular carcinoma (HCC) patients with hepatitis C (C+) versus B (B+) treated with sorafenib (abstract). Data preseted at the 2007 ASCO Gastrointestinal Cancers Symposium, January 19-21st, 2007, Orlando, FL. (abstract 173).

Hung WC, Chuang LY, Tsai JH, Chang CC. Effects of epidermal growth factor on growth control and signal transduction pathways in different human hepatoma cell lines. Biochem Mol Biol Int 1993; 30:319.

Huynh H, Nguyen TT, Chow KH, et al. Over-expression of the mitogen-activated protein kinase (MAPK) kinase (MEK)-MAPK in hepatocellular carcinoma: its role in tumor progression and apoptosis. BMC Gastroenterol 2003; 3:19.

Ihde DC, Kane RC, Cohen MH, et al: Adriamycin therapy in American patients with hepatocellular carcinoma. Cancer Treat Rep 61:1385-1387, 1977

Ikeda M, Okusaka T, Ueno H, et al. A phase II trial of continuous infusion of 5-fluorouracil, mitoxantrone, and cisplatin for metastatic hepatocellular carcinoma. Cancer 2005; 103:756.

Ito Y, Takeda T, Sakon M, et al. Expression and clinical significance of erb-B receptor family in hepatocellular carcinoma. Br J Cancer 2001; 84:1377.

Jia WD, Zhang CH, Xu GL et al. Octreotide therapy for hepatocellular carcinoma: a systematic review of the evidence from randomized controlled trials. Hepatogastroenterology; 2010 57(98);292-9.

Johnson PJ, Williams R, Thomas H, et al: Induction of remission in hepatocellular carcinoma with doxorubicin. Lancet 1:1006-1009, 1978

Kalayci C, Johnson PJ, Raby N, et al: Intraarterial adriamycin and lipiodol for inoperable hepatocellular carcinoma: A comparison with intravenous adriamycin. J Hepatol 11:349-353, 1990

Kalra M, Mayes J, Assefa S et al. Role of sex steroid receptors in pathobiology of hepatocellular carcinoma. World J Gastroenterol 2008;14(39):5945-61.

Kouroumalis E, Skordilis P, Thermos K, et al. Treatment of hepatocellular carcinoma wit h octreotide: a randomised controlled study. Gut 1998; 42:442.

Lai CL, Lau JY, Wu PC et al. Recombinant interferon-alpha in inoperable hepatocellular carcinoma: a randomized controlled trial.Hepatology 1993;17:389.

Lai CL, Wu PC, Lok AS et al. Recombinant alpha 2 interferon is superior to doxorubicin for inoperable hepatocellular carcinoam: a prospective randomized trial. Br J Cancer 1989;60:928.

Lai CL, Wu PC, Chan GC et al. Doxorubicin versus no antitumor threapy in inoperable hepatocellular carcinoma. A prospective randomized trial. Cancer 1988;62:479.

Lee J, Park JO, Kim WS, et al. Phase II study of doxorubicin and cisplatin in patients with metastatic hepatocellular carcinoma. Cancer Chemother Pharmacol 2004; 54:385.

Leung TW, Patt YZ, Lau WY, et al. Complete pathological remission is possible with systemic combination chemotherapy for inoperable hepatocellular carcinoma. Clin Cancer Res 1999; 5:1676.

Lind PA, Naucler G, Holm A et al. Efficacy of peglyated liposomal doxorubicin in patients advanced hepato cellular carcinoma. Acta Oncol 2007;46:230.

Liu I, Cao Y, Chen C et al.Sorafenib blocks the RAF/MEK/ERK pathway, inhibits tumor angiogenesis, and induces tumor cell apoptosis in hepatocellular carcinoma model PLC/PRF/5. Cancer Res 2006; 66(24):11851,2006.

Lin AY, Brophy N, Fisher GA et al. Phase II study of thalidomide in patients with unresectable hepatocellular carcinoma. Cancer 2005;103:119.

Llovet JM, Ricci S, Mazzaferro V, et al. Sorafenib in advanced hepatocellular carcinoma. N Engl J Med 2008; 359:378.

Llovet JM, Sala M, Castells L et al. Randomized controlled trial of interferon treatment for advanced hepatocellular carcinoma.Hepatology 2000;31:54.

Lombardi G, Zustovich F, Farinati F, et al. Pegylated liposomal doxorubicin and gemcitabine in patients with advanced hepatocellular carcinoma:results of a phase 2 study.Cancer 2011;117:125.

Louafi S, Boige V, Ducreux M, et al. Gemcitabine plus oxaliplatin (GEMOX) in patients with advanced hepatocellular carcinoma (HCC): results of a phase II study. Cancer 2007; 109:1384.

Louafi S, et al. Gemcitabine, oxaliplatin (GEMOX) and cetuximab for treatment of hepatocellular carcinoma (HCC): results of the phase II study ERGO (abstract). J Clin Oncol 2007; 25:221s.

Malka D, Dromain C, Farace F, et al. Bevacizumab in patients with advanced hepatocellular carcinoma (HCC): preliminarhy results of a phase II study with circulating endothelial cell (CEC) monitoring (abstract). J Clin Oncol 2007; 25:215s.

Melia WM, Johnson PJ, Williams R: Controlled clinical trial of doxorubicin and tamoxifen versus doxorubicin alone in hepatocellular carcinoma. Cancer Treat Rep 71:1213-1216, 1987

Melia WM, Johnson PJ, Williams R. Induction of remission in hepatocellular carcinoma. A comparison of VP-16 with adriamycin. Cancer 1983;51:206.

Miyaki M, Sato C, Sakai K, et al. Malignant transformation and EGFR activation of immortalized mouse liver epithelial cells caused by HBV enhancer-X from a human hepatocellular carcinoma. Int J Cancer 2000; 85:518.

Nagano H, Miyamoto A, Wada H, et al. Interferon-alpha and 5-fluorouracil combination therapy after palliative hepatic resection in patients with advanced hepatocellular carcinoma, portal venous tumor thrombus in the major trunk, and multiple nodules. Cancer 2007; 110:2493.

Nowak A, Findlay M, Culjak G, Stockler M. Tamoxifen for hepatocellular carcinoma. Cochrane Database Syst Rev 2004; :CD001024.

Olweny CL, Toya T, Katongole-Mbidde E et al. Treatment of Hepatocellular carcinoma with adriamycine. Preliminary communication.Cancer 1975;36:1250

O`Reilly EM, Stuart KE, Sanz-Altamira PM et al. A phase II study of irinotecan in patients with advanced hepatocellular carcinoma Cancer 2002;94:3186.

Ota H, Nagano H, Sakon M, et al. Treatment of hepatocellular carcinoma with major portal vein thrombosis by combined therapy with subcutaneous interferon-alpha and intra-arterial 5-fluorouracil; role of type 1 interferon receptor expression. Br J Cancer 2005; 93:557.

Parikh PM, Fuloria J, Babu G, et al. A phase II study of gemcitabine and cisplatin in patients with advanced hepatocellular carcinoma. Trop Gastroenterol 2005; 26:115.

Park SH, Lee Y, Han SH, et al. Systemic chemotherapy with doxorubicin, cisplatin and capecitabine for metastatic hepatocellular carcinoma. BMC Cancer 2006; 6:3.

Patt YZ, Hassan MM, Aguayo A et al. Oral capectibine for the treatment of hepatocellular carcinoma, cholongiocarcinoma and gallbladder carcinoma. Cancer 2004;101:578.

Patt YZ, Hassan MM, Lozano RD, et al. Phase II trial of systemic continuous fluorouracil and subcutaneous recombinant interferon Alfa-2b for treatment of hepatocellular carcinoma. J Clin Oncol 2003; 21:421.

Philip PA, Mahoney MR, Allmer C, et al. Phase II study of Erlotinib (OSI-774) in patients with advanced hepatocellular cancer. J Clin Oncol 2005; 23:6657.

Pohl J, Zuna I, Stremmel W et al. Systemic chemotherapy with epirubicin for treatment of advanced or multifocal hepatocellular carcinoma. Chemotherpay 2001;47:359.

Porta C, Moroni M, Nastasi G. et al. 5-Fluorouracil and d,l-leucovorin calcium are active to treat unresectable hepatocellular carcinoma patietns:preliminary results of a phase II study. Oncology 1995;52:487.

Qin, S, Bai, Y, Ye, J, et al. Phase III study of oxaliplatin plus fluorouracil/leucovorin (FOLFOX4) versus doxorubicin as palliative systemic chemotherapy in advanced HCC in Asian patients (abstract 4008). J Clin Oncol 2010; 28:303s.

Raderer M, Hejna MH, Muller C, et al. Treatment of hepatocellular cancer with the long acting somatostatin analog lanreotide in vitro and in vivo. Int J Oncol 2000; 16:1197.

Raderer M, Pidlich J, Müller C, et al. A phase I/II trial of epirubicin and high dose tamoxifen as a potential modulator of multidrug resistance in advanced hepatocellular carcinoma. Eur J Cancer 1996; 32A:2366.

Raoul J, Santoro A, Beaugrand M, et al. Efficacy and safety of sorafenib in patients with advanced hepatocellular carcinoma according to ECOG performance status: a subanalysis from the SHARP trial (abstract). J Clin Oncol 2008; 26:234s

Safran H, Charpentier K, Dubel Get al. Lenalidomide for advanced heaptocellular cancer in patients progressing or intolerant to sorafenib. ASCO 2010 Gastrointestinal Cancer Symposium. Abstract 228.

Sakon M, Nagano H, Dono K, et al. Combined intraarterial 5-fluorouracil and subcutaneous interferon-alpha therapy for advanced hepatocellular carcinoma with tumor thrombi in the major portal branches. Cancer 2002; 94:435.

Schiffer E, Housset C, Cacheux W, et al. Gefitinib, an EGFR inhibitor, prevents hepatocellular carcinoma development in the rat liver with cirrhosis. Hepatology 2005; 41:307.

Siegel AB, Cohen EI, Ocean A, et al. Phase II trial evaluating the clinical and biologic effects of bevacizumab in unresectable hepatocellular carcinoma. J Clin Oncol 2008; 26:2992.

Strumberg D, Richly H, Hilger RA, Phase I clinical and pharmacokinetic study of the Novel Raf kinase and vascular endothelial growth factor receptor inhibitor BAY 43-9006 in patients with advanced refractory solid tumors. J Clin Oncol 2005;23(5)965.

Stuart K, Tessitore J, Huberman M. 5-Fluorouracil and alpha-interferon in hepatocellular carcinoma. Am J Clin Oncol 1996; 19:136.

Thomas MB, Morris JS, Chadha R, et al. Phase II trial of the combination of bevacizumab and erlotinib in patients who have advanced hepatocellular carcinoma. J Clin Oncol 2009; 27:843.

Thomas MB, Chadha R, Glover K, et al. Phase 2 study of erlotinib in patients with unresectable hepatocellular carcinoma. Cancer 2007; 110:1059.

Thomas MB, Abbruzzese JL. Opportunities for targeted therapies in hepatocellular carcinoma. J Clin Oncol 2005; 23:8093.

Villa E, Ferretti I, Grottola A, et al. Hormonal therapy with megestrol in inoperable hepatocellular carcinoma characterized by variant oestrogen receptors. Br J Cancer 2001; 84:881.

Villa E, Dugani A, Fantoni E, et al. Type of estrogen receptor determines response to antiestrogen therapy. Cancer Res 1996; 56:3883.

Wu BW, Wu Y, Wang JL, et al. Study on the mechanism of epidermal growth factor-induced proliferation of hepatoma cells. World J Gastroenterol 2003; 9:271.

Yamaguchi K, Carr BI, Nalesnik MA. Concomitant and isolated expression of TGF-alpha and EGF-R in human hepatoma cells supports the hypothesis of autocrine, paracrine, and endocrine growth of human hepatoma. J Surg Oncol 1995; 58:240.

Yang TS, Chang HK, Chen JS, et al. Chemotherapy using 5-fluorouracil, mitoxantrone, and cisplatin for patients with advanced hepatocellular carcinoma: an analysis of 63 cases. J Gastroenterol 2004; 39:362.

Yang TS, Lin YC, Chen JS, Wang HM, Wang CH. Phase II study of gemcitabine in patients with advanced hepatocellular carcinoma. Cancer. 2000;89(4):750.

Yeo W, Mok TS, Zee B, et al. A randomized phase III study of doxorubicin versus cisplatin/interferon alpha-2b/doxorubicin/fluorouracil (PIAF) combination chemotherapy for unresectable hepatocellular carcinoma. J Natl Cancer Inst 2005; 97:1532.

Yuen MF, Poon RT, Lai CL, et al. A randomized placebo-controlled study of long-acting octreotide for the treatment of advanced hepatocellular carcinoma. Hepatology 2002; 36:687.

Zhu AX, Blaszkowsky LS, Ryan DP, et al. Phase II study of gemcitabine and oxaliplatin in combination with bevacizumab in patients with advanced hepatocellular carcinoma. J Clin Oncol 2006; 24:1898.

12

The Most Important Local and Regional Treatment Techniques of Hepatocellular Carcinoma and Their Effect over a Long Term Overall Survival

Federico Cattin, Alessandro Uzzau and Dino De Anna
Department of General Surgery, University of Udine School of Medicine
Italy

1. Introduction

During the last years, many local and regional techniques have been introduced, helping, together with surgery, to treat the hepatocellular carcinoma, and contributing to an important improvement of disease free survival and overall survival of patients affected by this disease. These techniques, suitable also for metastatic lesions, can be performed as exclusive ones or following surgery, and help controlling tumor progression even when it is over any possible surgical approach.

Local and regional therapies can be divided into two groups: in the first one we can consider the techniques using heat to obtain their effect, in the second one we consider those using chemotherapic drugs to obtain necrosis of the neoplastic tissue. Necrosis can be obtained through the energy produced by radiofrequency probes, through the alcohol or acetic acid injection or through the injection of embolyzing substances, also together with chemotherapic drugs, into the hepatic artery. Last but not least, the injection of yttrium labeled microspheres is available. These are injected into the hepatic artery and are able to cytoreduce the tumor through a local irradiation.

2. Description

The most important techniques nowadays available are:

2.1 Percutaneous ethanol injection

This is the oldest technique, and it consists in the percutaneous injection of absolute ethanol into the lesion using a fine needle provided with one or more infusion holes. Ethylic alcohol is able to induce a neoplasm coagulative necrosis through cellular dehydration and protein denaturing. Moreover, it causes vascular thrombosis with occlusion of the small vessels which normally feed the tumor. This is a feasible technique for small lesions under 2 centimeters of diameter. Considering these lesions, ethanol has demonstrated its ability to induce a necrosis of more than 95 % of the tumor volume. This result is absolutely similar to the one obtained with more recent techniques like radiofrequency ablation, which on the contrary gets better results if used on bigger nodules. In facts, in case of lesions 2-5 cm of diameter, PEI is able to produce a necrosis of just 50% of the neoplasm volume, and this percentage becomes inessential in case of even bigger cancers. On the contrary, even today PEI grants a curability percentage similar to that given by radiofrequency or advanced percutaneous techniques if we consider little HCCs.

Difficulties shown by PEI in treating medium and big lesions are characteristic of the injected drug: ethanol is not able to diffuse equally into the tumor, as it can not degrade the fibrous septa which are diffused into the nodule. In a 33% of cases these septa may cause a variable distribution of the drug in the lesion, and then a higher risk of relapse of disease. Moreover, big nodules are often well supplied of blood, and also blood circulation may determine a rapid ethanol wash out from the injected site, lowering the therapeutic effect of PEI. Even if PEI is a ultrasound-guided technique, the needle might be inserted in the peripheral part of the nodule, and then its farthest zones might not receive an adequate concentration of drug. In the end, percutaneous ethanol injection has a limited diffusion outside the lesion, and then it's not amenable to grant an adequate volume of oncologic safety based on healthy hepatic tissue around the tumor. This area has normally the highest probability to hide satellite nodules[1,2,3].

Percutaneous ethanol injection is a safe technique, easy, usually well tolerated and feasible also under local anesthesia in outpatients. Sometimes some sessions of therapy are required to achieve a positive oncologic result: most of the protocols schedule eight sessions, once or twice a week, for a whole amount of one or two months of treatment. Complications are linked to the particular kind of technique and to the treated organ: hepatic hematomas, hemoperitoneum, and alcohol diffusion in the blood vessels are the most probable of them, anyhow they are rare and easy to control. Worse complications are described in the Literature in a 0-2% of cases. Among them the tumor seeding along the needle path is included, and this event may happen during all the percutaneous treatments of neoplasm lesions[1,4].

3 years and 5 years survival after exclusive treatment are respectively 22% and 0%

2.2 Percutaneous acetic acid injection

Technically similar to the previous, acetic acid is able to enter easily into the cells, dissolve its lipids and destroy collagen. Acetic acid is used in a solution, and its efficacy rises as its concentration rises, until a plateau is reached when the concentration of drug is about 50%. This level has been defined during studies on mice, the exact one in humans has never been detected. Acetic acid has a cytotoxic effect three times higher than ethanol, and this is the reason why it reaches the same therapeutic result needing a lower number of sessions, improving patient's comfort and minimizing the risk of complications. PAI is in the end useful also for bigger lesions than those treated with PEI, as acetic acid spreads into the nodule through the collagen destruction[1,3].

In spite of these qualities, PAI is nowadays almost abandoned, turning to the advantage of modern techniques. There are many reasons for this: a remarkable risk of toxicity for intravascular diffusion of acid, considerably higher than the one linked to ethanol, risk of tumor seeding along the needle path[4], high level of pain (higher than the one linked to PEI) and then all the risks linked to the puncture of a high vascularized parenchyma, like the hepatic one, typical of every percutaneous treatment.

Percutaneous acetic acid injection seems more effective than PEI under a therapeutic point of view: the low pH characteristic of the acid is able to destroy any septum into the nodule, and so tumor necrosis is more homogeneous and safe. For this reason, PAI is healing as much as PEI and radiofrequency ablation if we consider small volume lesions, granting percentages of necrosis close to 95% if nodules are less than 2 cm of diameter[5,6]. In this case and in selected groups disease free survival rate is 100% and 92% respectively at 1 and 2 years (Ohnishi et al.), noticeably higher than the one linked to PEI.

3 years and 5 years survival, on the contrary, after exclusive treatment are respectively 40% and 0%[6].

2.3 Radiofrequency ablation

Radiofrequency ablation is a technique that induces tissue necrosis through cellular dehydration following a local heat growth. During this procedure, the patient is a part of a real and proper electric circuit, which comprises a generator, a needle to be inserted into the neoplasm, a wide surface plate to be used as an electric outflow, and of course patient's tissues. Heat growth is directly depending on tissue impedance against electric flow, measured in Ohm: as it is quite high, in the immediate surroundings of the entry point into the patient (the needle) a frictional verifiable thermic increase develops. It causes a coagulative necrosis of treated tissues, with a curative effect. Radiofrequency waves swing between 300 KHz and 2500 MHz, and the amount of necrotized tissue is depending on the heat, the time of exposure and the needle caliber.

A key point for a good radiofrequency procedure is the possibility to control the level of temperature reached during the treatment. In facts, a 55 degrees local temperature, kept for 4-6 minutes, is able to cause an irreversible cellular damage and then apoptosis. A 60-100 degrees local temperature causes an immediate tissue coagulation, as like as the one caused by an electrical scalpel during hemostasis, and then a mythocondrial and cytoplasmic enzymes damage, with a sudden cellular death. A temperature over 100 degrees induces tissue vaporization and carbonization[5].

These different reactions must be considered under the point of view of the different ability damaged tissues have to transmit electricity. At a first time a neoplastic carbonization might seem a valid and final result, but it's fundamental to consider that a carbonized tissue has a higher resistance to electric flow than a damaged or healthy one, and then it provides a protective effect to the surrounding structures, which are shielded from any electric exposure. This is the reason why the technique is ineffective if a tissue carbonization happens around the needle.

The system allows to control the temperature reached into the area under treatment, thus avoiding this event. The temperature effective to treatment ranges between 55 and 100 degrees. Needles contain a probe, and any thermic growths are recognized through the continuous measurement of system impedance, direct function of heat growth and tissue change of state. In case of growth, this may be controlled through reducing the energy given to the patient. Due to this, the complete time of treatment might grow up from 4-6 minutes. In our clinical experience, the medium length is about 10-12 minutes, but in some centers sessions lasting up to 30 minutes are performed.

Radiofrequency ablation therapy is a good option in hepatocellular carcinomas either alone, or in combination with surgery, and, even having different technical principles, it is a valid and modern alternative to percutaneous ethanol injection. It is able to reach the same results even through a lower number of treatment sessions, also for lesions more than 2 centimeters of diameter, or metastatic. Especially in these cases this technique has its best advantages in comparison to PEI, and represents a step forward in comparison to other percutaneous procedures.

Using a single needle, the volume of treated hepatic tissue is quite narrow, about 1.8 cm^3. This volume may be enhanced using more powerful generators and needles chilled with saline, which allows a tissue impedance reduction and a growth of heat diffusion and energy delivery. Then, the use of multiple needles or single hooked needles is possible[5,7].

Using these devices, the treated volume may rise up to 3 cm^3 and over. It's better in any case to use a single hooked needle, as it grants a similar treated volume if compared to multiple needles, but it has a bigger treatment evenness.

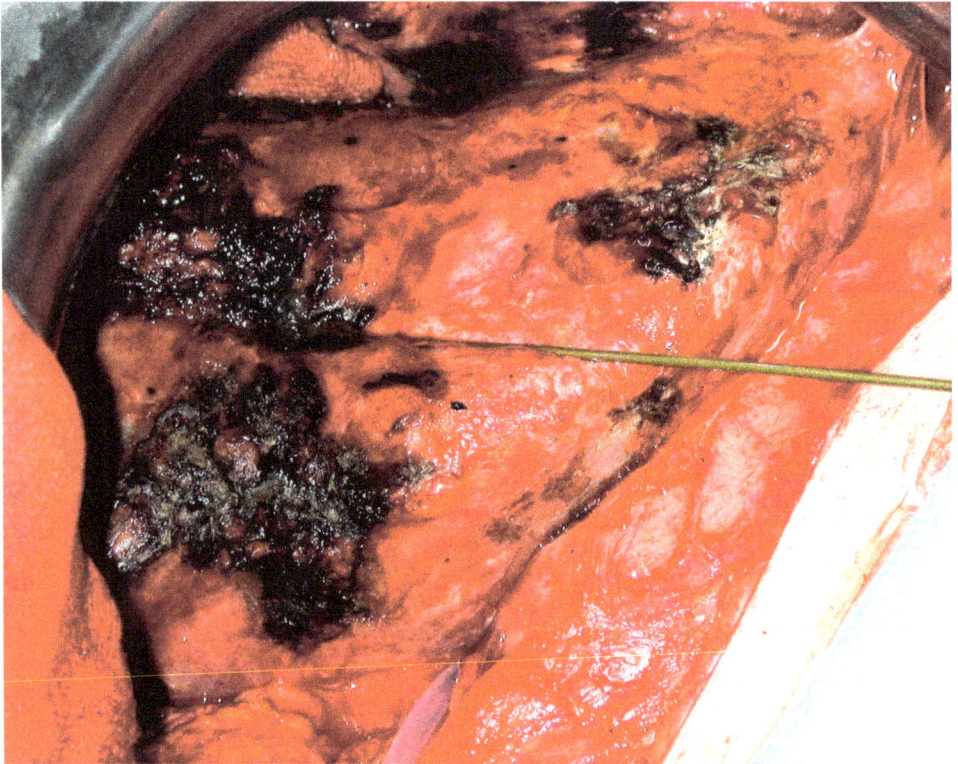

Fig. 1. Radiofrequency over resected liver

Radiofrequency is a versatile technique. It may be provided as an exclusive treatment, through percutaneous needle insertion, or it may follow surgery during an operation as a way to treat satellite lesions or to eliminate metastatic liver nodules during non hepatic surgery. Radiofrequency ablation as an exclusive technique may be provided under local anesthesia or conscious sedation. In some centers radiofrequency is used during surgery as a way to treat the surgical resection surface: it allows a coagulative necrosis of surface cells, thus providing a bigger oncologic safety than that obtained through resection itself.

Radiofrequency has a number of possible complications, linked to the needle insertion into the nodule and to the necrosis following the treatment. Complications described in Literature are, in order of probability, hepatic hematomas or hemoperitoneum needing blood supply, hepatic abscesses caused by necrosis infection and needing percutaneous drainage, thermic bile duct damages needing biliary drainage, hemothoraxes, bowel perforations caused by needle mispositioning, necrosis of organs close to liver due to thermic damage (especially when treating superficial liver lesions), hepatic failure. Neoplastic seeding along the needle path is quite high as a risk (about 2% of procedures), but it can be avoided keeping the system working during the needle extraction, and then performing a real and proper radiofrequency ablation over the tissues which have been in contact to the needle itself. To reach a good result, a temperature of about 75 degrees is important.

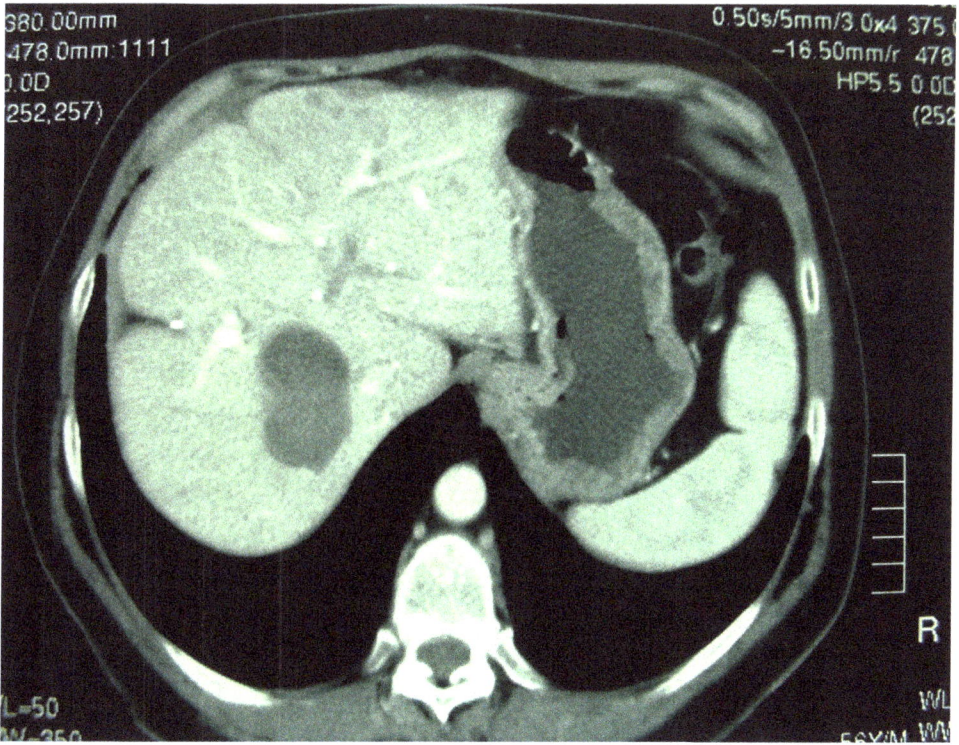

Fig. 2. A typical lesion suitable for radiofrequency during surgery

The strongest limit of this procedure is the presence of blood vessels more than 5 mm of diameter nearby the target lesion. Vessels can reduce the treatment efficacy through heat loss, and may be impossible to reach the 55 degrees temperature mandatory for the technique to be effective. Moreover, even if it's more effective than the previously described techniques, also radiofrequency is affected by the presence of collagen septa into the nodules: even if it's true that heat can destroy collagen, these septa can shield the tissue behind them form thermic effects. This is the reason why it's always impossible to predict the exact final amount of treated volume.

In the end, the only possibility to be certain to avoid any tumor relapse is to be sure to have destroyed every neoplastic cell. This is of course impossible. Heat damage induces the production of tissue growth factors by the cells surrounding the damaged ones, and these substances are the most important factors of disease relapse if any tumor cell survived the

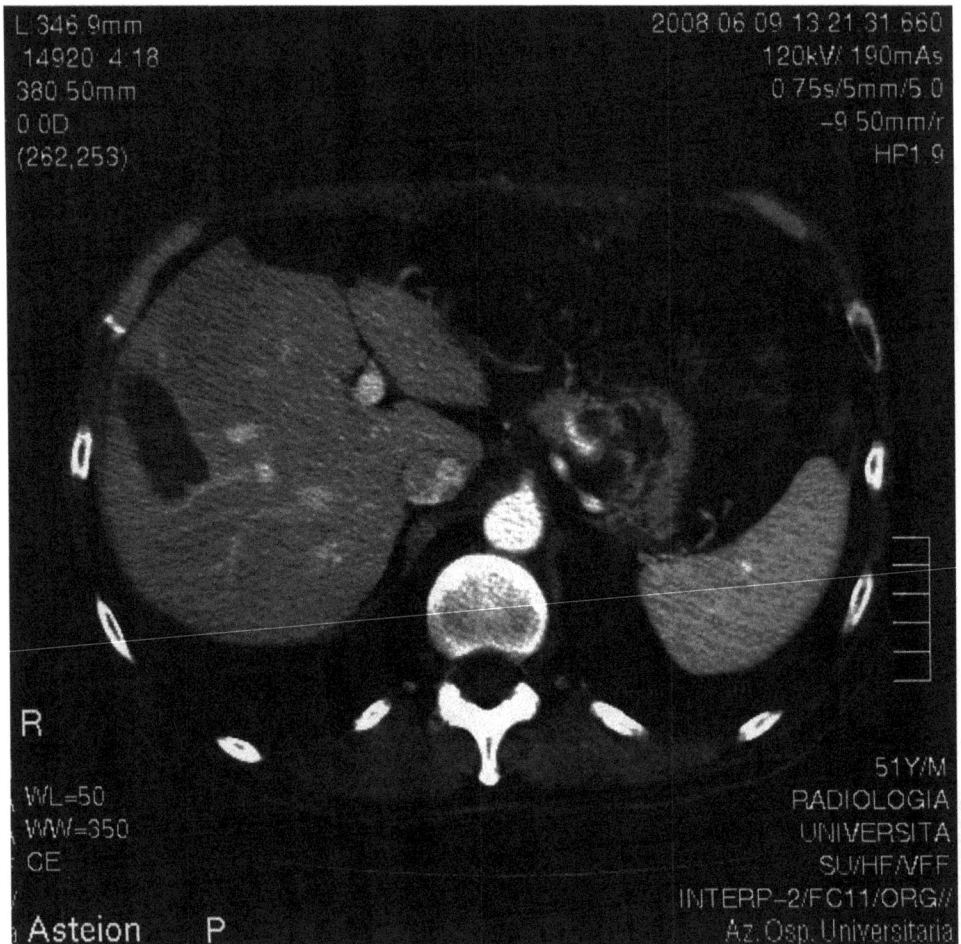

Fig. 3. A lesion suitable for percutaneous radiofrequency

procedure. This is the reason why 3 and 5 years survival rates after exclusive treatment are, respectively, 56-83% and 40-52%. Anyways, these rates are similar to surgical ones in case of surgery following disease relapse. This is the reason why, in these cases, nowadays radiofrequency ablation is a valid exclusive treatment[8].

2.4 Cryotherapy

It consists in positioning a cryogenic probe into the nodule and then in its freezing up to a temperature between -100 and -196 degrees by using liquid nitrogen. The procedure lasts about 15 minutes until the tumor and healthy surrounding tissue frostbite is reached, through the development of cytoplasmic ice crystals, the cellular volume growth and the break of cytoplasmic membranes. Cold as a therapeutic agent against hepatocellular carcinoma makes also use of a particular cellular response to temperature decrease: cryoablation is able to inhibit cellular growth by stimulating a sort of cryoimmunity and by producing cytokines activating the natural killer cells, able to control tumor proliferation. This activation, typical of cryotherapy, is not visible in any other therapy against HCC.

Cryotherapy allows to visualize with millimetric precision the limit between treated area and surroundings during routine radiologic controls. Low temperature action in facts is extremely zone-specific, and as it grows over the freezing limit for hepatic cells, it's possible to meet healthy tissue, not damaged and well distinguishable from the treated area. So knowing exactly how much volume has been treated allows to plan possible further procedures.

Cryotherapy, very promising, is now performed in the operatory room as a surgical time during hepatic resection. This is due to the dimension of probes, bigger than those of radiofrequency ablation. Technical evolution has brought to project and production of thinner probes, available for percutaneous use. This could make this technique available also for non-surgical patients in the immediate future[9].

Any of the two different approaches has of course pros and cons. Cryotherapy during surgery is made considering the possibility to explore all the parts of the abdomen and of the liver, looking for satellite nodules. Then, it's possible the exact positioning of the probe into the tumor, even if it is in areas not reachable through percutaneous puncture or close to other organs. Percutaneous cryotherapy is possible also for outpatients, allows a rapid recovery and an easy pain control. Percutaneous treatment requires two therapy sessions[9,10].

A real comparison between cryotherapy and the most used percutaneous technique – radiofrequency – is difficult to be done. The most important reason is the fact that nowadays radiofrequency is performed mostly as an exclusive and percutaneous technique, while cryotherapy is still a therapeutic option during surgery. Anyways, there is a number of capabilities which might make it even more effective once reached an adequate technical ability. First, cryotherapy induces the production of a group of cytokines inhibiting cellular growth, while radiofrequency induces the production of substances stimulating the relapse of disease. Second, cryotherapy shows an exact limit between treated and non-treated areas, and then allows to control the adequacy of treatment, while radiofrequency creates a shaded border. Third, during cryotherapy it's possible to verify, using ultrasounds, the blistering of ice crystals, and then assess the efficacy of therapy. Fourth, the procedure can be performed using multiple needles, without modifying the shape of the treated volume.

The most important complications typical of this procedure are the same of all the other percutaneous techniques. Using smaller probes than those used during intra-operatory approach (about 3.5 mm of diameter) has minimized the worst complication following cryotherapy, which is the rupture of the frozen area and then the following bleeding. Even if this event is possible after any cryogenic probe insertion, the probability of it is directly proportional to the dimension of the used needles. Another complication is the local and systemic thermic shock, with MOF and disseminated intravascular coagulation. In Literature this event has a risk of 1% of incidence using the old needles, close to 0% using the new smaller ones.

As this is a new technique, and as it is now performed during surgery, it's difficult to provide survival rates linked to its exclusive use. Anyways, in the Literature some Authors show a 3 years survival of about 35%[11].

2.5 Chemoembolization (TACE)

This technique is performed through puncture of the common femoral artery and retrograde reach of a selected branch of the hepatic artery, or percutaneously through puncture of an infuse-a-port previously inserted into the right vessel. It consists in injecting resin microspheres linked to a chemotherapic drug (a cocktail of Mitomycin C, Adriamycin and Cisplatinum) or alone (in this case is correct to call the procedure not chemoembolization but only "embolization"). These spheres close the artery which provides blood to the liver volume in which there is the tumor. Occlusion causes an ischemic necrosis of the nodule and of the healthy surrounding tissue, and the presence of the chemotherapic drugs allows a lasting treatment. This technique is indicated especially for multifocal neoplasms, normally more than four nodules, but is useful also for a lower number of big lesions, or in any case of non surgical disease[12].

The possibility of using TACE for treatment of all the non surgical patients makes it good for those who would have a light risk of liver failure in case of surgery, and this is the reason why this technique is a good option for all the Child B and C patients. More indications are the absence of vascular and periepatic infiltration and no extra-hepatic spread of disease. In all these cases, also according to the BCLC score, chemoembolization might be considered as a first line treatment for hepatocellular carcinoma.

During the first therapeutic trials, in order to gain a complete treatment, big volumes of hepatic healthy tissue were embolized together with the neoplasm. This could bring to a real risk of organ failure, especially in those patients with low liver function. This is the reason why technological evolution has helped physicians to embolyze liver arteries in an always more selective way, thus trying to perform selective procedures, even less invasive. The collaboration between CT scan techniques and intra-operatory angiography allows the selection of just the sub-segmentary arteries bringing blood to the lesion. Nowadays also the digital angiography is available, able to give clear images during the procedure, tridimensional if needed. Superselective chemoembolization, as it is performed in very little vessels, requires a new carrier of the chemotherapic drug. So, in this case it's impossible to use the standard resin microspheres, but a different material, once used in radiology for hepatic contrast images and no longer in use, which is Lipiodol. This material, thick and able to link to HCC cells, has a disposition to settle and stay into the treated area, and it can also be easily recognized also during a CT scan control without contrast because it is a radiological contrast by itself[13].

As said, chemoembolizing treatment is generally performed linking a drug to a resin microsphere. This process is obviously not necessary to obtain just the embolization of the blood vessel going to the tumor. There is a debate in the Literature whether there is a real need to link the drug to the resin, or not, as the resin alone is able to close the vessel and maybe to eliminate the lesion. Some studies show an almost comparable 3 years overall survival between the first and the second therapeutic option, some other suggest to perform a more complete procedure, and this is the reason why the discussion remains unresolved[13,14].

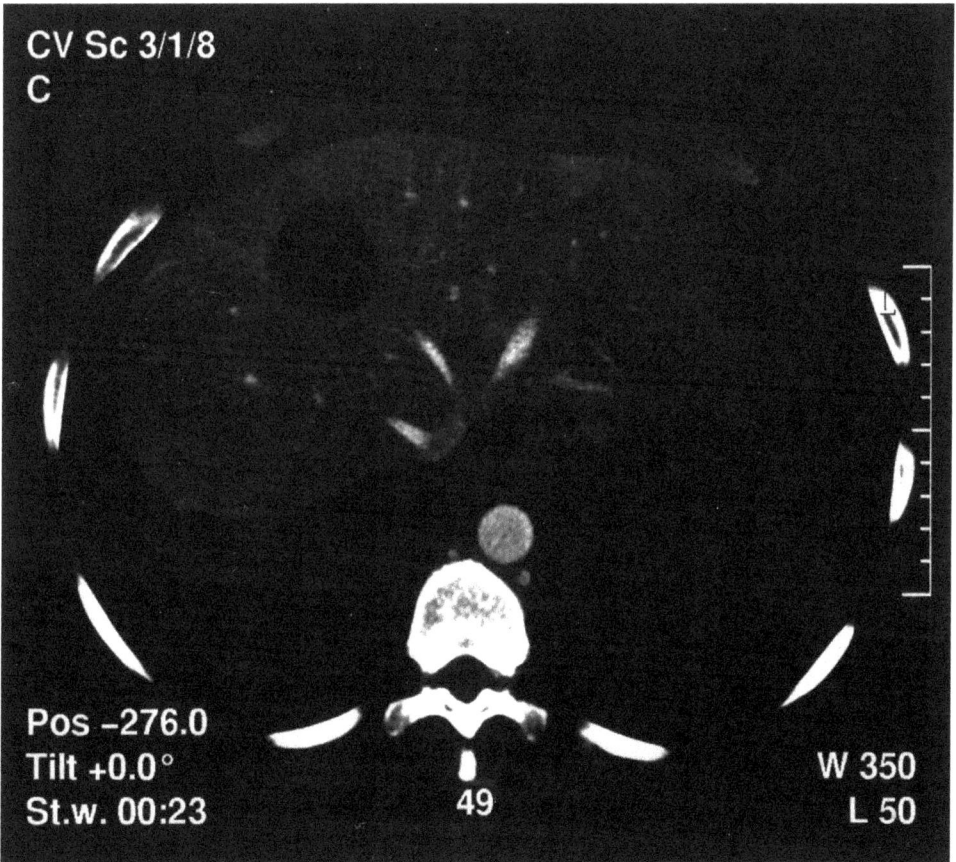

Fig. 4. A lesion following a TACE treatment seen with MR imaging

Chemoembolization does not show the complications typical of the percutaneous procedures with direct tumor puncture. Anyways, considering the loss of healthy liver tissue after TACE, it's mandatory to have a blood liver function test before performing the treatment, as destruction of a volume of liver, even if small in some cases, could bring to organ failure. Moreover a pre-treatment angiographic study is required, looking for vascular anatomic variations or aberrant vessels, which could keep the lesion fed also after the procedure and cause a drug wash out. A pre-treatment angiographic study is important also, on the contrary, to look for anatomic variations to avoid possible ischemic necrosis of other organs close to the liver and not directly involved in the treatment.

The characteristic possibility of TACE to treat also big lesions is the reason why survival after exclusive treatment is a direct consequence of neoplasm dimension. In case of small lesions a survival of 59% after 5 years is described. In case of nodules more than 5 centimeters in diameter, 3 years and 5 years survival are respectively of 27% and 20%, as reported in the Literature[15].

2.6 Yttrium microspheres embolization

This is a real and proper radioembolization, based on the finding that neoplastic liver tissue, as much as the metastatic one coming from other organs, is sensitive to therapeutic radiations. On the contrary, healthy liver tissue can be able to resist to cumulative doses even higher than 3000 Gy. Radioembolization is performed using two possible devices, which are resin microspheres covered with ^{90}Y, similar to those used for chemoembolization, or glass microspheres covered with the same radioactive material. In the USA, resin spheres are FDA authorized for any therapeutic use, while glass spheres are allowed only in case of non-surgical disease. In Europe both devices are allowed[16].

Procedures linked to the Yttrium microspheres treatment are strictly similar to those characteristic of chemoembolization, the only important difference is the fact the intra-arterial drug injection does not require the vessel embolization. In this way the production of some cytokines is avoided, among them there is also the factor 1α hypoxia induced and VEGF, able to stimulate the disease relapse over eventual not completely treated areas. This is the reason why there are some extended indications for this procedure in comparison with TACE: it's possible to perform it even in case of Portal Vein thrombosis, which is a contraindication for chemoembolization as it could bring to ischemic hepatitis, and it's particularly indicated for big lesions. Moreover, Yttrium microspheres appear easier to be tolerated than TACE, as they reduce post-treatment fever and post-chemotherapic diarrhea. On the contrary, patients who underwent this procedure often experience asthenia, and must be kept isolated for at least 24 hours as they are a source of ionizing dangerous waves. The general bearability of the treatment, anyways, makes it a valid option also for patients with a low performance status[16,17].

In the Literature there are always more papers trying to make a comparison between TACE and Yttrium microspheres. The two treatments are in facts quite similar, and results over disease free survival and overall survival are comparable. Today it's still difficult to project equivalence studies, as they require a very big sample population to give significant statistic results. It's demonstrated that radiometabolic treatment brings to an important improvement in terms of time to progression, which is the time between the treatment and the disease relapse. Moreover, if there is an adequate structure to accommodate them, older or weak people are some of the best patients to receive this treatment.

In the end, considering the wide amount of contact points between TACE and Yttrium microspheres treatment, technical evolution is moving towards the creation of a unifying method, creating a sort of radioembolization, able to present the good actions of the two procedures, avoiding the bad ones.

Survival curves characteristic of Yttrium microspheres treatment as an exclusive one are quite the same of chemoembolization[18].

3. Conclusions

Most of the techniques described have been performed in our institution, each one according to their indication, to treat hepatic lesions after surgery. We have noticed a growth of disease free survival and overall survival, experiencing how a combined approach to hepatocellular carcinoma is nowadays the most effective way to treat this disease.

4. References

[1] Germani, G. et al. (2010), Clinical outcomes of radiofrequency ablation, percutaneous alcohol and acetic acid injection for hepatocellular carcinoma: a meta-analysis. *Journal of hepatology*, 52 (3), 380-388

[2] Vilana, R. et al. (1992), Tumor size determines the efficacy of percutaneous ethanol injection for the treatment of small hepatocellular carcinoma. *Hepatology*, 16, 353-357

[3] Lencioni, R. et al. (1997), Long-term results of percutaneous ethanol injection therapy for hepatocellular carcinoma in cirrhosis: a European experience. *European journal of radiology*, 1997, 7, 514-519

[4] Stigliano, R. et al. (2007), Seeding following percutaneous diagnostic and therapeutic approaches for hepatocellular carcinoma. What is the risk and the outcome? Seeding risk for percutaneous approach of HCC. *Cancer treatment review*, 33, 437-447

[5] Lencioni, R. et al. (2004), Percutaneous ablation of hepatocellular carcinoma: state of the art. *Liver transplantation*, 10 (2), Suppl 1, S91-S97

[6] Ohnishi, K. et al. (1998), Prospective randomized controlled trial comparing percutaneous acetic acid injection and percutaneous ethanol injection for small hepatocellular carcinoma. *Hepatology*, 27, 67-72

[7] Goldberg, S.N. et al. (2000), Thermal ablation therapies for focal malignancies: a unified approach to underlying principles, techniques and diagnostic imaging guidance. *American journal of roentgenology*, 174, 323-331

[8] Choi, D. et al. (2007), Percutaneous radiofrequency ablation for recurrent hepatocellular carcinoma after hepatectomy: long-term results and prognostic factors. *Annals of surgical oncology*, 14 (8), 2319-29

[9] Chen, H.W. et al. (2011), Ultrasound-guided percutaneous cryotherapyof hepatocellular carcinoma. *International journal of surgery*, 9 (2), 188-191

[10] Han, B. et al. (2004), Improved cryosurgery by useof thermophysical and inflammatory adjuvants. *Technology cancer research and treatment*, 3, 103-111

[11] Adam, R. et al. (2002), A comparison of percutaneous cryosurgery and percutaneous radiofrequency for unresectable hepatic malignancies. *Archives of surgery*, 137, 1332-1339

[12] Takayasu, K. (2010), Chemoembolization for unresectable Hepatocellular carcinoma in Japan. *Oncology*, 78 (suppl.1), 135-141

[13] Matsui, O. et al. (1994), Subsegmental transcatheter arterial embolization for small hepatocellular carcinomas: Local therapeutic effect and 5-year survival rate. *Cancer chemotherapy and pharmacology*, 33 (suppl), 84-88

[14] Bronowicki, J.P. et al. (1994), Transcatheter oily chemoembolization for hepatocellular carcinoma: A 4-year study of 127 French patients. *Cancer*, 74, 16-24

[15] Coldwell, D. et al. (2010), Radioembolization in the treatment of unresectable liver tumors: experience across a range of primary cancers. *American journal of clinical oncology*, online first (November 30)

[16] Salem, R. et al. (2011), Radioembolization results in longer time-to-progression and reduced toxicity compared with chemoembolization in patients with hepatocellular carcinoma. *Gastroenterology*, 140, 497-507

[17] Leelawat, K. et al. (2008), The effect of doxorubicin on the changes of serum vascular endothelial growth factor (VEGF) in patients with hepatocellular carcinoma after transcatheter arterial chemoembolization (TACE). *Journal of medical association of Thailand*, 91, 1539-1543

[18] Virmani, S. et al. (2008), Comparison of hypoxia-induced factor 1α expression before and after transcatheter arterial embolization in rabbit VX2 liver tumors. *Journal of vascular interventional radiology*, 19, 1483-1489

13

Transcatheter Arterial Chemo-Embolization with a Fine-Powder Formulation of Cisplatin for Unresectable Hepatocellular Carcinoma

Kazuhiro Kasai and Kazuyuki Suzuki

Division of Gastroenterology and Hepatology, Department of Internal Medicine
Iwate Medical University
Japan

1. Introduction

Hepatocellular carcinoma (HCC) is the cancer with the sixth highest incidence in the world.[1] The incidence of this cancer has increased significantly in the United States, Japan and several European countries over the last two or three decades. HCC as a cause of death is also increasing throughout the world.[2-5] Development of new treatments for HCC has helped to improve patient prognosis.[6, 7] Transcatheter arterial chemoembolization (TACE) is one such treatment, and has been applied to patients with multiple or unresectable HCC.[8, 9] However, HCC has been reported to progress within the short period of multiple sessions of TACE into a complicated condition, even though the treatment is temporarily effective. In recent years, TACE using an emulsion of doxorubicin (ADM) with lipiodol (LPD) (ADM-LPD emulsion) followed by embolization with gelatin sponge has commonly been employed for HCC treatment.[10, 11] However, the tumors have been demonstrated to show a high frequency of recurrence after TACE.[9, 12, 13] Cisplatin (CDDP), a platinum compound, is an effective anticancer agent used in the treatment of various malignancies.[14] Researchers have recently reported that TACE using a suspension of CDDP in LPD may be more effective against unresectable HCC than that using ADM-LPD emulsion.[15, 16] Moreover, a fine-powder formulation of CDDP (DDPH, IA-call; Nipponkayaku, Tokyo, Japan) has also been available since 2004 as a therapeutic agent for intra-arterial infusion in Japan.

In this article, we report the results of a retrospective comparative review of TACE using a suspension of DDPH in LPD (DDPH-LPD suspension) and an emulsion of ADM in LPD, in terms of the response rate (RR), progression-free survival (PFS) and overall survival (OS). Moreover, we analyzed prognostic factors in patients undergoing TACE using DDPH-LPD suspension or ADM-LPD emulsion.

2. Methods

2.1 Patients

We reviewed 468 consecutive HCC patients who had undergone TACE using DDPH or ADM between April 2004 and September 2008 at the Hospital of Iwate Medical

University. HCC was diagnosed based on distinctive findings on ultrasonography (US), computed tomography (CT), magnetic resonance imaging (MRI) and angiography, and serum levels of des-γ-carboxy prothrombin (DCP) and α-fetoprotein (AFP). Histological examination was not always applied. Liver function was evaluated according to the Child-Pugh classification.[17]   Tumor stage was judged by the TNM classification established by the International Union Against Cancer.[18]   The extent of portal vein invasion was classified as follows: Vp0, no invasion of the portal vein; Vp1, invasion of the third or more distal branch of the left or right portal vein; Vp2, invasion of the second branch of the portal vein; Vp3, invasion of the first branch of the portal vein; and Vp4, invasion of the trunk of the portal vein.

We excluded 18 patients with serum bilirubin levels over 3.0 mg/dL, 12 patients with extra-hepatic metastasis, and 30 patients with uncontrolled ascites. In addition, we excluded 77 patients who had undergone repeated sessions of TACE using different regimens, and 44 patients who showed disease progression and received hepatic arterial infusion chemotherapy (HAIC) and/or systemic chemotherapy as additional therapy.

A final total of 287 HCC patients were enrolled in this study. All of the enrolled patients met the eligibility criteria for inclusion in the analysis described in the next paragraph. Patients were divided into two groups: one group consisting of 120 patients who had undergone TACE using DDPH-LPD suspension (DDPH group); and another group consisting of 167 patients who had undergone TACE using an emulsion of LPD with ADM (ADM group). Of the 120 patients in the DDPH group, 44 had also received various additional therapies such as radiofrequency ablation (RFA) or surgical operation (OPE) after TACE, and 76 patients had undergone TACE alone during the study period. Similarly, 79 patients of the ADM group had received various additional therapies such as RFA or OPE after TACE, and 88 patients had undergone TACE alone without any other therapies during the study period.

Informed consent was obtained from all patients. The study protocol was approved by the Ethics Committee of Iwate Medical University and the study was conducted in accordance with the Declaration of Helsinki 1975.

2.2 Eligibility criteria

Eligibility criteria for patients in this study were as follows: 1) no evidence of extrahepatic metastasis; 2) no evidence of active heart or renal diseases meeting the contraindications for ADM and CDDP therapy, respectively; 3) Eastern Cooperative Oncology Group (ECOG) performance status (PS)[19] level 0-2; 4) no uncontrolled ascites or pleural effusion; and 5) total serum bilirubin (T-Bil) less than 3 mg/dL. The presence of underlying liver disease such as hepatitis or cirrhosis was confirmed by laboratory, radiological examinations and pathological examinations. We classified chronic hepatitis patients into Child-Pugh class A, because chronic hepatitis is a known pre-cirrhotic condition.

2.3 Preparation of the agents for TACE

We used DDPH or ADM (Adriacin; Kyowa Hakko Kogyo, Tokyo, Japan) mixed with LPD (iodized oil; Andre Guerget, Aulnay-sous-Bois, France).

The DDPH/LPD suspension was prepared by mixing 50 mg of DDPH into 3-10 mL of LPD.

The ADM/LPD emulsion was prepared by the following procedure: 10-30 mg of ADM was dissolved in 1-2 mL of a contrast medium (Iomeron; Eisai, Tokyo, Japan) and then mixed with 3-10 mL of LPD.

The dosages of LPD and the anticancer drugs were adjusted depending on tumor size, number of tumors, degree of liver impairment and renal function, with the maximum dose of LPD not allowed to exceed 10 mL.

2.4 Treatment regimen

The patient enrolment period for the DDHP and ADM groups extended from May 2006 to September 2008 and April 2004 to September 2008, respectively. All patients provided fully informed consent prior to TACE. In terms of embolization agents, gelatin sponge particles (Gelpart; Nipponkayaku, Tokyo, Japan) were used for all patients.

After TACE, additional RFA or OPE therapy was provided to patients who met the following inclusion criteria: the presence of up to three tumors with none exceeding 30 mm in diameter or a solitary tumor less than 50 mm in diameter. Regardless of the additional therapy requirement, all patients were followed up with US, CT and/or MRI after 1 month, then every 3 months thereafter. TACE was undertaken again when relapse of treated lesions and/or new hepatic lesions were detected. These patients received additional TACE using the same agent during the follow-up period. TACE or TACE with additional therapy (RFA or OPE) was repeated until complete regression of the tumor was obtained, or until the patient could no longer be treated.

2.5 Post-treatment assessment

Tumor response was assessed by US, CT and/or MRI, conducted 1 month from the start of treatment and every 3 months thereafter. We regarded LPD accumulation in the tumor as representing a necrotic area, based on previous reports of such LPD retention areas corresponding to the necrotic areas on CT.[20-23] By measurement of the two largest perpendicular diameters of the tumor, we classified tumor response into four categories using the following criteria: complete response (CR), complete disappearance or 100% necrosis of all tumors; partial response (PR), reduction and/or necrosis, with a decrease of at least 50% in all measurable lesions; progressive disease (PD), an increase in tumor size exceeding 25% of all measurable lesions or appearance of a new lesion; stable disease (SD), disease not qualifying for classification as CR, PR, or PD.

Toxicity was evaluated using the National Cancer Institute–Common Terminology Criteria for Adverse Events, version 3.0 (CTCAE v3.0).

2.6 Evaluation of therapeutic effects

We analyzed outcomes in the DDPH and ADM groups in terms of RR, PFS and OS in September 2008. In addition, we also evaluated all patients for survival using uni- and multivariate analyses. Duration of response was calculated from the date of the start of treatment to the date of documented progression. Survival time was calculated from the date of the start of treatment to the date of death or last day of follow-up.

US, CT and/or MRI were performed as mentioned above. In addition, serum levels of biochemical parameters and tumor markers such as AFP and DCP were also measured before and after treatment. The same tests were repeated after completion of every session of treatment.

2.7 Statistical analysis

Differences in background clinical characteristics of patients between the DDPH and ADM groups were assessed using the Mann-Whitney U test, logistic regression test, or the χ^2 test, as appropriate.

PFS and OS were calculated from the date of the start of therapy to the date on which tumor progression was documented and the date of patient death, respectively. Both were assessed using the Kaplan-Meier life-table method, and differences between the two treatment groups were evaluated with the log-rank test. Univariate analysis to identify predictors of survival in patients was conducted with the Kaplan-Meier life-table method, and differences between groups were evaluated using the log-rank test. Multivariate analysis to identify predictors of survival was conducted using the Cox proportional hazards model. Statistical significance was defined as a value of $P<0.05$. All of the above analyses were performed using SPSS version 11 software (SPSS, Chicago, IL, USA).

3. Results

3.1 Patient profiles (table 1)

Characteristics of the 287 patients (200 men, 87 women) in both groups are summarized in Table 1. Mean age was 68.4 years (range, 21-90 years).

For the assessment of differences in patient characteristics, patients were divided into two groups based on each characteristic, and significant differences were observed between the DDPH and ADM groups in relation to the gender distribution, TNM classification, tumor size and number of tumors. That is, the DPHH group showed a significantly higher proportion of men ($P=0.030$), higher frequency of more advanced TNM classification ($P<0.001$), and larger tumor size and number ($P=0.004$, $P=0.026$, respectively) than the ADM group. No significant differences in any of the other characteristics were seen between groups.

In relation to differences in the characteristics of patients with no apparent history of additional therapy, significant differences in gender distribution and TNM classification were evident between groups, with higher proportions of men ($P=0.031$) and advanced TNM classification ($P=0.026$) in the DPHH group. No significant differences in any of the other characteristics were seen between groups.

On the other hand, with regard to differences in the characteristics of patients who received additional therapy, the DDPH group differed significantly from the ADM group in terms of TNM classification, tumor size and number of tumors. That is, TNM classification was more advanced ($P=0.003$), tumor size was larger ($P=0.007$) and number of tumors was greater ($P=0.050$) in the DDPH group. No significant differences in other patient characteristics were evident between groups.

	Overall		
Characteristics	DDPH	ADM	P value
No. of patients	120	167	
Age (years) [Median, (range)]	66 (32-87)	69 (21-90)	0.073
Gender (Male / Female)	92/28	108/59	0.030
Etiology (HBV/ HCV / NBNC)	17/83/20	21/119/27	0.911
Child- Pugh (A / B / C)	76/40/4	103/55/8	0.825
TNM classification (I-II / III-IV)	29/91	80/87	< 0.001
Tumor size (≤ 3.0/ >3.0 cm)	44/76	90/77	0.004
Number of tumors (1-3 / ≥4)	68/52	116/51	0.026
PVTT (Vp0-2 / Vp3-4)	106/14	158/9	0.053
Total bilirubin (≤ 1.5 / >1.5 mg/dL)	106/14	150/16	0.581
Albumin (≤ 3.5 / >3.5 g/dL)	54/66	73/93	0.863
AFP (≤ 1000 / >1000 ng/mL)	108/12	155/11	0.301
DCP (≤ 1000 / >1000 mAU/mL)	99/17	146/17	0.288

	According to additional therapy					
	Additional therapy (-)			Additional therapy (+)		
Characteristics	DDPH	ADM	P value	DDPH	ADM	P value
No. of patients	76	88		44	79	
Age (years) [Median, (range)]	67 (32-87)	69 (21-90)	0.093	63 (44-81)	68 (42-80)	0.143
Gender (Male/Female)	57/19	52/36	0.031	35/9	56/23	0.294
Etiology (HBV/HCV/NBNC)	11/50/15	8/64/16	0.508	7/32/5	15/53/11	0.818
Child- Pugh (A/B/C)	47/26/3	45/36/7	0.303	29/14/11	58/19/2	0.598
TNM classification (I-II/III-IV)	10/66	24/64	0.026	19/25	56/23	0.003
Tumor size (≤ 3.0/>3.0 cm)	21/55	30/58	0.373	23/21	60/19	0.007
Number of tumors (1-3/≥4)	35/41	46/42	0.427	33/11	70/9	0.050
PVTT (Vp0-2/Vp3-4)	62/14	80/8	0.080	44/0	78/1	0.454
Total bilirubin (≤ 1.5 / >1.5 mg/dL)	66/10	75/13	0.906	40/4	75/4	0.385
Albumin (≤ 3.5 / >3.5 g/dL)	38/38	45/42	0.822	16/28	28/51	0.919
AFP (≤ 1000 />1000 ng/mL)	68/8	79/8	0.776	40/4	76/3	0.225
DCP(≤ 1000/>1000 mAU/mL)	59/14	73/14	0.609	41/3	73/3	0.468

Table 1. Patient characteristics

Data are expressed as median with range values, or the number of patients. HBV, hepatitis B virus; HCV, hepatitis C virus; NBNC, negative for hepatitis B surface antigen and HCV antibody; PVTT, portal vein tumor thrombosis; AFP, α-fetoprotein; DCP, des-γ-carboxy prothrombin. Stages of HCC according to TNM classification were clustered into two groups (I–II and III–IV). Tumor characteristics and other parameters were classified as follows: tumor size, ≤ 3.0 vs. >3.0 cm; tumor number, 1-3 vs. >4; extent of PVTT, Vp0-2 vs. Vp3-4; serum bilirubin, ≤ 1.5 vs. >1.5 mg/dL; serum albumin, ≤ 3.5 vs. >3.5 g/dL; serum AFP levels, ≤ 1000 vs. >1000 ng/mL; and serum DCP levels, ≤ 1000 vs. >1000 mAU/mL.

3.2 Response to therapy (table 2)

3.2.1 Evaluation of the total subject population

RR for all 287 patients was evaluated after one session of therapy. Table 2 shows tumor responses in the two groups. In the DDPH group, 34 (28.3%), 49 (40.8%), 12 (10.0%) and 25 (20.9%) patients showed CR, PR, SD and PD, respectively. In the ADM group, 69 (41.4%), 23 (13.8%), 5 (2.9%) and 70 (41.9%) patients showed CR, PR, SD and PD, respectively. The objective response rate (CR + PR / all cases in each group) was thus significantly higher in the DDPH group (69.1%) than in the ADM group (55.2%; $P=0.0159$).

	Overall		
Response	DDPH (n=120)	ADM (n=167)	P value
CR(%)	34 (28.3%)	69 (41.4%)	
PR(%)	49 (40.8%)	23 (13.8%)	
SD(%)	12 (10.0%)	5 (2.9%)	
PD(%)	25 (20.9%)	70 (41.9%)	
CR+PR(%)	83 (69.1%)	92 (55.2%)	0.016

	Additional therapy					
	(-)			(+)		
Response	DDPH (n=76)	ADM (n=88)	P value	DDPH (n=44)	ADM (n=79)	P value
CR(%)	2 (2.7%)	5 (5.7%)		32 (72.7%)	64 (81.0%)	
PR(%)	39 (51.3%)	16 (18.2%)		10 (22.7%)	7 (8.9%)	
SD(%)	23 (30.2%)	5 (5.7%)		2 (4.6%)	0 (0%)	
PD(%)	12 (15.8%)	62 (70.4%)		0 (0%)	8 (10.1%)	
CR+PR(%)	41 (54.0%)	21 (23.9%)	<0.001	42 (95.4%)	71 (89.9%)	0.278

Table 2. Response

3.2.2 Evaluation of patients who reported no history of additional therapy

In the DDPH group, 2 (2.7%), 39 (51.3%), 23 (30.2%) and 12 (15.8%) patients showed CR, PR, SD and PD, respectively. In the ADM group, 5 (5.7%), 16 (18.2%), 5 (5.7%) and 62 (70.4%) patients showed CR, PR, SD and PD, respectively. The objective response rate was thus significantly higher in the DDPH group (54.0%) than in the ADM group (23.9%; $P<0.0001$).

3.2.3 Evaluation of patients who reported a history of additional therapy

In the DDPH group, 32 (72.7%), 10 (22.7%), 2 (4.6%) and 0 (0%) patients showed CR, PR, SD and PD, respectively. In the ADM group, 64 (81.0%), 7 (8.9%), 0 (0%) and 8 (10.1%) patients showed CR, PR, SD and PD, respectively. No significant difference in objective response rate was apparent between groups, with 95.4% in the DDPH group and 89.9% in the ADM group ($P=0.2778$).

Data are expressed as number of patients and percentages. CR, complete response; PR, partial response; SD, stable disease; PD, progressive disease.

3.3 PFS (fig. 1)

3.3.1 Evaluation of the entire subject population

Median PFS in the DDPH group and ADM group was 11.1 months and 5.0 months, respectively. PFS rates at 6, 12, 18 and 24 months were 70.0%, 47.0%, 27.2% and 24.5%, respectively, in the DDPH group. In contrast, corresponding values were 46.4%, 31.0%, 21.5% and 18.8%, respectively, in the ADM group. PFS rates were significantly higher in the DDPH group than in the ADM group ($P=0.0045$).

3.3.2 Evaluation of patients who reported no history of additional therapy

Median PFS was 7.6 months in the DDPH group and 3.0 months in the ADM group. PFS rates at 6, 12, 18 and 24 months were 56.5%, 32.2%, 15.3% and 15.3%, respectively, in the DDPH group. In contrast, corresponding values were 18.4%, 10.3%, 5.4% and 5.4%, respectively, in the ADM group. PFS rates were significantly higher in the DDPH group than in the ADM group ($P<0.0001$).

3.3.3 Evaluation of patients who reported a history of additional therapy

Median PFS was 17.7 months in the DDPH group and 12.9 months in the ADM group. PFS rates at 6, 12, 18 and 24 months were 90.7%, 74.9%, 42.1% and 42.1%, respectively, in the DDPH group, and 75.9%, 52.6%, 39.3% and 32.3%, respectively, in the ADM group. Although no significant differences in PFS rates were apparent between groups, rates tended to be higher in the DDPH group than in the ADM group ($P=0.1171$).

PFS rate was significantly higher in the DDPH group than in the ADM group in both assessment of the entire study population and assessment of patients who reported no history of receiving additional therapy (log-rank test: $P=0.05$, $P<0.001$, respectively). The difference in PFS rates between patients of the two groups who had received additional therapy was not significant, but a strong tendency was evident (log-rank test: $P=0.117$).

3.3.1) Evaluation of the entire study population

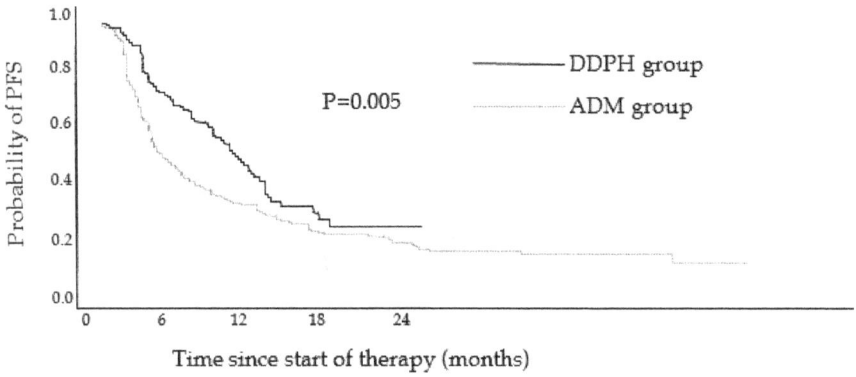

3.3.2) Evaluation of the patients who gave no history of additional therapy

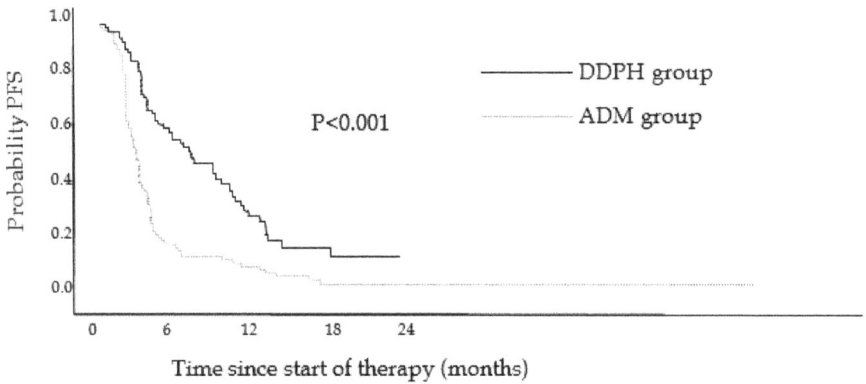

3.3.3.) Evaluation of the patients who gave a history of additional therapy

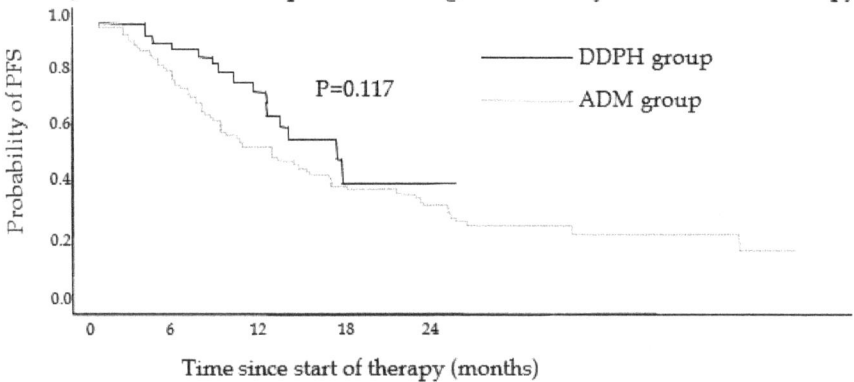

Fig. 1. Comparison of progression-free survival (PFS) rates between DDPH and ADM groups.

3.4 Survival (fig. 2, tables 3, 4)

3.4.1 Evaluation of the entire subject population

Median survival time (MST) in the DDPH and ADM groups was 'not reached' and 45.3 months, respectively. OS at 6, 12, 18, and 24 months were 94.7%, 86.3%, 82.3% and 77.5%, respectively, in the DDPH group. Corresponding values were 94.3%, 82.7%, 74.9% and 69.5%, respectively, in the ADM group. No significant differences in OS were seen between groups ($P=0.236$).

Univariate analysis to identify predictors of survival indicated seven possible factors affecting survival: Child-Pugh class; TNM classification; tumor size; number of tumors; PVTT; T-Bil; and DCP (Table 3). Multivariate analysis taking all of the factors identified by univariate analysis into account identified treatment regimen, Child-Pugh class, number of tumors, PVTT and DCP as independent factors affecting survival (Table 4).

3.4.2 Evaluation of patients who reported no history of additional therapy

MST in the DDPH and ADM groups was 'not reached' and 20.7 months, respectively. OS at 6, 12, 18, and 24 months were 91.6%, 78.9%, 73.4% and 67.3%, respectively, in the DDPH group. Corresponding values in the ADM group were 87.3%, 68.3%, 54.8% and 46.4%, respectively. OS was significantly higher in the DDPH group than in the ADM group ($P=0.046$).

3.4.3 Evaluation of patients who reported a history of additional therapy

MST in both groups was 'not reached'. OS at 6, 12, 18 and 24 months were 100%, 100%, 100% and 100%, respectively, in the DDPH group, compared to 100%, 95.9%, 94.5% and 90.1%, respectively, in the ADM group. No significant differences in OS were evident between groups ($P=0.456$).

OS was significantly higher in the DDPH group than in the ADM group in the assessment of the entire study population, as well as among patients who reported no history of receiving additional therapy (log-rank test: $P=0.046$). No significant difference in OS was seen between patients in the two groups who had received additional therapy (log-rank test: $P=0.236$, $P=0.456$, respectively).

HBV, hepatitis B virus; HCV, hepatitis C virus; NBNC, negative for hepatitis B surface antigen and HCV antibody; PVTT, portal vein tumor thrombosis; AFP, α-fetoprotein; DCP, des-γ-carboxy prothrombin.

3.5 Adverse effects (table 5)

Table 5 shows a summary of adverse effects in the two groups. Abdominal pain, nausea/vomiting, fever, and elevation of serum transaminase levels were observed in most patients of both groups, but these symptoms were mild and transient. The frequency of nausea/ vomiting was significantly higher in the DDPH group than in the ADM group ($P<0.0001$). In addition, frequencies of occlusion of the hepatic artery and leucopenia were significantly higher in the ADM group than in the DDPH group ($P<0.001$ and $P=0.002$, respectively). No other serious complications or treatment-related deaths were observed in either group.

3.4.1) Evaluation of the entire study population

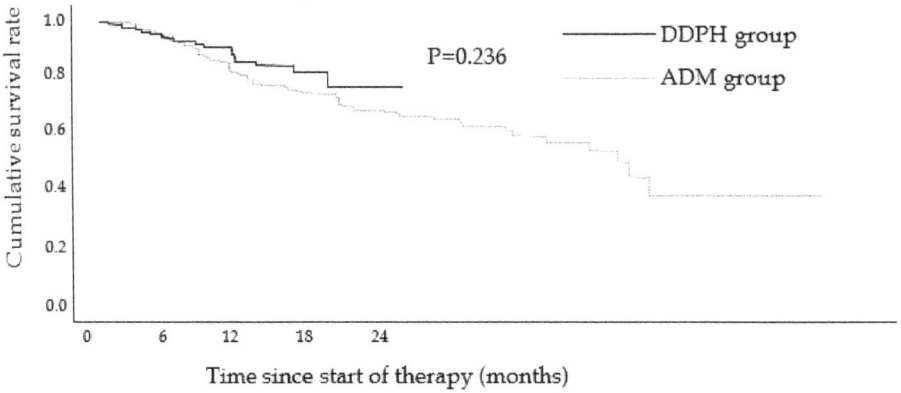

3.4.2) Evaluation of the patients who gave no history of additional therapy

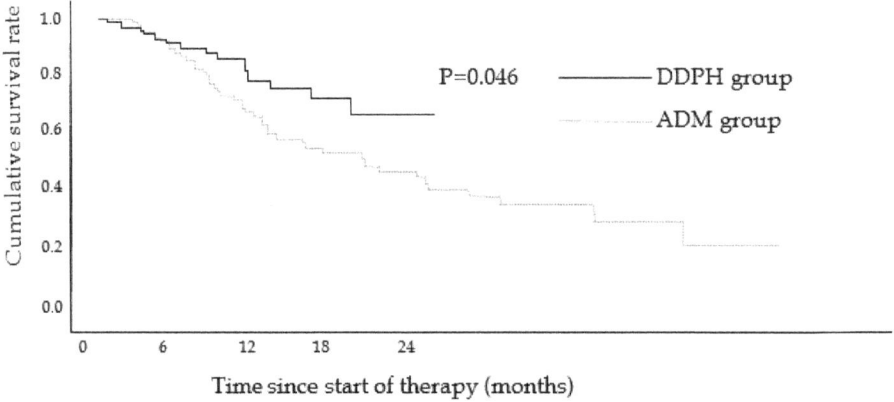

3.4.3) Evaluation of the patients who gave a history of additional therapy

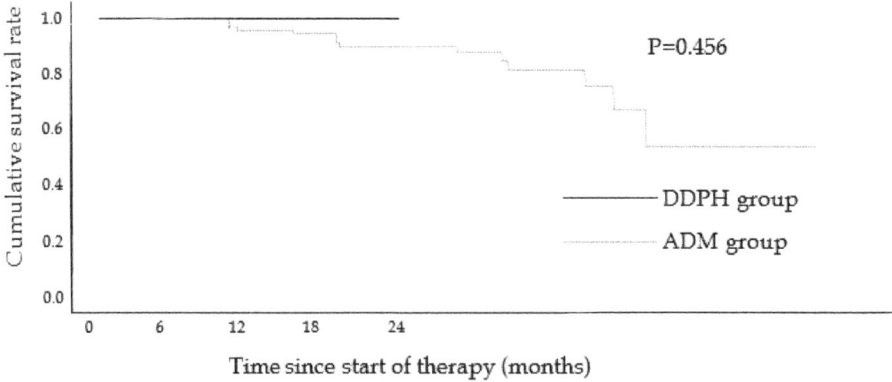

Fig. 2. Comparison of OS between DDPH and ADM groups.

Variable	Hazard ratio	95% confidence interval	P value
Treatment regimen (ADM vs. DDPH)	0.752	0.425-1.330	0.327
Age (≤65 years vs. >65 years)	1.466	0.895-2.400	0.129
Gender (Female vs. Male)	1.116	0.681-1.828	0.663
Etiology (NBNC vs. HBV/ HCV)	0.960	0.587-1.572	0.872
Child Pugh classification (A vs. B/C)	1.747	0.105-2.762	0.017
TNM classification (I-II vs. III-IV)	3.567	2.037-6.244	< 0.001
Tumor size (≤ 3.0 vs. >3.0 cm)	2.871	1.754-4.701	< 0.001
Number of tumors (1-3 vs. ≥4)	4.073	2.550-6.503	< 0.001
PVTT (Vp0-2 vs. Vp3-4)	6.951	3.804-12.703	< 0.001
Total bilirubin (≤ 1.5 vs. >1.5 mg/dL)	2.512	1.347-4.684	0.004
Albumin (≤ 3.5 vs. >3.5 g/dL)	0.633	0.400-1.002	0.051
AFP (≤ 1000 vs. >1000 ng/mL)	1.882	0.860-4.117	0.113
DCP (≤ 1000 vs. >1000 mAU/mL)	3.266	1.884-5.786	< 0.001

Table 3. Univariate analysis for identifying predictors of survival

Variable	Hazard ratio	95% confidence interval	P value
Treatment regimen (ADM vs. DDPH)	0.428	0.196-0.934	0.033
Child Pugh classification (A vs. B/C)	3.102	1.685-5.712	0.001
Number of tumors (1-3 vs. ≥4)	5.831	3.041-11.181	<0.001
PVTT (Vp0-2 vs. Vp3-4)	5.428	2.197-13.409	0.001
DCP (≤ 1000 vs. >1000 mAU/mL)	3.890	1.747-8.663	0.001

PVTT, portal vein tumor thrombosis; DCP, des-γ-carboxy prothrombin

Table 4. Multivariate analysis for identifying predictors of survival

| Adverse effect | Treatment group | | P value |
	DDPH group (n=120)	ADM group (n=167)	
Nausea / Vomiting	101 (84.2%)	103 (61.6%)	<0.001
Fever	96 (80.0%)	138 (82.6%)	0.571
Abdominal pain	83 (69.1%)	116 (69.4%)	0.957
Elevation of trans-aminase levels	87 (72.5%)	121 (72.4%)	0.993
Liver abscess	1 (0.8%)	2 (1.2%)	0.765
Hepatic artery occlusion	1 (0.8%)	28 (16.7%)	<0.001
Renal or liver failure	0 (0.0%)	2 (1.2%)	0.229
Leucopenia	5 (4.2%)	26 (15.6%)	0.002
Thrombocytopenia	7 (5.8%)	12 (7.2%)	0.650
Fatigue	38 (31.6%)	51 (30.5%)	0.839

Table 5. Adverse events

Data are expressed as number of patients, with percentages indicated in parentheses.

4. Discussion

TACE has been widely used for the treatment of unresectable HCC.[8, 9] The most commonly used agent in TACE for HCC treatment is an emulsion of LPD and ADM, followed by embolization with gelatin sponge particles,[10, 11] but tumors frequently recur[9, 12, 13] or residual tumors are observed at a high rate. CDDP is an effective anticancer agent used in the treatment of various malignancies.[14] Ono et al.[15] reported that TACE using a suspension of CDDP powder in LPD was more effective against unresectable HCC than that using an emulsion of ADM and LPD. Other investigators have also frequently reported favorable results obtained with TACE using a suspension of CDDP powder in LPD in HCC patients.[16, 24] However, the CDDP powder for this therapy was difficult to produce because of the characteristics of the drug formulation. CDDP powder thus had to be custom-made in individual institutions.[25] Consequently, when an institution was able to dispense CDDP powder in their own pharmacy department, TACE using a suspension of CDDP powder in LPD was undertaken.

A fine-powder formulation of CDDP, "DDPH", has been available for intra-arterial infusion for HCC treatment since 2004 in Japan. Dispensing of CDDP powder improved with the development of DDPH, and DDPH has now come to replace CDDP powder. The DDPH-LPD suspension for TACE in HCC patients was expected to yield better therapeutic outcomes, so TACE using DDPH has become widespread in Japanese institutions. Nevertheless, the efficacy of TACE using DDPH-LPD suspension has not yet been reported. We therefore compared the outcomes of TACE using DDPH-LPD suspension and an emulsion of LPD with ADM.

The antitumor activity of CDDP is closely associated with the serum concentration of the drug.[26] Antitumor activity can thus be enhanced by increasing the dose. LPD acts as a selective carrier of anticancer agents and as an embolic material;[20] the anticancer agent is gradually released from the iodized oil. Although the mechanism of topical accumulation of LPD in the tumor is not yet precisely understood, this approach is nonetheless used to achieve a targeted drug delivery system with long-lasting accumulation in the tumor and gradual drug release. Augmented antitumor efficacy and milder side-effects have therefore come to be expected with the use of this substance for TACE. In fact, Morimoto et al.[27] investigated the pharmacological advantages of TACE using DDPH for hypervascular hepatic tumors in animal experiments. They reported that the tumor concentration of platinum agent in the DDPH-LPD-TACE group was about 14-times higher than that in the DDPH-hepatic arterial infusion (HAI) group. In addition, they reported that plasma concentrations of the platinum agent at 5 and 10 min from start of infusion were lower in the DDPH-LPD-TACE group than in the DDPH-HAI group. Based on those findings, we decided to perform TACE using DDPH-LPD suspension.

Analysis of the results for the entire study population revealed that the objective response rate was significantly higher in the DDPH group than in the ADM group. Moreover, while no significant difference in OS was seen between groups, the OS of patients who had not received any additional therapy in the DDPH group was significantly higher than that of patients with no history of additional therapy in the ADM group. This could be explained as being due to the fact that TACE with ADM cannot be repeated as required, given the high frequency of adverse effects of ADM such as leucopenia, severe vascular changes and occlusion of the hepatic artery.[15, 28, 29] In fact, the incidences of leucopenia and occlusion of the hepatic artery were significantly higher in the ADM group in our study than in the DDPH group. Second, we concluded that anthracyclines such as ADM may be relatively less effective against HCC; this is attributable to high expression levels of P-glycoprotein, which transports antitumor agents such as anthracyclines and vinca alkaloids from cells with a highly active efflux mechanism in HCC tumors.[30]

On the other hand, Pelletier et al.[31] reported that TACE with CDDP sometimes caused severe complications, such as acute hepatic failure, without providing any significant improvement in survival rate. Severe complications could be expected with the high doses of CDDP used in that study. Modification of the CDDP dose used for the treatment to 50 mg of DDHP in our study resulted in lower severity of complications.

In terms of our results, no significant differences in objective response rate or OS were identified between DDPH and ADM groups in patients who reported a history of previous additional therapy. However, considering that the observation period for the DDPH group was shorter than that for the ADM group and that PFS tended to be longer in the DDPH group as compared with that in the ADM group, a significant difference in OS may be observed if the DDPH group was followed up for a longer period.

To avoid the confounding effects of any deviations in patient characteristics causing an impact on the results, such as the gender distribution, TNM classification, or larger size or number of tumors, we used multivariate analysis to compare efficacy between regimens. This analysis identified the treatment regimen employed for TACE as one of the most important prognostic factors.

5. Conclusion

We conclude that TACE using DDPH-LPD suspension could provide a useful treatment strategy for HCC patients, although further studies are required for a more thorough evaluation of the effectiveness of this therapy.

6. Acknowledgment

The authors wish to thank Ms. Kouko Motodate for preparing serum samples.

7. References

[1] Kamangar F, Dores GM, Anderson WF. Patterns of cancer incidence, mortality, and prevalence across five continents: defining priorities to reduce cancer disparities in different geographic regions of the world. J Clin Oncol. 2006 May 10;24: 2137-50.
[2] El-Serag HB, Mason AC. Rising incidence of hepatocellular carcinoma in the United States. N Engl J Med. 1999 Mar 11;340: 745-50.

[3] Fattovich G, Giustina G, Degos F, et al. Morbidity and mortality in compensated cirrhosis type C: a retrospective follow-up study of 384 patients. Gastroenterology. 1997 Feb;112: 463-72.

[4] La Vecchia C, Lucchini F, Franceschi S, Negri E, Levi F. Trends in mortality from primary liver cancer in Europe. Eur J Cancer. 2000 May;36: 909-15.

[5] Okuda K, Fujimoto I, Hanai A, Urano Y. Changing incidence of hepatocellular carcinoma in Japan. Cancer Res. 1987 Sep 15;47: 4967-72.

[6] Ohtomo K, Furui S, Kokubo T, et al. Transcatheter arterial embolization (TAE) in treatment for hepatoma--analysis of three-year survivors. Radiat Med. 1985 Jul-Sep;3: 176-80.

[7] Shiina S, Teratani T, Obi S, Hamamura K, Koike Y, Omata M. Nonsurgical treatment of hepatocellular carcinoma: from percutaneous ethanol injection therapy and percutaneous microwave coagulation therapy to radiofrequency ablation. Oncology. 2002;62 Suppl 1: 64-8.

[8] Kanematsu T, Furuta T, Takenaka K, et al. A 5-year experience of lipiodolization: selective regional chemotherapy for 200 patients with hepatocellular carcinoma. Hepatology. 1989 Jul;10: 98-102.

[9] Yamada R, Sato M, Kawabata M, Nakatsuka H, Nakamura K, Takashima S. Hepatic artery embolization in 120 patients with unresectable hepatoma. Radiology. 1983 Aug;148: 397-401.

[10] Shimamura Y, Gunven P, Takenaka Y, et al. Combined peripheral and central chemoembolization of liver tumors. Experience with lipiodol-doxorubicin and gelatin sponge (L-TAE). Cancer. 1988 Jan 15;61: 238-42.

[11] Takayasu K, Suzuki M, Uesaka K, et al. Hepatic artery embolization for inoperable hepatocellular carcinoma; prognosis and risk factors. Cancer Chemother Pharmacol. 1989;23 Suppl: S123-5.

[12] Takayasu K, Shima Y, Muramatsu Y, et al. Hepatocellular carcinoma: treatment with intraarterial iodized oil with and without chemotherapeutic agents. Radiology. 1987 May;163: 345-51.

[13] Kawai S, Okamura J, Ogawa M, et al. Prospective and randomized clinical trial for the treatment of hepatocellular carcinoma--a comparison of lipiodol-transcatheter arterial embolization with and without adriamycin (first cooperative study). The Cooperative Study Group for Liver Cancer Treatment of Japan. Cancer Chemother Pharmacol. 1992;31 Suppl: S1-6.

[14] Uchiyama N, Kobayashi H, Nakajo M, Shinohara S. Treatment of lung cancer with bronchial artery infusion of cisplatin and intravenous sodium thiosulfate rescue. Acta Oncol. 1988;27: 57-61.

[15] Ono Y, Yoshimasu T, Ashikaga R, et al. Long-term results of lipiodol-transcatheter arterial embolization with cisplatin or doxorubicin for unresectable hepatocellular carcinoma. Am J Clin Oncol. 2000 Dec;23: 564-8.

[16] Kamada K, Nakanishi T, Kitamoto M, et al. Long-term prognosis of patients undergoing transcatheter arterial chemoembolization for unresectable hepatocellular carcinoma: comparison of cisplatin lipiodol suspension and

      doxorubicin hydrochloride emulsion. J Vasc Interv Radiol. 2001 Jul;12: 847-54.

[17] Child CG, Turcotte JG. Surgery and portal hypertension. Major Probl Clin Surg. 1964;1: 1-85.

[18] Hermanek P, Scheibe O, Spiessl B, Wagner G. [TNM classification of malignant tumors: the new 1987 edition]. Rontgenblatter. 1987 Jun;40: 200.

[19] Oken MM, Creech RH, Tormey DC, et al. Toxicity and response criteria of the Eastern Cooperative Oncology Group. Am J Clin Oncol. 1982 Dec;5: 649-55.

[20] Nakakuma K, Tashiro S, Hiraoka T, et al. Studies on anticancer treatment with an oily anticancer drug injected into the ligated feeding hepatic artery for liver cancer. Cancer. 1983 Dec 15;52: 2193-200.

[21] Jinno K, Moriwaki S, Tanada M, Wada T, Mandai K, Okada Y. Clinicopathological study on combination therapy consisting of arterial infusion of lipiodol-dissolved SMANCS and transcatheter arterial embolization for hepatocellular carcinoma. Cancer Chemother Pharmacol. 1992;31 Suppl: S7-12.

[22] Imaeda T, Yamawaki Y, Seki M, et al. Lipiodol retention and massive necrosis after lipiodol-chemoembolization of hepatocellular carcinoma: correlation between computed tomography and histopathology. Cardiovasc Intervent Radiol. 1993 Jul-Aug;16: 209-13.

[23] Okusaka T, Okada S, Ueno H, et al. Evaluation of the therapeutic effect of transcatheter arterial embolization for hepatocellular carcinoma. Oncology. 2000 May;58: 293-9.

[24] Kasugai H, Kojima J, Tatsuta M, et al. Treatment of hepatocellular carcinoma by transcatheter arterial embolization combined with intraarterial infusion of a mixture of cisplatin and ethiodized oil. Gastroenterology. 1989 Oct;97: 965-71.

[25] Yamamoto K, Shimizu T, Narabayashi I. Intraarterial infusion chemotherapy with lipiodol-CDDP suspension for hepatocellular carcinoma. Cardiovasc Intervent Radiol. 2000 Jan-Feb;23: 26-39.

[26] Takahashi K, Ebihara K, Honda Y, et al. [Antitumor activity of cis-dichlorodiammineplatinum(II) and its effect on cell cycle progression]. Gan To Kagaku Ryoho. 1982 Apr;9: 624-31.

[27] Morimoto K, Sakaguchi H, Tanaka T, et al. Transarterial chemoembolization using cisplatin powder in a rabbit model of liver cancer. Cardiovasc Intervent Radiol. 2008 Sep-Oct;31: 981-5.

[28] Doroshow JH, Locker GY, Myers CE. Experimental animal models of adriamycin cardiotoxicity. Cancer Treat Rep. 1979 May;63: 855-60.

[29] Olson HM, Capen CC. Subacute cardiotoxicity of adriamycin in the rat: biochemical and ultrastructural investigations. Lab Invest. 1977 Oct;37: 386-94.

[30] Itsubo M, Ishikawa T, Toda G, Tanaka M. Immunohistochemical study of expression and cellular localization of the multidrug resistance gene product P-glycoprotein in primary liver carcinoma. Cancer. 1994 Jan 15;73: 298-303.

[31] Pelletier G, Ducreux M, Gay F, et al. Treatment of unresectable hepatocellular carcinoma with lipiodol chemoembolization: a multicenter randomized trial. Groupe CHC. J Hepatol. 1998 Jul;29: 129-34

14

Transarterial Chemoembolization for HCC with Drug-Eluting Microspheres

Maurizio Grosso, Fulvio Pedrazzini, Alberto Balderi,
Alberto Antonietti, Enrico Peano, Luigi Ferro and Davide Sortino
A. O. S. Croce e Carle, Cuneo
Italy

1. Introduction

HCC is the 5th most common cancer worldwide and the 3rd cause of cancer related deaths. Transarterial chemoembolization (TACE) is the mainstay therapy for intermediate non-resectable HCC, according to the BCLC Staging system. (Bruix & Sherman, 2011).

TACE significantly improves the overall rate of survival after 2 years compared with conservative treatment, but there is no evidence that TACE is more effective than transarterial embolization (TAE). However in more selected patients the 1 year survival rate

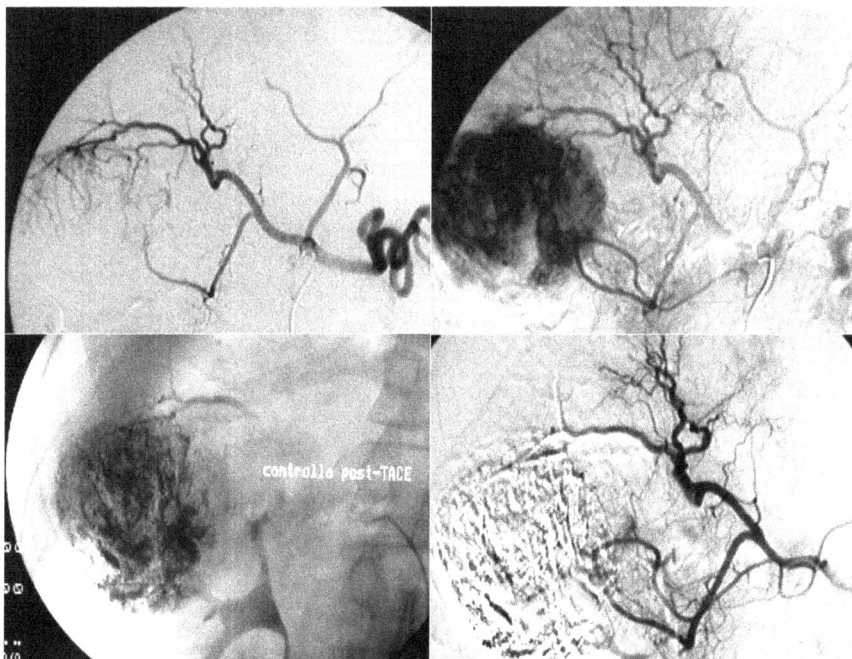

Fig. 1. TACE with Lipiodol.

is 82% after TACE, 75% after TAE and 63% after conservative treatment, while it is 63%, 50% and 27% respectively at 2 years (Llovet et al, 2002). Even if it is well known that Lipiodol stays for a prolongued period in the tumor after TACE, pharmacokinetic studies about traditional TACE with Lipiodol (Figure 1) and drug demonstrate that plasma levels of adriamycin are identical with intraarterial administration with or without Lipiodol.

With the aim of two different kind of drug-loaded carriers have been increasing the local concentration of the drugs and reducing systemic side effects introduced for transarterial treatment of HCC: HepaSphere™ Microspheres (BioSphere Medical, France) and DC Bead™ Microspheres (Biocompatibles, UK).

The aim of this study is to analyze the data recently published regarding DC Bead™ Microspheres and to present our experience with chemoembolization with HepaSphere™ Microspheres.

2. Conventional chemoembolization

Transarterial chemoembolization consists of the administration of chemotherapeutic drugs mixed with an embolizing material. It combines therapeutic effects of peripheral arterial occlusion with the local administration of chemoterapeutic agents. The target of arterial chemoembolization through the hepatic artery are to increase the local concentration of chemotherapeutic drugs in the tumor and reduce systemic side effects. The arterial system, mainly supplied vascularization of HCC unlike cirrhotic tissue, where vascularization is mainly supplied by the portal vein system. TACE can involve the whole hepatic parenchyma (embolization of the common hepatic artery or left/right hepatic artery) or can be selective (embolization of segmental/subsegmental hepatic artery) with better tumoral response and lower hepatic damage.

There is a great variability in the nature and description of transarterial techniques. There are at least four different kind of locoregional treatment: TACE (transarterial chemoembolization); TAE (transarterial embolization); TOCE (transarterial oily chemoembolization) and TAC (transarterial chemotherapy). TACE has been already described. TAE refers only to the last process, which may be preceded by the administration of Lipiodol (Lp-TAE), without using any chemotherapeutic agents. TOCE consists in the arterial administration of a mixture of anticancer drugs and Lipiodol without embolizzation. TAC is the locoregional infusion of chemotherapeutic agents through a catheter placed into the hepatic artery. (Marelli et al, 2007)

There is not yet a wide consensus about the characteristics of the patients suitable to undergo TACE. Selection criteria could be based on any combination of tumor dimension (tumor size, amount of liver replacement by tumor, serum α-phafetoprotein,portal vein thrombosis or obstruction), severity of liver disease (Child-Pugh score, serum bilirubin, serum albumin and ascites), health status (Karnofsky score, Performance Status test, and constitutional syndrome), and response to treatment. All these criteria have been found to be predictors of survival in patients undergoing TACE. The majority of studies included patients defined as having "unresectable HCC," that is HCC diagnosed according to the 2000 Barcelona EASL criteria, not suitable for curative treatments according to BCLC staging classification and treatment schedule. Exclusion criteria in different trials were: advanced liver disease (Child-Pugh C), active gastrointestinal bleeding, encephalopathy, refractory ascites, presence of vascular invasion or total portal vein occlusion due to liver tumor, extrahepatic metastases, any contraindication to an arterial procedure (impaired clotting tests and renal failure), WHO performance stage 3 or 4, and end-stage tumoral disease (Okuda III). (Marelli et al, 2007)

The indications have beeen explained by Barcelona Clinic Liver Cancer (BCLC) tumor staging; it combines the stage of liver disease, tumor stage, clinical performance, and treatment options and is certified by the European Association for the Study of Liver Disease(EASL) and the American Association for the Study of Liver Disease (AASLD). Actually, TACE is indicated in intermediate state (Bruix & Sherman, 2011).

Therefore absolute contraindications to TACE are Child C or Okuda III, tumor resecability or suitable for percuteneous ablations , sepsis, hepatic encephalopathy, uncorrectable contrast allergy or coagulation disorders, leucopenia (WBC<1000/µl), cardiac or renal insufficiency (serum creatinine>2 mg/dl) and complete portal vein thrombosis.

Relative contraindications are: serum bilirubin >3 mg/dl, LDH (lactate dehydrogenase) >425 U/l, AST (aspartate aminotransferase) >5X the upper limit of normal, extrahepatic metastases, tumor burden involving >50% of the liver, performance status (PS) >2, renal or cardiac insufficiency, recent variceal bleeding, or significant thrombocytopenia, intractable fav (arteriovenous fistula), ascites, surgical portocaval anastomosis, tumor invasion to inferior vena cava and right atrium, severe portal vein thrombosis. (Liapi & Geschwind, 2011)

Lipiodol (ethiodized oil) is an oily contrast medium which persists more selectively in tumor nodules for a few weeks or months when injected into the hepatic artery, due to the arterial hypervascularization and absence of Kupffer cells inside the tumor tissue, but it may also persist to a lesser extent in non-neoplastic nodules. Even if some investigators still believe in the embolic effect of lipiodol, nowadays it cannot be considered as an embolic agent since it does not result in arterial occlusion. It is used only as a vehicle to carry and localize chemotherapeutic agents inside the tumor. However, the major problem is how to combine anticancer drugs, which are water-based preparations, and lipiodol, which is an oil-based agent, in a stable formulation able to deliver drugs slowly over time. (Marelli et al, 2007)

The most common sole-agent anticancer drug used in literature is doxorubicin (36%), followed by cisplatin (31%), epi/doxorubicin (12%), mitoxantrone (8%), mitomycin C (8%), and SMANCS (5%). SMANCS is a chemical conjugate of a synthetic copolymer of styrene maleic acid (SMA) .

To date there is no evidence of superior efficacy of any chemotherapeutic agent alone or of monotherapy versus combination therapy. Anticancer drugs dosage was variable and not reported iaccording to standards: some studies used a fixed dose, some based the dosage on body surface area and others on patient weight, tumor size or bilirubin level. (Marelli et al, 2007)

The embolization endpoint is to achieve complete occlusion of the neo-vascularity, avoiding complete stasis in the afferent artery, which would lead to endothelial damage and subsequent thrombosis and would preclude future treatments. The embolized vessels are generally segmentary and subsegmentary branches.

Operative indications are:

1. Choose a delivery microcatheter based on the size of the target vessel.
2. Position the catheter tip as close as possible to the treatment site to avoid inadvertent occlusions of normal vessels and damage of "non-target" hepatic tissue. Large catheter causes "stop flow" with less selectivity and less accuracy in target embolization.

Undesirable reflux or passage of chemoembolic agent into normal arteries (adjacent to the target lesion or through the lesion into other arteries or arterial beds) can occur during embolization , with consequent non-target ischaemia (splenic, gastroduodenal, left, or right arteries embolization, etc.).

Post embolic syndrome (fever >38° C, nausea, vomiting, abdominal pain) frequently occurs after conventional TACE (90%), probably caused by inflammatory response and tissue ischemia. Liver ascess and acute liver failure occur in 2%, while ascites, transient abdominal pain, pleuric effusion, haemoperitoneum, splenic embolization, cardiac failure, thrombosis of hepatic artery, gastric ulcer bleeding, esophageal variceal bleeding, between 8 to 1% in the differents series.

The results of TACE in different series are reported in table 1-2-3. In randomized studies TACE improves survival in comparison with conservative treatments. Drug-eluting Microspheres increase the percentage of tumor tissue necrosis against the traditional TACE.

Authors	100%	99-88%	79-50%	< 50%
Hashimoto T *Nakamura H* *Hori S* *Tomoda K*	*29%*	*43%*	*12%*	*16%*
Morino M *Grosso M* *De Giuli M* *Bismuth H*	*27%*	*30%*	*19%*	*23%*

Table 1. Necrosis grading post-TACE

Authors	N. Pts	Survival		
		1 year	3 year	5 year
Atanaka	2159	65%	36%	18%
Savastano	57	75%	9 %	-
Shijo	110	79%	38%	14%
Ukida	1075	61%	15%	-
Grosso	340	59%	27%	17%

Table 2. TACE results.

Authors	N. Pts	Survival		
		1 year	3 year	5 year
Yamada	973	51%	12%	6 %
Bronowiki	127	65%		-
			27%	

Table 3. Segmental TACE results.

2.1 TACE with DcBead™ Microspheres

DC Bead™ Microspheres are Polyvinyl Alcohol polymer hydrogel N-Fil sulfonic acid Microspheres. They can be loaded with doxorubicin to provide accurate dosage of the drug and be suitable for superselective TACE. DC Bead™ primary embolic characteristics allow accurate, targeted delivery. They are available in a range of sizes associated to different colours (yellow: 100-300 µm; blue: 300-500 µm; red: 500-700 µm; green: 700-900 µm), while volume of Beads is 2 ml. The 100-300 µm microspheres are generally used in standard TACE, while 300-500 µm or 500-700 µm are used only in huge lesions or presence of arterial-portal fystulas

Choosing the appropriate size of microspheres best matches the pathology (i.e. tumour lesion/vessel size) provides the expected clinical outcome. Systemic plasma level of doxorubicin is 30 times lower in patients treated with DC Bead™ vs those treated with conventional TACE. DC Bead™ are hydrated and interaction of doxorubicin with SO3 groups displaces water from the hydration shells DC Bead™ drug delivery properties are explained as it follows: loads and elutes drugs relevant to clinical use; uniform distribution of drug throughout the loaded beads; consistent local delivery to the tumour, over an extended period. With DC Bead™ drug elution is dependent on ion exchange and is controlled and sustained – unlike the rapid separation of the drug from Lipiodol. DC Bead™ should enable delivery of drug to the tumour site over an extended period while minimising systemic release of doxorubicin and reducing the side effects associated with conventional TACE.

2.1.1 TACE with DcBead™ Microspheres: Preparation

DC Bead™ Microspheres can be loaded with Doxorubicin-HCl (up to 37.5 mg/mL; maximum dose/patient of 150 mg).

1. Reconstitute each 50mg doxorubicin vial with 2ml of sterile water for injection. Mix well to obtain a clear solution.
2. Remove as much saline as possible from DC Bead™ vial(s) using a syringe with a small gauge needle. Pierce bung with a second needle to eliminate vacuum. If a filter needle is not available, place flattened tip of needle against side of vial to prevent beads being drawn up the needle.
3. Using a syringe and needle add the reconstituted doxorubicin solution directly to the vial(s) of DC Bead™.
4. Agitate the DC Bead™/doxorubicin solution gently to encourage mixing then allow to stand until the beads are red and the solution is almost colourless.
5. DC Bead™ loading time is dependent on bead size.
6. Transfer the loaded beads into a 10ml syringe. Add an equal volume of non-ionic contrast media and mix gently (a 3-way connector and second syringe can be used).

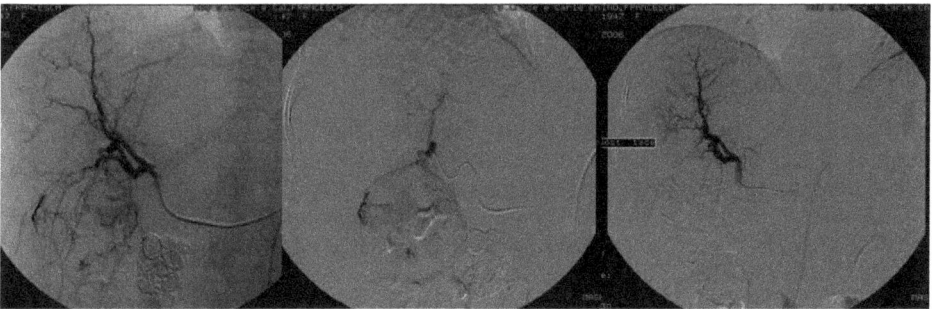

Fig. 2. TACE with DC Bead™ Microspheres.

Figures 2-3-4 demonstrate a case of HCC we treated with TACE with DC Bead™ Microspheres and the CT-follow-up at 1 and 6 months.

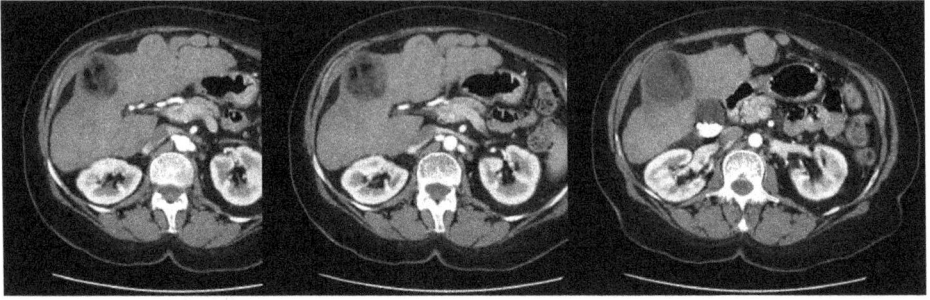

Fig. 3. 1-months CT follow-up of TACE with DC Bead™ Microspheres: complete necrosis of treated lesions.

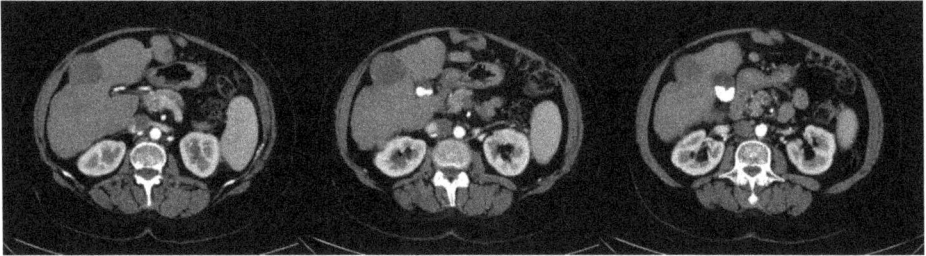

Fig. 4. 6-months CT follow-up of TACE with DC Bead™ Microspheres: complete necrosis of treated lesions.

2.1.2 TACE with DcBead™ Microspheres: Clinical experiences

Malagari presented the mid-term results of a single centre study from the 62 patients (cirrhotic with underlying hepatitis infection and documented unresectable HCC of 3-10 cm) Athenian Registry between December 2004 and March 2006. The aim of this study was to assess the safety and efficacy of doxorubicin loaded DC Bead in the treatment of unresectable HCC in cirrhotic patients. These patients were treated by selective or super-selective embolisation using two different sizes of DC Bead: 100-300μm and/or 300-500μm loaded with 37.5mg/mL of doxorubicin. Follow-up lasted 32 months. This shows that chemoembolization using doxorubicin-loaded DC Beads is a safe and effective treatment of HCC as demonstrated by the low complication rate, increased tumor response, and sustained reduction of alpha-fetoprotein levels". (Malagari et al, 2008)

The PRECISION V study (Lammer et al., 2010) support these results. It consists of a randomized trial comparing conventional TACE (cTACE) with TACE using DC Bead™ Microspheres for the treatment of cirrhotic patients with HCC. 212 patients with Child-Pugh A/B cirrhosis and large and/or multinodular, unresectable, N0, M0 HCCs were randomized to receive cTACE with doxorubicin or TACE with DC Bead™ Microspheres loaded with doxorubicin. Randomization was stratified according to performance status (ECOG 0/1), Child-Pugh status (A/B), bilobar disease (yes/no), and prior curative treatment (yes/no). The primary endpoint was tumor response (EASL) at 6 months following independent, blinded review of MRI studies. The drug-eluting bead group showed higher rates of complete response, objective response, and disease control compared with the cTACE group (27% vs. 22%, 52% vs. 44%, and 63% vs. 52%, respectively). The hypothesis of superiority was not found (one-sided P = 0.11). However, patients with Child-Pugh B, ECOG 1, bilobar disease, and recurrent disease showed a significant increase in objective response (P = 0.038) compared to cTACE. DC Bead was associated with improved tolerability, with a significant reduction in serious liver toxicity (P\0.001) and a significantly lower rate of doxorubicin-related side effects (P = 0.0001). This shows that TACE with DC Bead™ Microspheres and doxorubicin is safe and effective in the treatment of HCC and offers a benefit to patients with more advanced disease.

2.2 TACE with HepaSphere Microspheres

HepaSphere™ Microspheres are expandable microspheres approved for hepatic embolizations and chemoembolizations. They are Poly-sodium acrylate-vinyl alcohol Microspheres, developed in Japan by Dr Hori. They are available as 50 mg or 25 mg of dry powder, calibrated in 3 different dry sizes associated to different colours (yellow: 50-100 μm; blue: 100-150 μm; red: 150-200 μm), sterilized by irradiation. Their diameter expands x4 and volume x64.

They are negatively charged (anionic polymer), enabling strong interactions with positively charged drugs such as Doxorubicin reducing systemic toxicity.

2.2.1 TACE with HepaSphere Microspheres: Preparation

Prepare in Biohazard Hood

1. Using a 30 mL syringe and a 20G needle, reconstitute the 50 mg doxorubicin vial with 20 mL preservative-free 0.9% sodium chloride. Do not use pure sterile water.
2. Lift the cap from the HepaSphere™ vial to the vertical position taking care not to remove the cap or the metal retaining ring from the vial.
3. Roll the HepaSphere™ vial several times to disperse microspheres.
4. Using a new 30 mL syringe with a new 18 G needle, withdraw 20 mL (the intire contents) from the doxorubicin vial (50 mg) prepared in Step 1.
5. Inject 10 mL of doxorubicin from Step 4 to the HepaSphere™ vial. Note: there may be a vacuum in the HepaSphere™ vial.
6. Gently rotate and invert the HepaSphere™ vial back and forth 5 to 10 times so that the liquid contacts the grey stopper (do not shake vigorously). Let the vial stand for 10 minutes; invert every few minutes to continue to mix the spheres with the doxorubicin.
7. After the 10 minutes from Step 6, withdraw the entire contents of the HepaSphere™ vial into the 30 mL syringe containing the remaining doxorubicin (25 mg/10 mL) prepared in Step 4. (Do not attempt to extract every red colored sphere). Gently agitate the syringe back and forth to completely mix and disperse the contents.
8. Remove the needle and cap the syringe. Note the time and wait 60 minutes to optimize the uptake of the doxorubicin into the spheres before administering.
9. Do not begin this step until at least 60 minutes has elapsed from Step 8. Attach syringe to a 3-way stopcock. Allow the spheres to settle at the bottom. Purge 10 mL of the supernatant and discard. Add/replace with 10 mL of non-ionic contrast.
10. Invert this syringe several times to disperse and mix the contents in the syringe until suspension is achieved.

2.2.2 TACE with HepaSphere Microspheres: Clinical experiences

We have reported the early results of a multicentre Italian trial using HepaSphere™ Microspheres loaded with chemotherapeutic agents (doxorubicin or epirubicin) for TACE in patients with unresectable hepatocellular carcinoma (December 2005 – March 2007; 50 patients, 36 male – 14 female, mean age 68.4 years). The diameter of the treated lesions ranged from 20 to 100 mm (mean 42.5; maximum of 4 tumor nodules). Tumor response was evaluated by CTaccording to the World Health Organization criteria as modified by the European Association for the Study of Liver Diseases. Technical success was performed in all procedures without major complications. At 1-month CT follow-up, complete tumor response was observed in 24 of 50 (48%), partial response in 18 of 50 (36%), and stable disease in 8 of 50 (16%) patients without cases of disease progression. At 6-month follow-up (31/50 patients) complete tumor response was obtained in 16/31 (51.6%), partial response in 8/31 (25.8%), and progressive disease in 7/31 (22.6%) patients. Within the initial 9-month follow-up, TACE with HepaSphere™ Microspheres was successfully repeated twice in 3 patients, while 3 patients underwent the procedure 3 times. Our initial multicentre experience demonstrates that TACE using HepaSphere is feasible, is well tolerated, has a low complication rate, and is associated with promising tumor response. When complete tumor response in not achieved, additional treatments can be performed.

Longer follow-up on larger series is mandatory to confirm these preliminary results. (Grosso et al., 2008)

We compared our experience using HepaSphere™ microspheres (Biosphere Medical) loaded with Doxorubicin in patients with unresectable Hepatocellular Carcinoma with our precedent series of traditonal TACE: TACE with Lipiodol and Gelfoam (340 pts treated from December 1991 to April 1996) and TACE with Lipiodol and Embosphere (46 pts treated from February 2000 to November 2005). From December 2005 to December 2010, we treated 111 patients (83 male, 28 female, mean age 71 years; 70% with a minimum follow-up of 6 months) by selective TACE using HepaSphere™ loaded with Doxorubicin in 173 procedures. The diameter of the lesions ranged from 25 to 176 mm (mean diameter: 61.5 mm; maximum: multifocal lesions). Technical success rate was 100%, with complete devascularization of the lesions at the end of all procedures. One month CT follow-up shows complete necrosis (90-100%) of lesions in 39.9%, partial necrosis (50-89%) in 44.2%, progression disease (0-49%) in 15.9%. 6 month follow-up shows complete necrosis in 32.4%, partial in 44.5%, progression disease in 23.1%. 39 patients underwent RFA (29 pre-TACE; 10 post-TACE); 12 were lost at follow-up, 5 died. Survival at 6 months was 93.8% in HepaSphere™, 91.3% in Embosphere,

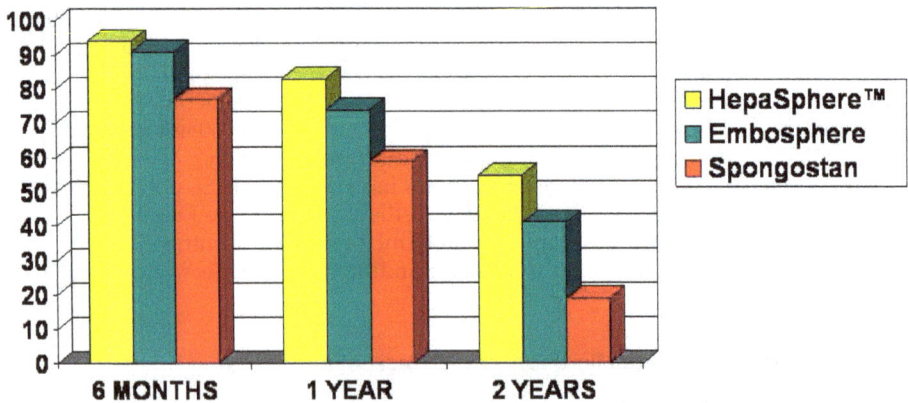

Fig. 5. Personal experience A.S.O. S. croce e Carle – Cuneo. Survival %.

77% in Gelfoam group; at 12 months it was 83.3% in HepaSphere™, 73.9% in Embosphere, 59.1% in Gelfoam group; at 24 months was 55% in HepaSphere™, 41% in Embosphere, 19% in Gelfoam group (Figure 5).

This comparison demonstrates that TACE using HepaSphere™ is feasible, with low complication rate and promising efficacy.

Figures 5-6 demonstrate a case of HCC we treated with TACE with HepaSphere™ Microspheres and 1 months US-follow-up.

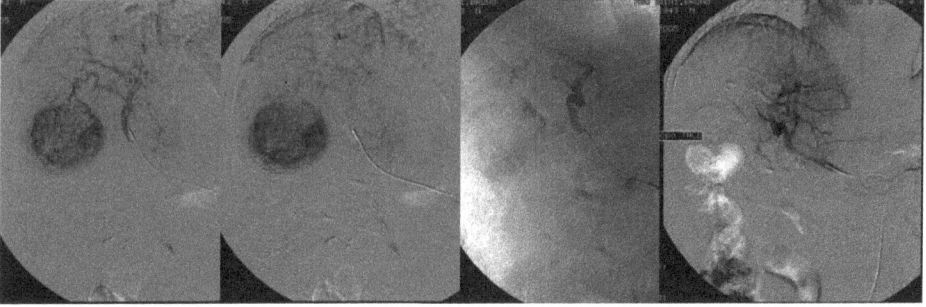

Fig. 6. TACE with HepaSphere™.

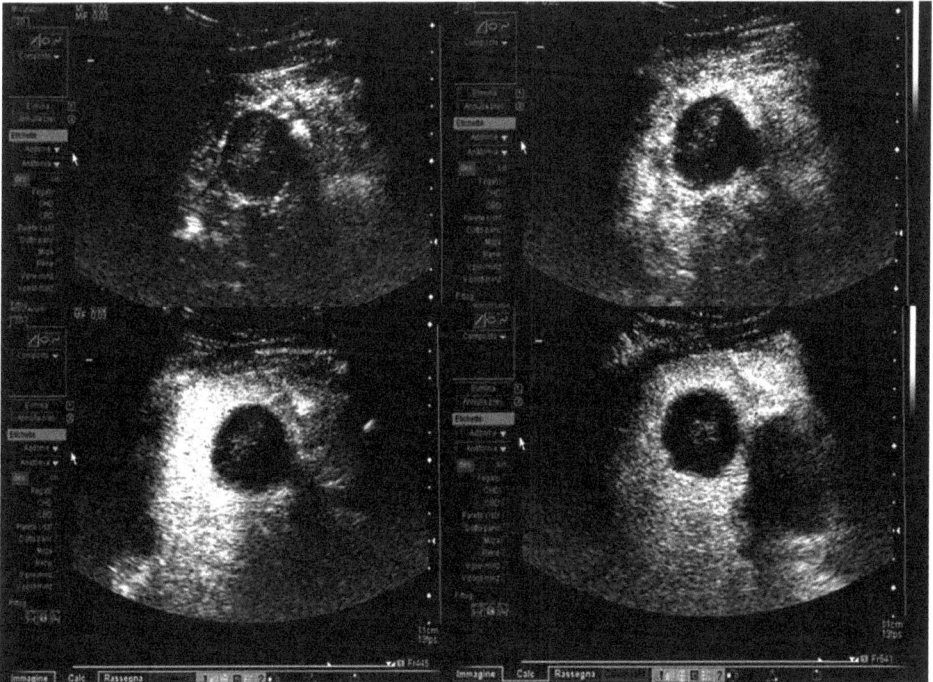

Fig. 7. 1-month US follow-up after TACE with HepaSphere™: complete necrosis of nodule of HCC we treated.

3. Conclusions

TACE is the most successful treatment of intermediate HCC or HCC not suitable for resection and percutaneous ablation, improving the life quality an medium/long survival rates in patients with intermediate HCC.

The results of TACE using Microspheres, compared with results of conventional TACE, are promising less side-effects, complications and especially seems to offer benefit to patients with advanced tumor.

4. References

Bruix J. and Sherman M. (2011) Management of Hepatocellular Carcinoma: An Update. *Hepatology*, Mar;53(3):1020-2.

Grosso M., Vignali C., Quaretti P., Nicolini A., Melchiorre F., Gallarato G., Bargellini I., Petruzzi P., Massa Saluzzo C., Crespi S., Sarti I. (2008). Transarterial chemoembolization for hepatocellular carcinoma with drug-eluting microspheres: preliminary results from an Italian multicentre study. *Cardiovasc Intervent Radiol.* Nov-Dec;31(6):1141-9.

Lammer J., Malagari K., Vogl T., Pilleul F., Denys A., Watkinson A., Pitton M., Sergent G., Pfammatter T., Terraz S., Benhamou Y., Avajon Y., Gruenberger T., Pomoni M., Langenberger H., Schuchmann M., Dumortier J., Mueller C., Chevallier P., Lencioni R.; PRECISION V Investigators.. (2010) Prospective randomized study of doxorubicin-eluting-bead embolization in the treatment of hepatocellular carcinoma: results of the PRECISION V study. *Cardiovasc Intervent Radiol.* Feb ;33(1):41-52.

Liapi E., Geschwind J.F. (2011). Transcatheter arterial chemoembolization for liver cancer: is it time to distinguish conventional from drug-eluting chemoembolization? *Cardiovasc Intervent Radiol.* Feb;34(1):37-49.

Llovet J.M, Real M.I, Montana X, Planas R, Coll S, Aponte J, Ayuso C, Sala M, Muchart J, Sola R, Rodes J and Bruix J. (2002) Arterial embolisation or chemoembolisation versus symptomatic treatment in patients with unresectable hepatocellular carcinoma: a randomised controlled trial. *Lancet*; ; 359 (9319): 1734-1739.

Malagari K., Chatzimichael K., Alexopoulou E., Kelekis A., Hall B., Dourakis S., Delis S., Gouliamos A., Kelekis D. (2008). Transarterial chemoembolization of unresectable hepatocellular carcinoma with drug eluting beads: results of an open-label study of 62 patients. *Cardiovasc Intervent Radiol.* Mar-Apr; 31(2):269-80.

Marelli L., Stigliano R., Triantos C., Senzolo M., Cholongitas E., Davies N., Tibballs J., Meyer T., Patch D.W., Burroughs A.K. (2007). Transarterial therapy for hepatocellular carcinoma: which technique is more effective? A systematic review of cohort and randomized studies. *Cardiovasc Intervent Radiol.* Jan-Feb; 30(1):6-25.

15

Radiofrequency Ablation for Hepatocellular Carcinoma at the Dome of the Liver: A Review

Kiyoshi Mochizuki

Department of Gastroenterology and Hepatology, Kansai Rousai Hospital, Hyogo
Japan

1. Introduction

Hepatocellular carcinoma is the third-leading cause of global cancer-related mortality. Major causes of this disease are hepatotropic viruses including hepatitis B and C viruses, nonalcoholic steatohepatitis, alcohol, autoimmunity, primary biliary cirrhosis, primary sclerosing cholangitis, vascular disorders and so on (Olsen et al., 2010). These factors related to hepatitis lead the patients to the high-risk group for decompensated liver cirrhosis and hepatocellular carcinoma during their clinical course in 20–30 years. Interferon or other medical therapy for each disease have been accommodating better conditions of the liver and make it possible to prolong their lives. However, the possibility of the occurrence of hepatocellular carcinoma could not have been completely avoided in these patients during their lifetime.

Recently, the improvements of surveillance techniques and disease awareness have led to earlier diagnosis and more appropriate treatment for liver tumors. Surgical therapy could be curative treatment to avoid local recurrence, but many patients are unable to undergo surgical resection due to severely compromised liver function or multiple tumors. Moreover, frequent recurrence of heparocellular carcinoma makes it hazardous for the patients to undergo surgical therapy repeatedly to maintain the liver function after the treatment. Thus, non-surgical interventional therapy has been introduced to control hepatocellular carcinoma and have played an important role in the treatment of hepatocellular carcinoma (Livraghi et al, 1999; Poon et al, 2002). These locoregional therapies including transcatheter arterial chemoembolization, percutaneous ethanol injection therapy, percutaneous radiofrequeny ablation therapy and others, have been making significant contributions to reduce the decrease of the liver function and to maintain the condition of the patients (Poon et al, 2002; Buix et al, 2004; Orland et al, 2009). Radiofrequency ablation has provided one of the greatest recent advances in the treatment of hepatocellular carcinoma because of the improvement of the local control and the patient survival. Radiofrequency ablation is reported as a minimally invasive and effective treatment for small hepatocellular carcinoma and now this treatment is the most widely used technique of the therapy for hepatocellular carcinoma worldwide. Many studies have established the effectiveness of radiofrequency ablation in treating hepatocellular carcinoma (McGhana &Dodd, 2001; Livraghi et al, 2003; Lencioni et al, 2005; Tateishi et al, 2005; Choi et al, 2007) and have achieved to expand the indications for radiofrequency ablation.

However, one of the most characteristic complications of this therapy is that related to the thermal effect. We experienced a case that developed diaphragmatic hernia due to the thermal effect of radiofrequency ablation twenty months after the treatment for a tumor located in the segment VIII area of his liver. Patients who have undergone radiofrequency ablation for hepatic tumors adjacent to the diaphragm should be carefully followed up for possible damage of the diaphragm, even after the long postoperative intervals. Recently, the artificial ascites technique has been developed and introduced in this field. This technique could be approved for the prevention of the diaphragmatic damage and the thermal complications of the surrounding organs.

2. Radiofrequency ablation for hepatocellular carcinoma

Radiofrequency ablation includes the methods of tumor necrosis through the direct placement of the needles into the tumor under the ultrasonographical guide and the usage of alternating electrical current to create ionic agitation and frictional heating leading to the tissue damage. The benefits of this therapy include excellent local control comparable to surgical resection, low morbidity, repeatability for recurrence, preservation of liver function, and few complications (Livraghi et al, 1999; Poon et al, 2002).

Although radiofrequency ablation is considered safe (Curley et al, 2000; Livraghi et al, 2000; Wood et al, 2000), some serious complications have been reported. These include bleeding from costal or hepatic artery, pneumothorax or puncture of surrounding organ, infection, pain, nausea or vomiting, and so on (Curley et al, 2000; Livraghi et al, 2000; Wood et al, 2000). One of the most characteristic and unpredictable complications of this therapy is that induced by heat conduction. Even though the needle could be inserted into the appropriate lesion under the ultrasonographic guide, because the ablated area should be larger than the tumor and involving the whole tumor, it is difficult to grasp the ablated area around the tumor and the environmental situation precisely during the treatment. The ablation produce microbubbles due to heating up in the tissue surrounding the tumor resulting in occurrence of difficulty in grasping the precise ablated area. If the physicians could release the needle from the ultrasonographic transducer during the treatment, it could be possible to grasp roughly the area from other view points. However, high echoic area of microbubbles is not always identical to ablated area and sometimes expands beyond the thermal margin of the effective thermal area. Three-dimensional analysis with radiological study should be helpful to evaluate the ablated area, but it is impossible to predict before the treatment because of the existence of environmental factors of the ablated area including blood flow and respiratory movement of the liver.

3. Technical difficulties for hepatocellular carcinoma situated at the dome of the liver

Because all of the procedures for the liver diseases under ultrasonographic guidance need to be performed with the fully clear detection of the target site, insufficient and poor imaging of ultrasonography means the hardly successful treatment. However, ultrasonographic visualization of the whole tumor under the diaphragm is not always possible due to the atrophy of the right lobe of the cirrhotic liver and the normal respiratory expansion of the lung over the liver causing the acoustic shadow. Therefore, the deformity or the atrophy of the liver due to the chronic inflammation and the damage would make ultrasonographically undetectable region in the liver and lead the physicians to have difficulties in such treatment. Hepatocellular carcinoma can locate in every lobe of the liver, and sometimes locates under the diaphragm dome and this could often be the key factor affecting the effectiveness or the insufficiency of this treatment (Koda et al, 2003; Kang et al, 2009). It may be unavoidable in such cases to make unintended burns to the diaphragm neighboring or close to the target tumor because physicians should burn larger area including hepatocellular carcinoma in order to gain the safety margin around it.

4. Reported complications including a diaphragmatic hernia in the literature, and the case report

4.1 A review of diaphragmatic hernia reported in the literature

Mulier et al. reviewd the complication of radiofrequency ablation from 82 reports of 3670 cases and reported that the prevalence of diaphragm burn was estimated as 0.1% (5 out of 3670) (Mulier et al, 2002). However, Head HW et al. reported that 5 (17%) in 29 radiofrequency ablation cases of hepatocellular carcinoma adjacent to the diaphragm had right shoulder pain and 3 cases showed thickening of the diaphragm induced by the thermal effect of radiofrequency ablation (Head et al, 2007). It is also reported that the symptom of diaphragm injury manifests as referred right shoulder pain that occurs during the treatment and can last up to 2 weeks after the ablation (Livraghi et al, 2003). It may be unavoidable in cases that hepatocellular carcinomas locate under the diaphragm dome to make unintended burn to the diaphragm because of the environmental and technical factors (Kang et al, 2009). The unintended burn of the limited area of the diaphragm may not induce any significant phenomena in the short term except in a few cases, but Curly et al. analyzed the data of 608 cases and emphasized the risk of the late complications of the radiofrequency ablation treatment (Curley et al, 2004). It should be known that radiofrequency ablation could induce serious combined diseases more than several months after the treatment.

4.2 Case report: Diaphragmatic hernia twenty months after percutaneous radiofrequency ablation for hepatocellular carcinoma

In August, 2006, we experienced one case of a 50-year-old man with hepatitis B virus infection who underwent radiofrequency ablation for hepatocellular carcinoma of 2.2 cm in diameter located in the segment VIII area of his liver adjacent to the diaphragm (Figure 1a). The tumor could be almost fully scanned ultrasonographically and it was located just under the costal region close to the costpleural angle. Laboratory tests showed his liver function as Child-Pugh class A liver cirrhosis.

Ultrasound-guided radiofrequency ablation was performed using RITA Medical System 1500 RF generator attached to a 15-gauge Starburst XL model 90 probe needle for 20 minutes and the needle was expanded to 4cm in a stepwise manner. There was no technical problem and enough ablation area around hepatocellular carcinoma could be achieved with a safety margin of the necrotic area (Figure 1b). He did not feel nausea and did not complained about a thermal effect like right shoulder pain which could be a sign of diaphragm damage (Livraghi et al, 2003). After the procedure, he was discharged in a week without any adverse effects. He had been under observation in our hospital regularly and medicated by entecavir to control hepatitis B virus replication. Since multiple recurrence lesions were detected in the segment VIII later, he was treated with transcatheter arterial chemoembolization therapy in April, 2007 and in February, 2008.

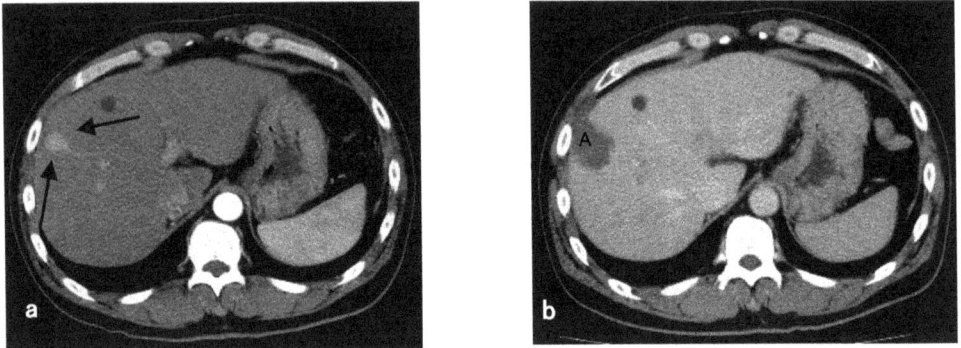

Fig. 1. 50-year-old man with hepatocellular carcinoma. (adapted from Nawa T et al).
a. Arterial phase computed tomography scan obtained prior to the radiofrequency ablation shows enhancing nodule (black arrows) in the segment VIII of the liver.
b. Portal phase computed tomography scan obtained after the radiofrequency ablation shows the ablation zone (A).

Twenty months later after the radiofrequency ablation treatment in April 2008, he was admitted to our hospital emergency department because of severe right hypochondralgia and dyspnea.

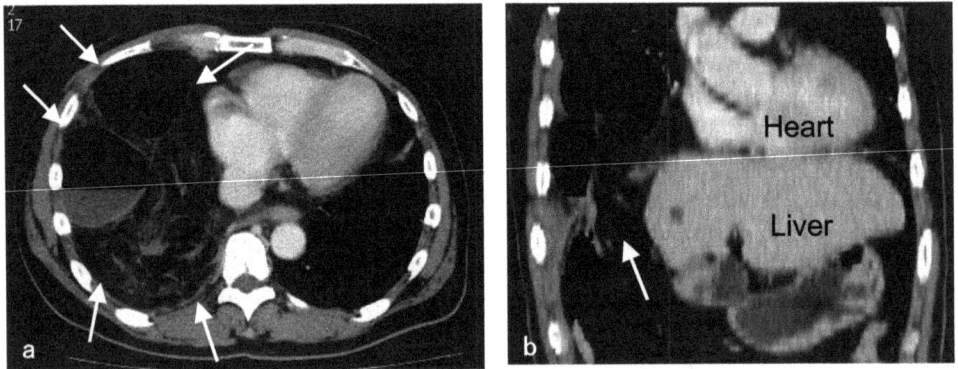

Fig. 2. Computed tomography scan obtained at the hospital emergency department twenty months later after the radiofrequency ablation therapy. (adapted from Nawa T et al).
a. Computed tomography scan shows the prolapsed large intestine and the omentum in his right pleural cavity (white arrows).
b. Coronal multidetector computed tomography image of his chest shows the portion of the large intestine in the right lower thorax, indicating the anatomic relationship of the diaphragmatic defect (white arrow) and the surrounding organs.

Computed tomography revealed the prolapsed large intestine and the omentum through a defect on the right diaphragm (Figure 2a, 2b), and emergency surgery was performed to close the hole in the diaphragm following the diagnosis of diaphragmatic hernia. The operation showed that the ascending and transverse colon had been herniated into the right pleural cavity through the diaphragmatic hole which measured 5x3 cm in diameter (Figure 3) and no apparent invasion of hepatocellular carcinoma around the hole was observed. Although the colon was perforated in the pleural cavity and induced pyothorax after the operation, he recovered with the intense care using antibiotics and drainage (Nawa et al, 2010).

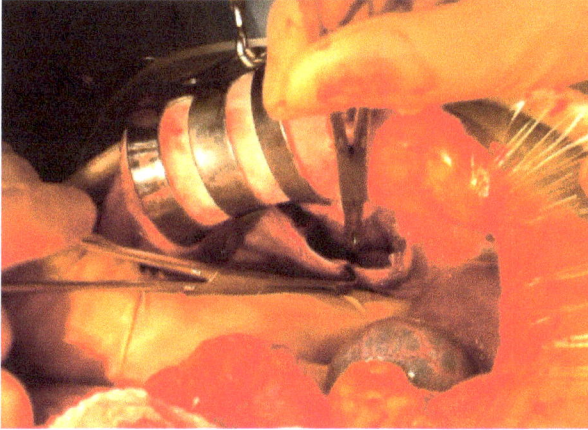

Fig. 3. The photograph taken during the surgery. (adapted from Nawa T et al).
This photograph is showing the hole in the diaphragm.

In our case, the location of the diaphragm defect was apparently different from that of congenital diaphragmatic hernia and his clinical history showed that nothing other than the radiofrequency ablation could be the cause of the diaphragmatic perforation. The repeated treatments of transcatheter arterial chemoembolization against hepatocellular carcinoma recurrence during twenty months might accelerate the atrophy of the right lobe of his liver (Figure 4, a-d). This atrophic change could be thought to make the space between the liver and the diaphragm for his large intestine to access to the hole.

It is often a problem of radiofrequency ablation using an expandable electrode that all of the multiple tips of the needle cannot always be detected under ultrasonography because the tips are multidirectional meaning there is a risk of puncture of vessels or other organs close to a tumor beyond the possible scan area. However, diaphragmatic hernia was reported not only in the case of expandable electrodes but also in the case of a single straight electrode. Therefore, the thermal effect for the diaphragm could not always be induced by the direct puncture of expandable electrode.

Because this complication was observed in the cases of hepatocellular carcinoma located in the segment IV, VII or VIII close to the diaphragm, it should be recommended to follow carefully such cases, especially with the apparent atrophic change of the right lobe of the liver, as the high-risk groups of diaphragmatic hernia.

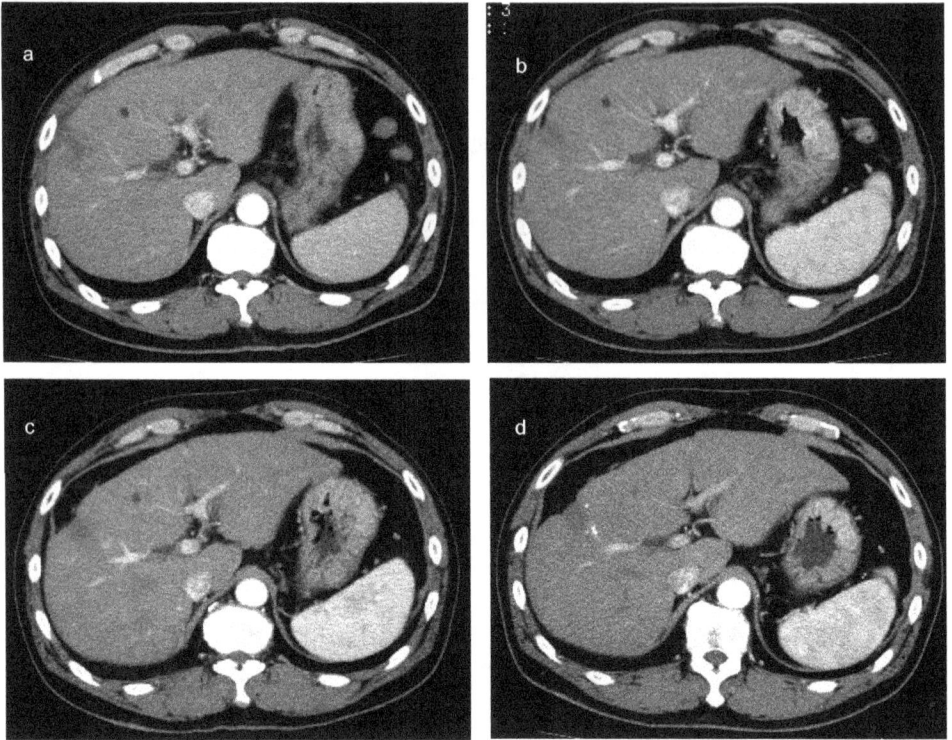

Fig. 4. Computed tomography scan obtained after the radiofrequency ablation therapy. (adapted from Nawa T et al).
Computed tomography obtained in August, 2006, (a); in November, 2006,(b); in March, 2007, (c); in May, 2007, (d). The serial computed tomography scans are showing the gradual atrophic change of the liver causing to space between the diaphragm and the liver.

5. Technical solution for radiofrequency ablation for hepatocellular carcinoma at the dome of the diaphragm: The techniques of artificial ascites

5.1 The purpose of the artificial ascites technique

Radiofrequency ablation is difficult to perform if a tumor is located under the diaphragm because this region is often invisible or is poorly visible on ultrasonography. Local ablation therapy under laparoscopy or thoracoscopy could be a possible treatment in such case, but it is more invasive than percutaneous procedure and other special equipment would be needed. The artificial pleural or peritoneal effusion has been explored as a beneficial treatment option that offers excellent local control through visualization of hepatocellular carcinoma under the diaphragm (Katayama et al, 2002; Uehara et al, 2007; Rhim et al, 2008). It was meaningful that this method has been reported to be effective to keep enough space between the liver and the adjacent organs including the diaphragm by a solution that can cool down the local ablated area by circulating in the peritoneal space. The procedure of artificial ascites technique is briefly shown below.

5.2 Procedure of artificial ascites

1. The location of the puncture site should be defined first as a clearly visible point in the liver with ultrasonography usually at the sixth to eighth intercostal space along the anterior to middle axillary line. It is necessary to avoid around the radiofrequency ablation puncture site for the artificial ascites puncture site since radiofrequency ablation treatment should be started during the artificial ascites procedure before the ascites spreads to other or lower abdominal cavity. If it is difficult to avoid the ablation puncture site for the artificial ascites puncture site, it is able to start making the artificial ascites at that site and try other sites after gaining a solution space in the abdominal cavity since there should be more puncture sites to make the ascites after gaining it.

2. After the administration of the local anesthesia at the skin of the puncture site, an 18-gauge sheathed needle would be prepared to insert into the peritoneal space. If the outer sheath has a side hole for infusion, it would be much easier and faster to achieve enough volume of ascites. The pneumoperitoneum needle can be used for the puncture of the appropriate site instead of the sheathed needle for this procedure.

3. Patients are asked to perform inspiration to move the liver downward and then to hold the breath for a while. Oxygen administration could be helpful for the patients to hold the breath. The physician inserts the 18-gauge sheathed needle into the parenchyma of the liver (Figure 5a) and removes the inner stylet of the sheathed needle (Figure 5b).

4. Next, the patients are asked to perform full expiration so that the needle sheath can slip away from the hepatic capsule and located in the perihepatic intraperitoneal space (Figure 5c). If the needle sheath could not slip away from the liver, further deep inspiration and expiration could help a successful placement of the sheath.

5. After the placement of the outer sheath into the peritoneal cavity, 500-1500 ml of 5% glucose solution could be infused until the tumor is fully visualized and the path for the radiofrequency ablation electrode could be clearly developed (Figure 5d). In case of diabetic patients, saline could be used instead of glucose solution.

5.3 The other issues of artificial ascites technique

5.3.1 Learning of the knack of artificial ascites procedure

a. The puncture directed in the dorsal space of the liver without direct puncture of the liver parenchyma could be selected, but it may take longer time to achieve enough volume of ascites above ventral side of the target liver surface.

b. Even though the needle sheath could not slip away from the liver parenchyma at step 4), the solution infusion could be started slowly. Sometimes, a blood back flow is seen after stylet removal through the needle sheath, but if the blood flow does not come from a hepatic artery, usually the solution infusion can be started. The back flow of the solution infusion from the liver parenchyma would make the ultrasonographically visible thin layer of the solution showing faint blinking streams around the liver (Figure 4e, 4f). At that time, respiratory movement might affect the drip infusion while it stops during the time of the expiration and it starts during the time of the inspiration due to the change of abdominal pressure.

c. If an outflow of the blinking stream through hepatic vein could be observed (Figure 4g), the physician should stop infusion and retry the puncture.

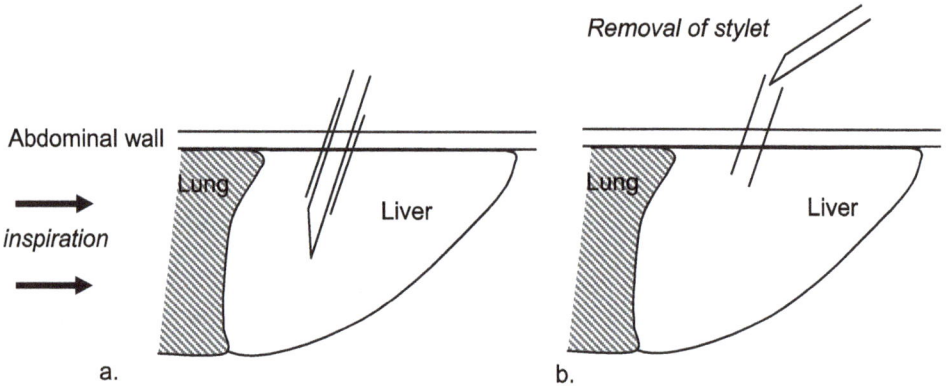

a.

b.

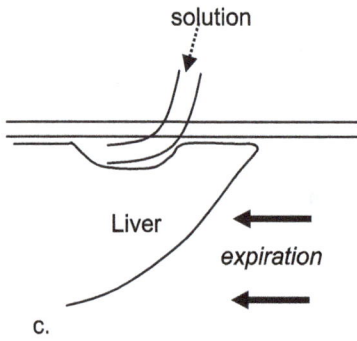

c.

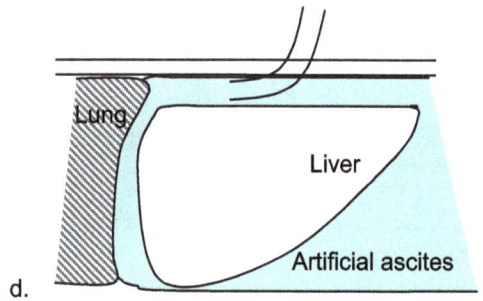

d.

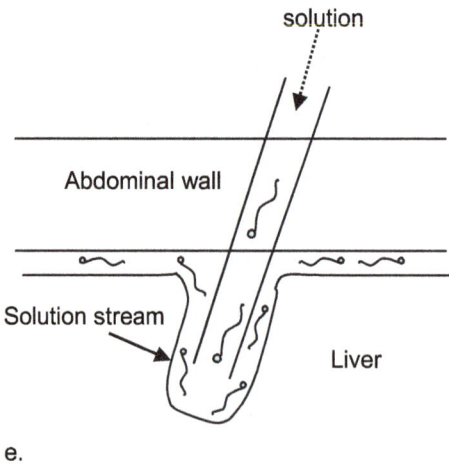

e.

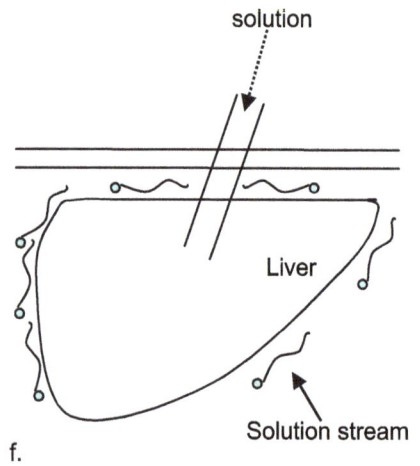

f.

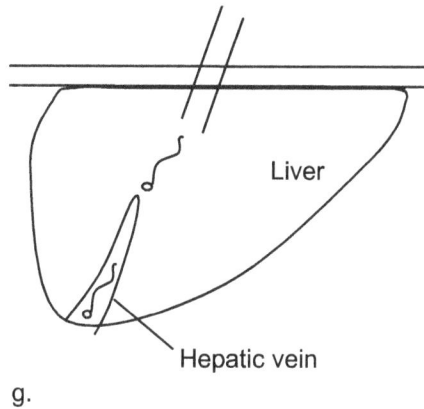

g.

Fig. 5. The diagrams show the procedure to obtain artificial ascites during radiofrequency ablation.

a. The insertion of the 18-gauge sheathed needle into the parenchyma of the liver.
b. The removal of the inner stylet of the sheathed needle.
c. The placement of the outer needle sheath in the perihepatic intraperitoneal space.
d. The achievement of the artificial ascites that can visualize the whole tumor and the path for the RFA electrode.
e. The faint blinking streams of the back flow of the solution infusion from the outer sheath needle in the liver parenchyma.
f. The faint blinking streams around the liver.
g. The unsuccessful streams of solution outflowing to the hepatic vein

d. It is reported that oxygen saturation decreased by only 2.3% even in performing artificial pleural effusion (McGhana & Dodd, 2001) and most of the solution infused into the peritoneal cavity would disappear in 3 to 7 days in our experience.
e. Artificial ascites technique can be used in the cases that hepatocellular carcinoma is located at ventral or dorsal side beneath the liver capsule in order to avoid the thermal effect to the abdominal wall or gastrointestinal tract (Kondo et al, 2006).

5.3.2 Technical pitfalls of artificial ascites procedure

The infusion should not be vigorously performed until enough thickness (about 2 to 5 mm) of the layer could be detected because such infusion often causes the sheath dislocation from the first placed site and produces an unintended inflow to the abdominal wall. The physicians often notice such inflow with the swelling of the puncture site or an ultrasonographic thickening of the abdominal wall. In this case, the physicians should also remove the sheath as soon as possible and retry the puncture, but it often becomes more difficult to insert from the same site because the abdominal wall becomes thicker than the distance that the puncture needle can reach. Therefore, the physicians should try to find another appropriate site for a puncture or try it again another day.

5.3.3 Out of the indication of artificial ascites

If the patients have histories of abdominal operation or peritonitis, the adhesions between the liver and the abdominal wall might be hazardous to have successful artificial ascites. In those cases, the other locoregional treatments like transcatheter arterial chemoembolization, percutaneous ethanol injection therapy, or computed tomography guided radiofrequency ablation could be suitable procedures to treat the patients.

6. Conclusion

The patients who have undergone radiofrequency ablation for hepatic tumors adjacent to the diaphragm should be carefully followed up for possible diaphragmatic hernia, even after the long postoperative intervals. The artificial ascites technique can be used not only to visualize the whole HCC under the diaphragm, but also to reduce the unavoidable and unintended thermal complications of the diaphragm and the surrounding organs if successfully performed.

7. References

Bruix J, Sala M, Llovet JM. (2004). Chemoembolization for hepatocellular carcinoma. Gastroenterology 127. 5, (Nov 2004), S179-188, 0016-5085.

Choi D, Lim HK, Rhim H, Kim YS, Lee WJ, Palk SW, Koh KC, Lee JH, Choi MS, Yoo BC. (2007). Percutaneous radiofrequency ablation for early-stage hepatocellular carcinoma as a first-line treatment: long-term results and prognostic factors in a large single-institution series. Eur Radiol 17. 3, (Mar 2007), 684-692, 0938-7994.

Curley SA, Izzo F, Ellis LM, Nicolas Vaughey J, Vallone P. (2000). Radiofrequency ablation of hepatocellular cancer in 110 patients with cirrhosis. Ann Surg 232. 3, (Sep 2000), 381-391, 0003-4932.

Curley SA, Marra P, Beaty K, Ellis LM, Vauthey JN, Abdalla EK, Scalfe C, Raut C, Wolff R, Choi H, Loyer E, Vallone P, Flore F, Scordino F, De Rosa V, Orlando R, Pignata S, Daniele B, Izzo F. (2004). Early and late complications after radiofrequency ablation of malignant liver tumors in 608 patients. Ann Surg 239. 4, (Apr 2004), 450-458, 0003-4932.

Head HW, Dodd III GD, Dalrymple NC, Prasad SR, El-Merhi FM, Freckleton MW, Hubbard LG. (2007). Percutaneous radiofrequency ablation of hepatic tumors against the diaphragm: frequency of diaphragmatic injury. Radioilogy 243. 3, (Jun 2007), 877-884, 0033-8419.

Kang TW, Rhim H, Kim EY, Kim Ys, Choi D, Lee Wj, Lim HK (2009). Percutaneous radiofrequency ablation for the hepatocellular carcinoma abutting the diaphragm: assessment of safety and therapeutic efficacy. Korean J Radiol 10. 1, (Jan-Feb 2009), 34-42, 1229-6929.

Katayama K, Ohka Y, Uemura A, Shinzaki S, Egawa S, Naito M, Ishibashi K, Kamoi R. (2002). Saline injection into the pleural cavity to detect tumors of the hepatic dome with sonography; A new approach for treatment of hepatocellular carcinoma. AJR Am J Roentgenol 179. 1, (Jul 2002), 102-104. 0361-803X.

Koda M, Ueki M, Maeda N, Murawaki Y. (2003). Diaphragmatic perforation and hernia after hepatic radiofrequency ablation. AJR Am J Roentgenol 180. 6, (Jun 2003), 1561-1562. 0361-803X.

Kondo Y, Yoshida H, Shiina S, Tateishi R, Teratani T, Omata M. (2006). Artificial ascites technique for percutaneous radiofrequency ablation of liver cancer adjacent to the gastrointestinal tract. Br J Surg 93. 10, 1277-1292, 0007-1323.

Lencioni R, Cioni D, Crocetti L, Franchini C, Pina CD, Lera J, Bartolozzi C. (2005). Early-stage hepatocellular carcinoma in patients with cirrhosis: long-term results of percutaneous image-guided radiofrequency ablation. Radiology 234. 3, (Mar 2005), 961-967, 0033-8419.

Livraghi T, Golberg SN, Lazzaroni S, Meloni F, Solbiati L, Gazelle GS. (1999). Small hepatocellular carcinoma: treatment with radio-frequency ablation versus ethanol injection. Radiology 210. 3, (Mar 1999), 655-661, 0033-8419.

Livraghi T, Goldberg SN, Lazzaroni S, Meloni F, Ierace T, Solbiati L, Gazelle GS. (2000). Hepatocellular carcinoma: radio-frequency ablation of medium and large lesions. Radiology 214. 3, (Mar 2000), 761-768, 0033-8419.

Livraghi T, Solbiati L, Meloni MF, Gazelle GS, Halpern EF, Goldberg SN. (2003). Treatment of focal liver tumors with percutaneous radio-frequency ablation: complications encountered in a multicenter study. Radiology 226. 2, (Feb 2003), 441-451, 0033-8419.

McGhana JP, Dodd GD 3rd. (2001). Radiofrequency ablation of the liver; current status. AJR Am J Roentgenol 176. 1, (Jan 2001), 3-16, 0361-803X.

Mulier S, Mulier P, Ni Y, Miao Y, Dupas B, Marchal G, DeWever I, Michel L. (2002). Complications of radiofrequency coagulation of liver tumorurs. Br J Surg 89. 10, (Oct 2002), 1206-1222. 0007-1323.

Nawa T, Mochizuki K, Yakushijin T, Hamano M, Itose I, Egawa S, Nishida T, Tsutsui S, Hiramatsu N, Kanto T, Takehara T, Hayashi N. (2010). A patient who developed diaphragmatic hernia 20 months after percutaneous radiofrequency ablation for hepatocellular carcinoma. Nippon Shokakibyo Gakkai Zasshi 107. 7, (Jul 2010), 1167-1174. 0446-6586.

Olsen SK, Brown RS, and Siegel AB. (2010). Hepatocellular carcinoma: review of current treatment with a focus on targeted molecular therapies, *Therap Adv Gatroenterol*, 3. 1, (Jan 2010), 55-66, 1756-283X

Orlando A, Learndro G, Olivo M, Andriulli A, Cottone M. (2009). Radiofrequency thermal ablation vs. percutaneous ethanol injection for small hepatocellular carcinoma in cirrhosis: meta-analysis of randomized controlled trials. Am J Gastroenterol 104. 2, (Feb 2009), 514-524, 0002-9270.

Poon RT, Fan ST, Tsan FH, Wong J. (2002). Locoregional therapies for hepatocellular carcinoma: a critical review from the surgeon's perspective. Ann Surg, 235. 4, (Apr 2002), 466-486, 0003-4932.

Rhim H, Lim Hk, Kim YS, Choi D. (2008). Percutaneous Radiofrequency ablation with artificial ascites for hepatocellular carcinoma in the hepatic dome : initial experience. AJR Am J Roentgenol. 190. 1, (Jan 2008), 91-97. 0361-803X.

Tateishi R, Shiina S, Teratani T, Obi S, Sato S, Koike Y, Fujishima T, Yoshida H, Kawabe T, Omata M. (2005). Percutaneous radiofrequency ablation for hepatocellular carcinoma: an analysis of 1000 cases. Cancer 103. 6, (Mar 2005), 1201-1209, 0008-543X.

Uehara T, Hirooka M, Ishida K, Hiraoka A, Kumagi T, Kisaka Y, Hiasa Y, Onji M. (2007). Percutaneous ultrasound-guided radiofrequency ablation of hepatocellular carcinoma with artificially induced pleural effusion and ascites. J Gastroenterol 42. 4, (Apr 2007), 306-311, 0944-1174.

Wood TF, Rose DM, Chung M, Allegra DP, Foshag LJ, Bilchik AJ. (2000). Radiofrequency
    ablation of 231 unresectable hepatic tumors: indications, limitations, and
    complications. Ann Surg Oncol 7. 8, (Sep 2000), 593-600, 1068-9265.

Therapy of Hepatocellular Carcinoma with Iodine-131-Lipidiol

Hojjat Ahmadzadehfar[1,*], Amir Sabet[1],
Hans Jürgen Biersack[1] and Jörn Risse[2]
[1]Department of Nuclear Medicine, University Hospital Bonn
[2]Radiology and Nuclear Medicine Institute, Bad Honnef
Germany

1. Introduction

Therapy in nuclear medicine practice has a long distinguished history. Nuclear medicine therapy is required to be highly specific and targeted, since it always involves administration of unsealed sources of radioactivity. Most therapy agents utilize ß-particle emissions for their ability to penetrate tissues. This deposition of energy in tissue by ß emitters results in cellular damage. Among the ß emitters there are several choices with respect to energy of the ß emission. Lower energy ß particles can travel a few cell diameters, or at most in the sub-millimeter range. Higher energy ß particles such as those emitted by Y-90 have an excellent tissue penetration with a range beyond the source of several millimeters. The physical half-life of the therapeutic radionuclide is an important consideration and underlying principle for therapy planning. Rarely, except in thyroid treatment, is the simple salt form of the radionuclide used. It is most likely attached to a drug or particle that controls its biodistribution. The ideal therapeutic radiopharmaceutical is one that remains attached to the parent drug or its metabolites, and is excreted rapidly through a known simple route[1].

For selected patients with HCC, confined to the liver but not amenable to resection or transplantation, both systemic and locoregional therapies can be considered. These include

1. Percutaneous interventions (ethanol injection, radiofrequency thermal ablation),
2. Transarterial interventions
a. Embolization (TAE), chemoperfusion (TAC), or chemoembolization (TACE),
b. Radioembolization (RE) or radioactive agent perfusion such as 131Iodine-Lipiodol or 188RE-Lipiodol
3. External radiation therapy and
4. Chemotherapy, including gene and immune therapy.

In this chapter we focus only on the therapeutic indications, usefulness and methods of treatment with 131-Iodine Lipiodol (131I-Lipiodol). Its rationale comes from the anatomical

---

* Corresponding Author

and physiological aspects of HCC being exploited for the delivery of the therapeutic agent. The liver has a dual blood supply: the hepatic artery and the portal vein. Observations on vascular supply to hepatic malignancies have demonstrated that metastatic hepatic tumours >3 mm derive in contrast to healthy hepatic cells 80–100% of their blood supply from the arterial rather than the portal hepatic circulation[2].

2. Basic characteristics of 131 I-Lipiodol

131I is a beta emitting radionuclide with a physical half life of 8.04 days. The maximum and mean beta particle energies are 0.61MeV and 0.192MeV respectively. Additionally, 131I emits a principal gamma photon of 364 keV (81% abundance). The Beta radiation of I131 is responsible for its therapeutic effects while gamma radiation makes the distribution of the radiopharmaceutical visible.

Lipiodol is a mixture of iodized esters of poppy seed oil fatty acids used as a contrast medium for the detection of HCC which remains in these tumours for a longer period compared to normal liver or in other tissues. Isotopic exchange is used to label iodine-rich Lipiodol with 131I (Lipiocis®, CIS Bio International/ member of IBA group). Lipiocis® is licensed in France for the treatment of patients with HCC and portal vein thrombosis (PVT)[3]. It was developed in the 1990s and was the first radiolabeled vector to be used in this setting. According to biodistribution data, more than 75% of the 131I-Lipiodol stays following the arterial administration in the liver and the remainder reaches the lungs[4]. Other tissues, including the thyroid gland, receive very little radiation.

An in vitro assessment [5] showed an unspecific uptake of Lipiodol in non-malignant endothelial cells apart from its concentration in cancer cell lines. Lipiodol alone does not appear to have any cytotoxic effect against any of the studied cell lines. However, 131I-Lipiodol is highly and only selectively cytotoxic for the cancer cell lines. Inability of tumourous cells unlike non-malignant ones to expel Lipiodol, revealed by quantification methods using computer-assisted image analysis, may further enhance the cytotoxic effect of 131I-Lipiodol in cancer cells. There is no separation of the 131I from Lipiodol during the uptake process by the cancer cells, as Lipiodol is a naturally iodinated oil compound with an iodine content of 38–40%. 131I-Lipiodol shows cytotoxic effects against the cancer cell lines even in doses as small as a quarter of the radioactivity of the 131I alone[5].

The tumour/ non tumour uptake ratio is about 15–20:1 and increases with time, while the effective half life within the HCC tissue is also longer than that in healthy tissues (almost 6 days versus 4 days). Generally, more than 10 % of the injected Lipiodol remains within the tumour [6]. The retention of 131I-Lipiodol in HCC tumours after intra-arterial infusion is related not only to embolization in the micro vessels of the tumour, but also to the entry into the interstitium and the tumour cells themselves. This retention can be assessed by tomodensitometric examination and inversely relates to the tumour size. Indeed, 88% of the HCCs smaller than 5 cm exhibit a high retention (of type 3 or 4 according to the criteria of Maki et al.[7]) whereas 74% of the HCCs larger than 10 cm exhibit only a weak retention of less than 50% (of type 1 or 2 according to the criteria of Maki) [8, 9]. Moreover, the clearance of Lipiodol from the tumour lasts longer than from the normal liver or from the lungs, possibly because of a lack of macrophagic cells in the tumour [3]. 131I-Lipiodol is eliminated mainly through the urinary tract, reaching 30–50% of the injected activity at day 8, but also to a small extent by way of the faeces (<3% at day 5) [4].

The required therapy activity for the intended tumour dose can be calculated for a given tumour mass according to its size. For instance producing 120 Gy in a tumour with a diameter of 1 cm requires less than 3 MBq I-131 while the same dose in a tumour with a fivefold larger diameter requires hundredfold more activity [10].

The radionuclide is supplied in 2 ml solution for injection and stored in a 4 ml cone shaped glass vial. The specific activity at calibration date is 1.1 GBq/ml and its shelf life from this time is 3 days [11, 12].

The conjunction of lipiodol with TACE, also called TOCA (transarterial oily chemoembolization), has also been used allowing the delivery of locally concentrated therapy due to the selective retention of the agent in the tumours for an extended period [13].

3. Basics of interventional nuclear medicine therapies of HCC with I131-Lipiodol

Radiation is tumoricidal if sufficient doses can be delivered selectively to the tumour without damaging adjacent normal tissue [14]. Normal hepatocytes have a lower tolerance to the effects of radiation than neoplastic tissue. The dose required to destroy solid tumors, estimated at ≥70 Gy, is far greater than the liver tolerance dose of 35 Gy when delivered to the whole liver in 1.8 Gy/d fractions [15]. If the whole liver is exposed to external-beam radiation at a mean radiation dose of 43 Gy, more than 50% of patients develop liver dysfunction [16]. Conformal and stereotactic radiation therapy techniques can be used to deliver much higher radiation doses in cases with focal involvement [17]; however, since primary neoplasms are often multifocal and irregular in shape and potentially replace large parts of the liver volume, only a small minority of patients are optimal candidates for such therapies [18]. Internal radiation aims at improving the selectivity of the radiation by targeting the radioisotopes to the tumour cells. To achieve this targeting, the therapeutic radiopharmaceuticals such as 90Y microspheres or 131I-Lipiodol may be administered via the hepatic artery [19].

Based on studies considering biodistribution of intraarterial 131I-Lipiodol in humans [4, 20, 21], radiation doses for every mCi (37 MBq) of administered activity were estimated to be 31 cGy for the normal liver, 22 cGy for the lungs, and 239 cGy for a tumor with a greatest diameter of 4 cm using the formula:

$$\text{Dose (cGy)} = 73.8 \times E \times Te \times \frac{A_0}{M} + 0.0346 \times \Gamma \times g \times \frac{A_0}{M}$$

where E is the average beta energy (MeV), Te is the effective half-life (days), Γ is the specific gamma ray constant (cGy cm^2/mCi hr), Ao is the initial activity (µCi), M is the mass(g), and g is the geometric factor (cm).

4. Contraindications

Absolute contraindications

1. Pregnancy and breastfeeding, 2. life expectancy less than 1 month, 3. hepatic encephalopathy, 4. tumour Stage OKUDA III[11, 12].

Relative contraindications

1. High extrahepatic tumor burden, 2. acute or severe chronic pulmonary disease, 3. The presence of contraindications for hepatic artery catheterisation [11, 12].

5. Therapeutic indications for 131I-Lipiodol

5.1 Palliative treatment of inoperable hepatocellular carcinoma

An improved survival rate is readily documented for those treated with 131I-Lipiodol, comparing to those receiving only medical support [22]. The treatment is more effective for small, solitary and well encapsulated tumors and the response rate decreases with increasing tumor size. Its main limitation is its ineffectiveness in large (>5 cm) tumours. However, transarterial therapy with 131I-Lipiodol is superior to systemic therapy in tumours up to 5 cm in diameter[23].

The data on therapy efficacy have remained non-uniform. A decrease in tumour size has been reported in about 50 % to 60 % of patients; two early studies with seven and nine patients showed response in all tumours [24, 25]. In larger studies classifying therapy success according to the WHO criteria, the response rate decreases to about 30 % [26]. This is in agreement with our own data [27]. Reported response rates in different studies are summarised in table 1; only reports with more than ten patients, data on changes in tumour size and follow-up studies of at least one month, are considered.

First author, year, reference	Number of evaluable patients	CR	PR	MR	SD	PD	AFP decrease
Yoo 1991[29]	24	0	3	5	8	8	13/16
Raoul 1992[30]	30	0	18	4	6	2	22/29
Leung 1994[31]	22	1	3	-	12	6	13/25
Bhattacharya 1995[32]	22	0	7	-	8	7	2/22
Raoul 1997[28]	25	1	15	4	3	2	20/40
De Baere 1999[26]	23	0	3	-	12	8	-
Risse 2000 [27]	13	0	2	3	4	4	-
Rindani 2002 [33]	12	0	6	-	5	1	5/7
Borbath 2005 [34]	19	1	0	-	7	11	2/24
Risse 2006 [35]	17	0	4	1	7	5	-
Boucher 2007[36]	40	1	18	-	19	2	

CR: complete response, PR: partial response (tumour reduction > 50 %), MR: minimal response (tumor reduction between 25 an 50 %, AFP alpha-fetoprotein, SD: stable disease (tumour size change between - 25 % - +25 %), PD: progressive disease (tumour increase > 25 %)

Table 1. Efficacy of 131I-Lipiodol therapy in patients with unresectable HCC

131I-Lipiodol is also comparatively favourable to other regional therapy procedures for palliative treatment of HCC. A multicentre randomised trial by Raoul et al[28] showed that 131I-Lipiodol therapy (n=73) was associated with a better patient tolerance and fewer vascular complications than TACE (n=69), although no survival advantage was demonstrated[28].

In a published study from our group 38 courses of intra-arterial 131I-Lipiodol therapy with a total activity up to 6.7 GBq were performed in 18 patients with HCC (6 with PVT)[35]. Tumour volume decreased in 20/32 index nodules (63%) after the first course. Repeated therapy frequently resulted in further tumour reduction. Partial response was seen in 11 nodules while 4 nodules showed a minor response. Stable disease was found in 12 patients and progressive disease in 5. Significant response was associated with pre-therapeutic nodule volume up to 150 ml (diameter of 6.6 cm). Survival rate after 3, 6, 9, 12, 24 and 36 months was 78, 61, 50, 39, 17, and 6% respectively. Matched-pairs analysis of survival revealed 131I-Lipiodol to be superior to medical treatment. The most important side effect was a pancreatitis-like syndrome while overall tolerance was very acceptable.

The median survival in patients with unresctable HCC undergoing 131I-Lipiodol therapy has been reported between 7 and 27 months [34, 36-38]. Chua et al reported the factors associated with survival in a newly published study including the AJCC stage (1-2 vs 3-4), Barcelona Clinic Liver Cancer stage (A-B vs C), Cancer of the Liver Italian Program score (< 2 vs >2), maximum tumor size (<4 vs >4 cm), extrahepatic disease, previous surgery and response to treatment (favorable vs unfavourable).[38] Considering response rate, AJCC stage 1-2 and Cancer of the Liver Italian Program score < 2 were found to be independent predictors for a favorable response in this study[38].

5.1.1 Palliative treatment of HCC with Portal vein thrombosis (PVT)

Although the PVT prohibits any attempt of TACE, 131I-Lipiodol has proved to be an effective therapy option in patients with HCC and PVT[39]. Raoul et al. compared 131I-Lipiodol therapy and best supportive care in patients with HCC and PVT. The survival rates at 3, 6 and 9 mo was 71%, 48% and 7% for the treated group; and 10%, 0% and 0% for the group receiving only supportive care. The authors concluded that 131I-Lipiodol is a safe and effective palliative treatment of HCC in the presence of portal vein thrombosis [22]. However it should be noted that radioembolization (RE) with 90Y-Microspheres has proved to be a feasible alternative treatment for HCC patients with PVT as discussed in following section.

5.1.2 131I-Lipiodol versus radioembolisation with 90Y-Microspheres

90Y radioembolization (RE), or selective internal radiation therapy (SIRT), is a promising catheter-based liver-directed modality approved by the Food and Drug Administration for patients with primary and metastatic liver cancer[40]. In a meta-analysis of 14 published articles Venti et al showed almost 80% any response (AR = [CR +PR +SD]) for a total of 325 patients with HCC. According to this meta-analysis, treatment with resin microspheres was associated with a significantly higher proportion of AR than with glass microsphere (0.89 vs 0.78 [P <0.02])[41].

Although RE is currently the preferred method for treating HCC compared to 131I-Lipiodol, its embolic nature makes severe liver dysfunction a theoretic contraindication for this technique, as in TACE. In addition, techniques using 90Y-labeled products tend to cost up to 10 times more than therapy with 131I-Lipiodol [42], affecting the therapeutic approach especially in the countries with a poor insurance system.

PVT is not an absolute contraindication for RE any more. Although resin microspheres could pose the patient at risk for significant liver dysfunction based on the embolic treatment effect, therasphere has been shown to be safe even when the portal vein has been invaded by tumor[14]. However, recent studies describe safe performance of RE with resin microspheres even in PVT. There is no prospective study which compares these two methods (RE vs 131I-Lipiodol) in patients with PVT in HCC considering response rate, time-to-progression, and survival.

5.1.3 131I-Lipiodol-therapy versus TAE and TACE

131I-Lipiodol therapy in patients with cirrhosis and HCC has an efficacy similar to that of TACE/TAE therapy [28, 32, 42]. However 131I-Lipiodol appears to be of more benefit in patients with advanced disease, for example, in those with Okuda stage III disease or BCLC stage D as well as in patients with PVT [42]. PVT patients receiving 131I-Lipiodol lived on average almost a year longer than those treated with TACE or TAE. Moreover, 131I-Lipiodol is much better tolerated than chemoembolization, both in terms of clinically expressed side effects and arteriographic findings [28].

5.2 Performing 131I-Lipiodol as an adjuvant or neo-adjuvant therapy

Early intrahepatic recurrence is common after curative resection of hepatocellular carcinoma, frequently due to microscopic metastatic disease or less commonly, metachronous multicentric carcinoma within the liver remnant not detected before or during resection by conventional imaging [43] and has led to attempts at adjuvant or neoadjuvant therapies.

5.2.1 131I-Lipiodol as an adjuvant therapy

It has been thought that when the postsurgical liver starts to regenerate, small microscopic daughter tumours can be stimulated to grow. If these were pre-cleared the chances of a recurrence would be lowered. Thus,131I-Lipiodol has been used in an adjuvant setting after curative surgical resection [44]. A single dose of 1.85 GBq 131I-Lipiodol administered 6 weeks after curative resection of hepatocellular carcinoma could significantly decrease the rate of recurrence and increased disease-free and overall survival in a study by Lau et al. [43]. In their recent published paper the same authors confirmed their results after a longer follow up [45]. These findings were also confirmed by Boucher et al. administering 2.4 GBq 131I-Lipiodol 8-12 weeks after surgery [46]. NG et. al.[47] also reported a good overall survival with 1.7 GBq I131-Lipiodol 1-8 months after surgery. It seems that there is no clinically significant adverse effect of adjuvant therapy by intra-arterial131I-Lipiodol after curative liver resection for HCC [48]. These results were also confirmed in a recent published study from Chua et. al. [49]. It is necessary to perform more randomized controlled trials with more patients to confirm the role of 131I-Lipiodol as an adjuvant treatment especially considering the timing and the administered dose.

5.2.2 Neo-adjuvant 131I-Lipiodol administration before liver transplantation/resection

In a study by Raoul et. al[50] curative resection of hepatocellular carcinoma or liver transplantation was preceded by 2 injections of 2.4 GBq 131I-Lipiodol (5 weeks preoperative) to reduce intrahepatic recurrence. The procedure was well tolerated and associated with an objective tumour response in 56 % and a complete histological response in 24 % of 34 treated patients. An objective tumour response or necrosis of more than 90 % of the tumour mass was observed in three-quarters of these patients. Brans et. al. treated 10 HCC patients with almost 1.8 GBq 131I-Lipiodol in a pilot study followed by liver transplantation within 1–9 months [51]. The evidence of an anti-tumoural effect of 131L-Lipiodol was observed in 50% of patients. However, performing randomized comparisons between surgery alone *versus* surgery after intra-arterial injection of 131I-labelled Lipiodol in patients with large but technically resectable tumours is needed.

6. Imaging before performing the therapy

The work-up includes a three-phase contrast computed tomography (CT) and gadolinium-enhanced magnetic resonance imaging (MRI) of the liver for the assessment of tumour and non-tumour volume, portal vein patency, and the extent of extra-hepatic disease. Although FDG-PET is suitable for tumours showing high glucose metabolism such as colorectal carcinoma, melanoma, head and neck, and breast cancers, malignancies such as HCC or neuroendocrine tumours, except for their aggressive types show no or a very low-grade FDG uptake[40].

The suboptimal sensitivity of FDG-PET for the detection of HCC, ranging between 50% and 70% makes it an unsatisfactory imaging choice for the pre- and post-treatment evaluation in this group of patients; however, it adds valuable prognostic information (metabolic grading) as patients with a negative FDG-PET show a better prognosis than those with high FDG uptake. Choline PET/CT may also play a role in imaging of specific types of HCC in the near future [40, 52-54].

7. Intervention technique

Treatment with 131I-Lipiodol serves as an example for multidisciplinary management including the patient selection and care, the detailed anatomical study and dose calculation, the post-interventional treatment including timing and selection of systemic treatment, adequate follow-up of the patient as well as the management of possible complications. Prior to the therapy, patients should receive both written and verbal information about the procedure and the palliative nature of the treatment [12]. The renal functional status should be adequate for the use of contrast agents during the pre-therapeutic angiogram. Haemodialysis patients may be treated with 131I-Lipiodol, however, dialysis has to be planned and timed before and after the intervention. Patients should be given a peri-interventional drug regimen with slow intravenous infusion of 24 mg dexamethasone and 8 mg ondansetrone during the whole procedure and intraarterial injection of 50 mg pethidine immediately before application of the radiopharmaceutical. After blocking the thyroid with perchlorate, diagnostic angiography of the liver vessels should be performed with special attention to collateral arteries to other organs. Occasionally, computed tomography with arterioportography (CT-AP) via the catheter could be added, partly with the injection of small amounts of "cold" Lipiodol (Guerbet®). In patients with "normal" hepatic arterial anatomy the catheter can be positioned in the main hepatic artery for nonselective injection of 131I-Lipiodol. In cases with multiple nodules or variable arterial blood supply, the liver lobe containing the largest tumour mass is treated in the first session and the remaining masses in the following ones.

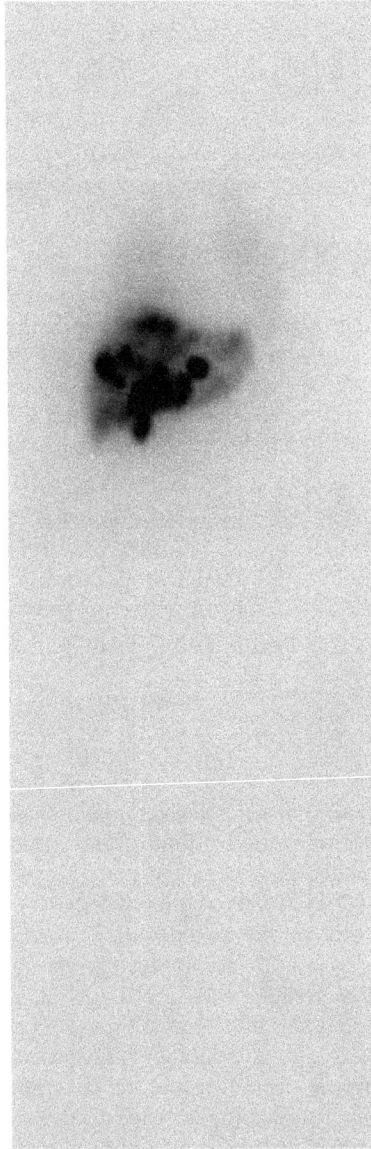

Fig. 1. Quantitative whole body scintigraphy obtained 7 days post therapeutic in a 52-year-old man showing significant activity in the HCCs and only a faint lung uptake.

131I-Lipiodol (2.22 GBq in 2 ml / ampulla) should be prepared in an appropriately ventilated cabinet in the department of Nuclear Medicine to avoid radioiodine aerosol inhalation. Injection should take at least some minutes to ensure good tolerance by the patient. The procedure and special radiation protection measures have been readily published in detail [55]. The applied activity should be determined as the difference between activity in the last receptacle before injection and the remaining activity of last receptacle and the catheter-system after flushing with saline. After the procedure the patients are transferred to the station and isolated until radiation exposure to their environment becomes low enough to be discharged (e.g in Germany < 1mSv/year) [35].

Dexamethasone and tamoxifen could increase the tumoral uptake of Lipiodol and could be combined with 131I-Lipiodol to improve the therapy effectiveness [56].

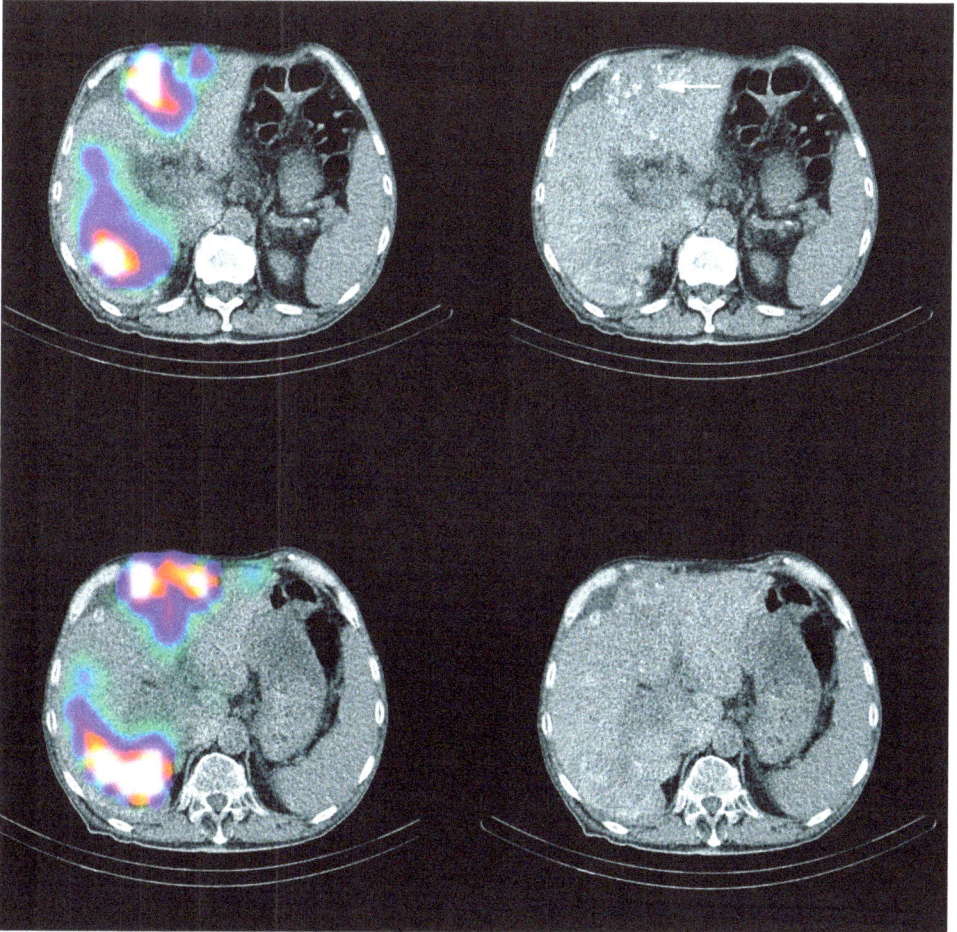

Fig. 2. SPECT/CT of the liver could be used for a better quantification of the radioactive distribution as well as dosimetry simultaneously. Note the distribution of 131I-Lipiodol in the HCCs showed with arrow.

For certain patients, in particular those presenting with a relatively large tumour several injections in 2-3 months interval may be necessary to obtain an effective response.

As Garin et. al. stated, nuclear medicine specialist receives an average dose between 140 and 443 µSv at the level of the fingers(according to the fingers) and about 17 µSv at the thorax. For the radiologists, the average doses received are 215 µSv and 15 µSv at the level of the fingers and at the thorax respectively. The authors showed that the administration of high therapeutic activities of 131I-Lipiodol can be carried out with a dose much lower than the European regulatory limit of 500 mSv at the level of the fingers for the exposed personnel [57].

8. Follow-up

Definitions of the appropriate length of the follow-up and the time points required for technical success are not well established and post treatment follow-up schedules vary depending on the treatment plan of each patient. For the evaluation of response, abdominal imaging should be performed 4 weeks and 2-3 months after each therapy [12]. Follow-up should be performed with the same modality used pre-therapeutic such as MRI, 3 phase CT, 18F-FDG, 11C-/18F-Cholin or 11C-/18F-Acetate PET/CT. AFP should be tested for patients with initially increased AFP.

9. Dosimetry

Becker et al. performed a dosimetric evaluation using SPECT/CT [58], applied to a series of 41 patients who received one or more injections of 131I-Lipiodol for treatment of HCC using a standard activity of 2220 MBq. They found a mean tumoural absorbed dose of 248±176 Gy for the first treatment, compared with 152±122 Gy for the second treatment, and pointed out a correlation between the tumoural absorbed dose, calculated in tomographic mode, and morphological response to first treatment alone. These results pleaded in favour of increasing the administered activity at the first treatment. A tumoral absorbed dose of 280 Gy was found to represent an effective threshold absorbed dose. While 84% of the patients above this value were responders, no one appeared to respond at lower absorbed doses [58]. Tumour response adversely correlates with tumour size. High response rates have been found in tumour nodes with diameters below 6 cm in which an absorbed dose of up to 288 Gy has been calculated [25, 30, 59]. However, it must be considered that a reduction in tumour mass does not necessarily correlate with improved survival[6].

10. Safety of 131I-Lipiodol therapy

A phase I study [24] and a multi centric phase II trial [30] could not demonstrate any specific toxic effects of 131I-Lipiodol. The main limiting factor was the long patient isolation required for the purpose of radioprotection. Consequently, a fixed injected activity of 2.2 GBq is proposed as a good compromise to achieve the desired efficacy while reducing the hospital stay to 1 week. Serious adverse effects are very rare. Undesirable effects observed fairly frequently consist of moderate and temporary fever (29%), moderate and temporary disturbances of the biological liver test (20%) and hepatic pain on injection (12.5%).

Moderate and reversible leukopenia (7%) and serious interstitial pneumopathies (2%) are observed more rarely [11, 12, 60]. Interstitial pneumonia has been reported in an estimated prevalence of 15.5 cases per 1000 treated patients with a median respiratory symptoms delay of 30 days[61].

Some authors have expressed their concern about hypothyroidism despite the very low thyroid uptake [62]. Using potassium iodide premedication can significantly decrease thyroid iodide uptake and consequently probability of hypothyroidism [63].

11. Conclusion

The effectiveness of 131I-Lipiodol treatment is proven both in the treatment of HCC with portal thrombosis and as an adjuvant to surgery after the resection of HCCs. It is at least as effective as chemoembolization and is tolerated much better. Severe liver dysfunction represents theoretic contraindication for radioembolization as well as for TACE. In such cases 131I-Lipiodol is an alternative therapy option especially in tumors smaller than 6 cm.

12. References

[1] Eary J. Principles of Therapy with Unsealed Sources. In: Eary J, Brenner W, eds. *NUCLEAR MEDICINE THERAPY* 2007.

[2] Lien WM, Ackerman NB. The blood supply of experimental liver metastases. II. A microcirculatory study of the normal and tumor vessels of the liver with the use of perfused silicone rubber. *Surgery.* Aug 1970;68(2):334-340.

[3] Raoul JL, Boucher E, Rolland Y, Garin E. Treatment of hepatocellular carcinoma with intra-arterial injection of radionuclides. *Nat Rev Gastroenterol Hepatol.* Jan 2010;7(1):41-49.

[4] Raoul JL, Bourguet P, Bretagne JF, et al. Hepatic artery injection of I-131-labeled lipiodol. Part I. Biodistribution study results in patients with hepatocellular carcinoma and liver metastases. *Radiology.* Aug 1988;168(2):541-545.

[5] Al-Mufti RA, Pedley RB, Marshall D, et al. In vitro assessment of Lipiodol-targeted radiotherapy for liver and colorectal cancer cell lines. *Br J Cancer.* Apr 1999;79(11-12):1665-1671.

[6] Risse JH, Menzel C, Grunwald F, Strunk H, Biersack HJ, Palmedo H. Therapy of hepatocellular cancer with iodine-131-Lipiodol. *Rom J Gastroenterol.* Jun 2004;13(2):119-124.

[7] Maki S, Konno T, Maeda H. Image enhancement in computerized tomography for sensitive diagnosis of liver cancer and semiquantitation of tumor selective drug targeting with oily contrast medium. *Cancer.* Aug 15 1985;56(4):751-757.

[8] Brans B, Bacher K, Vandevyver V, et al. Intra-arterial radionuclide therapy for liver tumours: effect of selectivity of catheterization and 131I-Lipiodol delivery on tumour uptake and response. *Nucl Med Commun.* Apr 2003;24(4):391-396.

[9] Garin E, Bourguet P. Intra-arterial Therapy of Liver Tumours. In: Biersack HJ, Freeman LM, eds. *Clinical Nuclear Medicine:* Springer-Verlag Berlin Heidelberg; 2007:491-508.

[10] Yoo HS, Park CH, Suh JH, et al. Radioiodinated fatty acid esters in the management of hepatocellular carcinoma: preliminary findings. *Cancer Chemother Pharmacol.* 1989;23 Suppl:S54-58.

[11] Guidelines for 131I-ethiodised oil (Lipiodol) therapy. *Eur J Nucl Med Mol Imaging.* Mar 2003;30(3):BP20-22.

[12] Giammarile F. EANM procedure guideline for the treatment of liver cancer and metastases with intra-arterial radioactive ligands. *23rd ANNUAL CONGRESS OF THE EUROPEAN ASSOCIATION OF NUCLEAR MEDICINE.* Vol Vienna2010:40-41.

[13] Thomas MB, Jaffe D, Choti MM, et al. Hepatocellular carcinoma: consensus recommendations of the National Cancer Institute Clinical Trials Planning Meeting. *J Clin Oncol.* Sep 1 2010;28(25):3994-4005.

[14] Salem R, Lewandowski R, Roberts C, et al. Use of Yttrium-90 glass microspheres (TheraSphere) for the treatment of unresectable hepatocellular carcinoma in patients with portal vein thrombosis. *J Vasc Interv Radiol.* Apr 2004;15(4):335-345.

[15] Kennedy A, Nag S, Salem R, et al. Recommendations for radioembolization of hepatic malignancies using yttrium-90 microsphere brachytherapy: a consensus panel report from the radioembolization brachytherapy oncology consortium. *Int J Radiat Oncol Biol Phys.* May 1 2007;68(1):13-23.

[16] Dawson LA, Normolle D, Balter JM, McGinn CJ, Lawrence TS, Ten Haken RK. Analysis of radiation-induced liver disease using the Lyman NTCP model. *Int J Radiat Oncol Biol Phys.* Jul 15 2002;53(4):810-821.

[17] Greco C, Catalano G, Di Grazia A, Orecchia R. Radiotherapy of liver malignancies. From whole liver irradiation to stereotactic hypofractionated radiotherapy. *Tumori.* Jan-Feb 2004;90(1):73-79.

[18] Murthy R, Nunez R, Szklaruk J, et al. Yttrium-90 microsphere therapy for hepatic malignancy: devices, indications, technical considerations, and potential complications. *Radiographics.* Oct 2005;25 Suppl 1:S41-55.

[19] Ho S, Lau WY, Leung TW, Johnson PJ. Internal radiation therapy for patients with primary or metastatic hepatic cancer: a review. *Cancer.* Nov 1 1998;83(9):1894-1907.

[20] Nakajo M, Kobayashi H, Shimabukuro K, et al. Biodistribution and in vivo kinetics of iodine-131 lipiodol infused via the hepatic artery of patients with hepatic cancer. *J Nucl Med.* Jun 1988;29(6):1066-1077.

[21] Madsen MT, Park CH, Thakur ML. Dosimetry of iodine-131 ethiodol in the treatment of hepatoma. *J Nucl Med.* Jun 1988;29(6):1038-1044.

[22] Raoul JL, Guyader D, Bretagne JF, et al. Randomized controlled trial for hepatocellular carcinoma with portal vein thrombosis: intra-arterial iodine-131-iodized oil versus medical support. *J Nucl Med.* Nov 1994;35(11):1782-1787.

[23] Lau WY, Lai EC. Hepatocellular carcinoma: current management and recent advances. *Hepatobiliary Pancreat Dis Int.* Jun 2008;7(3):237-257.

[24] Bretagne JF, Raoul JL, Bourguet P, et al. Hepatic artery injection of I-131-labeled lipiodol. Part II. Preliminary results of therapeutic use in patients with hepatocellular carcinoma and liver metastases. *Radiology.* Aug 1988;168(2):547-550.

[25] Kobayashi H, Hidaka H, Kajiya Y, et al. Treatment of hepatocellular carcinoma by transarterial injection of anticancer agents in iodized oil suspension or of radioactive iodized oil solution. *Acta Radiol Diagn (Stockh).* Mar-Apr 1986;27(2):139-147.

[26] de Baere T, Taourel P, Tubiana JM, et al. Hepatic intraarterial 131I iodized oil for treatment of hepatocellular carcinoma in patients with impeded portal venous flow. *Radiology.* Sep 1999;212(3):665-668.

[27] Risse JH, Grunwald F, Kersjes W, et al. Intraarterial HCC therapy with I-131-Lipiodol. *Cancer Biother Radiopharm.* Feb 2000;15(1):65-70.

[28] Raoul JL, Guyader D, Bretagne JF, et al. Prospective randomized trial of chemoembolization versus intra-arterial injection of 131I-labeled-iodized oil in the treatment of hepatocellular carcinoma. *Hepatology.* Nov 1997;26(5):1156-1161.

[29] Yoo HS, Lee JT, Kim KW, et al. Nodular hepatocellular carcinoma. Treatment with subsegmental intraarterial injection of iodine 131-labeled iodized oil. *Cancer*. Nov 1 1991;68(9):1878-1884.

[30] Raoul JI, Bretagne JF, Caucanas JP, et al. Internal radiation therapy for hepatocellular carcinoma. Results of a French multicenter phase II trial of transarterial injection of iodine 131-labeled Lipiodol. *Cancer*. Jan 15 1992;69(2):346-352.

[31] Leung WT, Lau WY, Ho S, et al. Selective internal radiation therapy with intra-arterial iodine-131-Lipiodol in inoperable hepatocellular carcinoma. *J Nucl Med*. Aug 1994;35(8):1313-1318.

[32] Bhattacharya S, Novell JR, Dusheiko GM, Hilson AJ, Dick R, Hobbs KE. Epirubicin-Lipiodol chemotherapy versus 131iodine-Lipiodol radiotherapy in the treatment of unresectable hepatocellular carcinoma. *Cancer*. Dec 1 1995;76(11):2202-2210.

[33] Rindani RB, Hugh TJ, Roche J, Roach PJ, Smith RC. 131I lipiodol therapy for unresectable hepatocellular carcinoma. *ANZ J Surg*. Mar 2002;72(3):210-214.

[34] Borbath I, Lhommel R, Bittich L, et al. 131I-Labelled-iodized oil for palliative treatment of hepatocellular carcinoma. *Eur J Gastroenterol Hepatol*. Sep 2005;17(9):905-910.

[35] Risse JH, Rabe C, Pauleit D, et al. Therapy of hepatocellular carcinoma with iodine-131-lipiodol. Results in a large German cohort. *Nuklearmedizin*. 2006;45(4):185-192.

[36] Boucher E, Garin E, Guylligomarc'h A, Olivie D, Boudjema K, Raoul JL. Intra-arterial injection of iodine-131-labeled lipiodol for treatment of hepatocellular carcinoma. *Radiother Oncol*. Jan 2007;82(1):76-82.

[37] Kanhere HA, Leopardi LN, Fischer L, Kitchener MI, Maddern GJ. Treatment of unresectable hepatocellular carcinoma with radiolabelled lipiodol. *ANZ J Surg*. May 2008;78(5):371-376.

[38] Chua TC, Chu F, Butler SP, et al. Intra-arterial iodine-131-lipiodol for unresectable hepatocellular carcinoma. *Cancer*. Sep 1 2010;116(17):4069-4077.

[39] Raoul JL, Boucher E, Roland V, Garin E. 131-iodine Lipiodol therapy in hepatocellular carcinoma. *Q J Nucl Med Mol Imaging*. Jun 2009;53(3):348-355.

[40] Ahmadzadehfar H, Biersack HJ, Ezziddin S. Radioembolization of liver tumors with yttrium-90 microspheres. *Semin Nucl Med*. Mar 2010;40(2):105-121.

[41] Vente MA, Wondergem M, van der Tweel I, et al. Yttrium-90 microsphere radioembolization for the treatment of liver malignancies: a structured meta-analysis. *Eur Radiol*. Apr 2009;19(4):951-959.

[42] Marelli L, Shusang V, Buscombe JR, et al. Transarterial injection of (131)I-lipiodol, compared with chemoembolization, in the treatment of unresectable hepatocellular cancer. *J Nucl Med*. Jun 2009;50(6):871-877.

[43] Lau WY, Leung TW, Ho SK, et al. Adjuvant intra-arterial iodine-131-labelled lipiodol for resectable hepatocellular carcinoma: a prospective randomised trial. *Lancet*. Mar 6 1999;353(9155):797-801.

[44] Buscombe JR. Interventional nuclear medicine in hepatocellular carcinoma and other tumours. *Nucl Med Commun*. Sep 2002;23(9):837-841.

[45] Lau WY, Lai EC, Leung TW, Yu SC. Adjuvant intra-arterial iodine-131-labeled lipiodol for resectable hepatocellular carcinoma: a prospective randomized trial-update on 5-year and 10-year survival. *Ann Surg*. Jan 2008;247(1):43-48.

[46] Boucher E, Bouguen G, Garin E, Guillygomarch A, Boudjema K, Raoul JL. Adjuvant intraarterial injection of 131I-labeled lipiodol after resection of hepatocellular carcinoma: progress report of a case-control study with a 5-year minimal follow-up. *J Nucl Med*. Mar 2008;49(3):362-366.

[47] Ng KM, Niu R, Yan TD, et al. Adjuvant lipiodol I-131 after curative resection/ablation of hepatocellular carcinoma. *HPB (Oxford)*. 2008;10(6):388-395.

[48] Partensky C, Sassolas G, Henry L, Paliard P, Maddern GJ. Intra-arterial iodine 131-labeled lipiodol as adjuvant therapy after curative liver resection for hepatocellular carcinoma: a phase 2 clinical study. *Arch Surg*. Nov 2000;135(11):1298-1300.

[49] Chua TC, Saxena A, Chu F, et al. Hepatic resection with or without adjuvant iodine-131-lipiodol for hepatocellular carcinoma: a comparative analysis. *Int J Clin Oncol*. Nov 9 2010.

[50] Raoul JL, Messner M, Boucher E, Bretagne JF, Campion JP, Boudjema K. Preoperative treatment of hepatocellular carcinoma with intra-arterial injection of 131I-labelled lipiodol. *Br J Surg*. Nov 2003;90(11):1379-1383.

[51] Brans B, De Winter F, Defreyne L, et al. The anti-tumoral activity of neoadjuvant intra-arterial 131I-lipiodol treatment for hepatocellular carcinoma: a pilot study. *Cancer Biother Radiopharm*. Aug 2001;16(4):333-338.

[52] Kwee SA, DeGrado TR, Talbot JN, Gutman F, Coel MN. Cancer imaging with fluorine-18-labeled choline derivatives. *Semin Nucl Med*. Nov 2007;37(6):420-428.

[53] Talbot JN, Gutman F, Fartoux L, et al. PET/CT in patients with hepatocellular carcinoma using [(18)F]fluorocholine: preliminary comparison with [(18)F]FDG PET/CT. *Eur J Nucl Med Mol Imaging*. Nov 2006;33(11):1285-1289.

[54] Yamamoto Y, Nishiyama Y, Kameyama R, et al. Detection of hepatocellular carcinoma using 11C-choline PET: comparison with 18F-FDG PET. *J Nucl Med*. Aug 2008;49(8):1245-1248.

[55] Risse JH, Ponath C, Palmedo H, Menzel C, Grunwald F, Biersack HJ. Radiation exposure and radiation protection of the physician in iodine-131 Lipiodol therapy of liver tumours. *Eur J Nucl Med*. Jul 2001;28(7):914-918.

[56] Becker S, Ardisson V, Lepareur N, et al. Increased Lipiodol uptake in hepatocellular carcinoma possibly due to increased membrane fluidity by dexamethasone and tamoxifen. *Nucl Med Biol*. Oct 2010;37(7):777-784.

[57] Garin E, Laffont S, Rolland Y, et al. Safe radiation exposure of medical personnel by using simple methods of radioprotection while administering 131I-lipiodol therapy for hepatocellular carcinoma. *Nucl Med Commun*. Jun 2003;24(6):671-678.

[58] Becker S, Laffont S, Vitry F, et al. Dosimetric evaluation and therapeutic response to internal radiation therapy of hepatocarcinomas using iodine-131-labelled lipiodol. *Nucl Med Commun*. Sep 2008;29(9):815-825.

[59] Lui WY, Liu RS, Chiang JH, et al. Report of a pilot study of intra-arterial injection of I-131 lipiodol for the treatment of hepatoma. *Zhonghua Yi Xue Za Zhi (Taipei)*. Sep 1990;46(3):125-133.

[60] Lambert B, Van de Wiele C. Treatment of hepatocellular carcinoma by means of radiopharmaceuticals. *Eur J Nucl Med Mol Imaging*. Aug 2005;32(8):980-989.

[61] Jouneau S, Vauleon E, Caulet-Maugendre S, et al. 131I-Labeled Lipiodol-Induced Interstitial Pneumonia: A Series of 15 Cases. *Chest*. Oct 14 2010.

[62] Toubeau M, Touzery C, Berriolo-Riedinger A, et al. 131I thyroid uptake in patients treated with 131I-Lipiodol for hepatocellular carcinoma. *Eur J Nucl Med*. May 2001;28(5):669-670.

[63] Bacher K, Brans B, Monsieurs M, De Winter F, Dierckx RA, Thierens H. Thyroid uptake and radiation dose after (131)I-lipiodol treatment: is thyroid blocking by potassium iodide necessary? *Eur J Nucl Med Mol Imaging*. Oct 2002;29(10):1311-1316.

17

Future Trends in the Management of Advanced Hepatocellular Carcinoma (HCC)

Dimitrios Dimitroulopoulos and Aikaterini Fotopoulou

Gastroenterology Dpt., "Agios Savvas" Cancer Hospital
Radiation-Oncology Dpt., "Hygia" Hospital, Athens
Greece

1. Introduction

Liver Cancer is the 6th most common cancer worldwide. It is the 3rd most common cause of cancer-related death and accounts for 85% to 90% of primary liver cancers. It is 2.4 times more common in men than women. The worldwide incidence of the disease is 626,162 per year and the worldwide mortality 598,321 persons per year, making HCC the most common cause of cancer related death in the world. (Parkin et al., 2005)

Most patients with HCC also suffer from coexisting cirrhosis, which is the major clinical risk factor for hepatic cancer and is correlated to hepatitis B virus or hepatitis C virus (HCV) infection. However, cirrhosis from non-viral causes such as alcoholism, hemochromatosis and primary biliary cirrhosis are also associated with an elevated risk of HCC. Furthermore, concomitant risk factors such as

HCV infection in addition to alcoholism, tobacco use, diabetes or obesity increase the relative risk of HCC development, as numerous studies in humans and animal models have shown. The incidence of HCC varies by geographic area worldwide. Research has shown that Southeast Asia and sub-Saharan Africa have an incidence rate of HCC that ranges from 150 to 500 per 100 000 population, primarily because of the endemic nature of hepatitis B and C in those regions.

Patients at the early stage are those who present with an asymptomatic single HCC with the nodule < 5 cm in diameter or ≤ 3 in number. Patients exceeding these limits, but free of cancer-related symptoms and vascular invasion or extrahepatic spread, are considered at the intermediate stage. The patients with the cancer-related symptoms and vascular invasion or extrahepatic spread are deemed at the advanced stage. HCC is frequently diagnosed at the late stage and has a high mortality rate. Surgical resection is a potentially curative therapy for HCC, however, only a minority of HCC patients are eligible for curative hepatectomy. Comprehensive therapy for HCC has become the focus of interest in recent years.

In HCC patients the prediction of prognosis is more complex than in patients with other solid tumors because the underlying liver function also affects prognosis.

Several staging systems that separate patients into prognostic groups and serve to select appropriate treatment have been developed. Historically, HCC was classified by tumor, node, metastasis (TNM) staging or the Okuda classification, but they do not distinguish between early and advanced stages. In the recent years 5 new classifications have been developed (Table 1):

- Japan Integrated Staging (JIS)
- Group d'Etude de Traitement du Carcinoma Hepatocellulaire (GRETCH)
- Cancer of the Liver Italian Program (CLIP)
- Barcelona Clinic Liver Cancer staging (BCLC)
- Chinese University Prognostic Index (CUPI)

but none of these staging systems has received universal acceptance.

Parameter	Okuda	CLIP	CUPI	TNM6	JIS	GRETCH	BCLC
Cirrhosis-related parameters							
Albumin	X	X			X		X
Bilirubin	X	X	X		X	X	X
Ascites	X	X	X		X		X
PT/INR		X			X		X
Encephalopathy		X			X		X
Alkaline phosphatase			X			X	
Tumor-related parameters							
Tumor stage/ disease extent	X	X	X	X	X		X
Portal vein thrombosis		X				X	X
Alpha fetoprotein		X	X			X	
Asymptomatic			X				
Performance status						X	X

INR = international normalized ratio; PT = prothrombin time;
TNM-6 = tumor, node, metastasis classification, 6th ed.

Table 1. Comparison of Staging Systems for HCC

The BCLC staging system was first introduced at 1999 and constitutes an evolving approach as it has regularly incorporated changes that have emerged since its first publication. (Llovet et al., 1999) On the other hand, links five stages of the disease with the appropriate therapeutic options and has been endorsed by the American Association for the Study of Liver Diseases (AASLD) and the European Association for the Study of Liver (EASL) (Forner et al., 2010).

2. The current management

Historically, the diagnosis of HCC was almost always made when the disease was in advanced stage and when patients were symptomatic and presented with a variable degree of liver function impairment. At this stage, no treatment had any chance to be effective or to significantly improve survival rates. Additionally, the morbidity associated with therapeutic options was extremely high.

Today, many patients are diagnosed at an early stage when liver function is well preserved and there are no cancer related symptoms. On the other hand, there are several active treatment modalities available that will potentially improve survival.

2.1 Surgical treatment options for very early-stage HCC

The only curative approach for HCC is surgery (resection or transplantation). Surgical treatments are applicable in 10% to 15% of patients with HCC at first diagnosis, and only in 2% to 5% of those with recurrent HCC.

Although, surgical resection is the treatment of choice for HCC non cirrhotic patients, these people account only 5% of the HCC cases in Western countries and almost 40% in Asia. These patients will tolerate major resections with low morbidity. On the other hand, cirrhotic candidates for resection must to be carefully selected because of the high risk of postoperative liver failure and the increased risk of death.

Surgical resection historical 5-year survival rate is 30% to 40% and the 5-year progression free survival (PFS) rate as high as 48%, but the vast majority of these patients develop recurrence or secondary primary tumors. For patients who undergo resection, recurrence rates can be as high as 50% at 2 years. (Liu et al., 2004)

Liver transplantation is now part of the conventional armamentarium for the treatment of HCC.

Although survival rate was improved to 61.1% from 1996-2001 and the 5-year overall survival (OS) rates of 58% to 74%, the morbidity and death rates in the early and intermediate follow up period are higher than in resection surgery in optimal candidates. (Mazzaferro et al., 2009)

But unfortunately, the vast majority of HCC patients present with advanced or unresectable disease. No surgical treatments are applicable in 70% to 85% of patients with HCC at first diagnosis and in 50% to 70% of those with recurrent HCC. The 3-year survival rate for these patients is 10% to 40% . (Bruix J& Sherman, 2011)

2.2 Local ablative therapy for early-stage HCC

The two most widely used local ablative techniques are radiofrequency ablation (RFA) and percutaneous ethanol injection (PEI) and are used in small (< 3 cm) solitary tumors.

RFA induces temperature changes by using a high-frequency alternating current applied via electrodes placed within the tissue to generate areas of coagulative necrosis and tissue desiccation. During RFA treatment, heat energy generated by high-frequency alternating currents targeted at the living tissues causes protein denaturation at a temperature of 60-110℃ through ionic vibration, resulting in coagulative necrosis of the target lesion. In addition, RFA treatment stimulates the immune system and provides an easy way to achieve in vivo vaccination against tumoral antigens. RFA can be performed intraoperatively or under image guidance.

Intraoperatively RFA is generally indicated for HCC patients who are not candidates for either liver resection or transplantation. HCC patients are required to have ≤ 5 nodules, each < 3 cm in diameter, no evidence of vascular invasion or extrahepatic spread, 0 score performance status of the Eastern Cooperative Oncology Group (ECOG), and liver cirrhosis in Child-Pugh class A or B. The more versatile radiofrequency probes allow ablation of nodule > 5 cm. When complete resection by major hepatectomy is dangerous because of difficult nodule location, selective use of intraoperative RFA will be helpful. The integration of intraoperative RFA into resection surgery contributes to complete removal of nodules with adequate margin, diminishes the extent of parenchymal resection, and improves the resectability rate for patients with advanced HCC.

Ultrasound or CT guided (percutaneous) RFA is now the first choice treatment to inoperable HCC.

Depending on the type of electrode used, ablation diameters up to between 5 and 7 cm are now possible.

PEI involves a needle being inserted into a liver tumor and absolute or 95% ethanol slowly injected into the lesion to induce nonselective protein degradation and cellular dehydration leading to necrosis. RFA has been shown to be superior to PEI in tumor response and long-term survival.

Response rate for RFA is 91% vs 82% for PEI and the 1- and 2-year local recurrence-free survival rates are 98% and 96% for RFA vs 83% and 62% for PEI. The 4-year survival rate is 74% vs 57%. RFA present a 46% lower risk of death, a 43% lower risk of overall occurrence, and an 88% lower risk of local tumor progression than PEI.

Other techniques such as laser, microwave, high intensity ultrasound, cryotherapy or acetic acid injection are less common or validated in terms of efficacy and safety.

2.3 Regional therapy for intermediate-stage HCC: Transarterial chemoembolization (TACE)

The portal vein supplies 75% to 85% of the blood to the liver, while the hepatic artery provides 20% to 25%. In HCC, the hepatic artery supplies 90% to 100%.

Enough evidence exists on the effectiveness of conventional TACE in prolonging survival in intermediate HCC patients with well preserved liver function (Child-Pugh A class). (El-Serag et al., 2008).

Candidates for TACE should not have advanced HCC, should be no major portal vein invasion, and liver function should be preserved.

Embolization agents (generally gelatin or microspheres) are administered with a high-viscosity mixture of lipiodol and chemotherapy (doxorubicin, mitomycin, or cisplatin), blocking blood flow to the tumor.

At 1 and 2 years, the survival probabilities are 82% and 63% for chemoembolization with doxorubicin or cisplatin versus 63% and 27% for supportive care (P =0.009). Is reported 3-year survival rates of 26% vs 3% for supportive care.

A meta-analysis has shown a beneficial effect on 2-year survival (odds ratio = 0.53, P = 0.017) and a median survival of 20 vs 16 months for conventional therapies.

There is no good evidence for the best chemotherapy agent and the optimum treatment strategy.

The improved survival rates with TACE have led to its use as a bridge therapy to liver transplantation or resection. TACE may increase the chance of a patient staying on the transplant list and acquiring an organ, as well as decrease recurrence and prolong survival.

TACE was investigated in combination with RFA and was compared with TACE alone and showed increased 1-year survival (100% vs 67%, P = 0.04) and mean survival (25.3 mo ± 15.9 vs 11.4 mo ± 7.3, P < 0.05).

TACE combined with RFA in HCC patients after hepatectomy was compared with single TACE or RFA treatment. The intrahepatic recurrence rate was lower in the combination group vs TACE (20.7% vs 57.1%, P = 0.002) and vs RFA (20.7% vs 43.2%, P = 0.036). The overall 1-, 3-, and 5-year survival rates were 88.5%, 64.6%, and 44.3% for the combination, 65.8%, 38.9%, and 19.5% for TACE, and 73.9%, 51.1%, and 28.0% for RFA.

Neoadjuvant and adjuvant TACE have shown little effect (Raul at al., 2011).

2.4 Systemic therapy for advanced-stage HCC

No significant survival advantage has been demonstrated with systemic chemotherapy. Most published studies report response rates of 0% to 25%. Of the single agents, doxorubicin is perhaps most widely used. Gemcitabine plus Oxaliplatine (GEMOX) appears to be more active than gemcitabine alone (Table 2). Tamoxifen showed no antitumoral effect or survival benefit. The presence of estrogen receptors in advanced HCC was the rationale for antiestrogen treatment.

Agent	Year	2008	Pts	Response Rate, %	Median Survival, mo
Doxorubicin	2005	III	94	11	6.8
PIAF	2005	III	94	21	8.7
Nolatrexed	2007	III	222	1	5.6
Paclitaxel	1998	II	20	0	3.0
Capecitabine	2000	II	37	13	6.0
Irinotecan	2001	II	14	7	8.2
Gemcitabine	2002	II	30	0	6.9
GEMOX	2007	II	34	18	11.5
XELOX	2007	II	50	6	9.3
Capecitabine/cisplatin	2008	Cohort *	178	20	10.5

* Retrospective analysis.
PIAF = cisplatin, interferon, doxorubicin, 5-fluorouracil; GEMOX = gemcitabine and oxaliplatin; XELOX = capecitabine (Xeloda), oxaliplatin.

Table 2. Summary of Responses to Systemic Chemotherapy in HCC

2.5 Sorafenib (Nexavar)

Sorafenib (Nexavar) is a multikinase inhibitor (RAF-tyrosine kinase/VEGF/c-KIT/PDGFR-β inhibitor) and is a new treatment approach for HCC.

Is an oral VEGF- PDGF inhibitor with activity against RAF/MEK/ERK pathway that block both tumor cell proliferation and angiogenesis.

Preclinical studies reported antitumor activity in HCC cells and xenograft models.

Results of a phase II study involving patients with advanced HCC and Child-Pugh class A and B cirrhosis with a dose of 400 mg twice daily induced a PR in 2.2% of patients, a minor response in 5.8%, and stable disease lasting 16 weeks in 34%. Median time to progression (TTP) was 4.2 months, and median OS was 9.2 months.

The SHARP study, a randomized placebo controlled phase III trial, showed improved overall survival for the Sorafenib group (44% vs 33% for the placebo group). Median survival (MS) was 10.7 months vs 7.9 months. Drug related adverse events were more frequent in the Sorafenib group than in the placebo group (80% vs 52%) and included diarrhea, weight loss, hand-foot skin reaction, anorexia, alopecia, and voice changes. The majority of these were grade 1 or 2 in severity. (Llovet et al., 2008). A similar design phase III Asian Pasific study revealed a survival benefit of similar magnitude, mostly for patients with hepatitis B virus infection, but the median overall survival was significantly lower (6.5 months for the Sorafenib group vs 4.2 for the placebo group). (Liu et al., 2009).

Thus, Nexavar is approved from 2007 in U.S.A. and E.U. for the treatment of advanced HCC in Child-Pugh A cirrhotic patients.

The results of SHARP trial was a milestone in the treatment of HCC and stimulated the search for similar compounds targeting other molecular alterations, in particular because combination treatments are postulated to be a promising approach through synergistic anti-tumoral effects (Rimassa & Santoro, 2010)

3.The future trends

3.1 Sorafenib in cirrhosis stage B and C

Recently published papers report data of patients with HCC in different stages of liver cirrhosis treated with Sorafenib. Small benefit and only for patients without extrahepatic metastatic disease was observed.

3.2 Sorafenib as adjuvant treatment

An important goal of HCC research and therapy is the prevention of tumor recurrence in patients previously treated with resection or local ablation, since 70% of this population will develop HCC recurrence within 5 years. Recurrence could result from intrahepatic metastases that remain after incomplete treatment of primary tumor or through formation of new tumors, caused by the persistence of the carcinogenic field present in the cirrhotic liver. The molecular features of each recurrent tumor type are likely to differ. Sorafenib is tested now an adjuvant treatment in the STORM trial.

3.3 Sorafenib in several combinations

The efficacy of Sorafenib in patients with advanced HCC was also tested in combination with several chemotherapeutic agents. At the moment there are 65 registered trials testing Sorafenib (alone or in combination with other agents), in phases I-IV.

3.3.1 Sorafenib + doxorubicin vs placebo + doxorubicin (phase II study)

Although a higher response rate and acceptable safety profile have been reported from several small studies, the combination of this drugs is not yet been approved for the treatment of advanced HCC.

Patients with Eastern Cooperative Oncology Group performance status of 0–2, Child-Pugh A cirrhosis, and no prior systemic therapy received Doxorubicin at 60 mg/m^2 intravenously every 21 days (cycle) plus either Sorafenib at 400 mg orally twice daily or placebo, for a maximum of six cycles of Doxorubicin. Patients could continue with single-agent Sorafenib or placebo afterward. The primary end point was TTP by independent review. The median OS and TTP were 13.7 and 8.6 months for the Doxorubicin plus Sorafenib arm and 6.5 and 4.8 months for the Doxorubicin plus Placebo arm, respectively. The response rate was 4% in the Doxorubicin plus Sorafenib arm and 2% for the Doxorubicin plus Placebo arm. The safety profiles seemed to be comparable for both groups, including grade 3-4 neutropenia in almost 50% of patients . (Abou-Alfa et al., 2010).

3.3.2 Sorafenib + erlotinib vs sorafenib + placebo (as first line treatment)

Erlotinib is an orally administered inhibitor of tyrocine kinase activity of the epidermal growth factor receptor (EGFR). Results from two small, Erlotinib monotherapy studies, in patients with advanced HCC have been reported overall survival rates ranging between 6.25 and 13 month and time to tumor progression rates raging between 6.5 and 3.2 months. At the moment, a randomized, double-blind, phase III study comparing Sorafenib with the combination of Sorafenib and Erlotinib is ongoing.

Furthermore, ongoing and planed clinical studies will evaluate the benefit of combining molecular-targeted therapies that block complementary pathways that are activated in HCC (Villanueva & Llovet, 2011).

3.3.3 Sorafenib in real-life setting studies

In addition to randomized controlled trials (RCTs,) because the treatment of HCC is complex and confounded by comorbidities, studies evaluating therapy in the real-life setting are also essential to allow physicians to make fully informed treatment decisions. Among these is the Global Investigation of therapeutic DEcisions in hepatocellular carcinoma and Of its treatment with sorafeNib (GIDEON) study. This is an international, prospective, open-label, multicenter, noninterventional study of patients with unresectable HCC for whom the decision has been taken to treat with sorafenib. The aim of the GIDEON study is to compile a large robust database of information from sorafenib treated patients that can be analyzed to gain a detailed understanding of the local, regional, and global factors influencing the management of patients with HCC. As such, detailed medical information from 3000 patients globally over 5 years will be obtained, and information regarding the practice patterns of the treating physicians will also be collected, making it potentially the largest study of its kind in this patient population. The primary objective of this study is to evaluate the safety of sorafenib in the real-life clinical setting. Secondary objectives include: efficacy evaluations (OS, progression-free survival, time to progression, response rate, and rate of stable disease); duration of therapy; regional and global methods of patient evaluation, diagnosis, and follow-up; evaluation of comorbidities and their influence on treatment and outcome; and evaluation of regional and global practice patterns of the physicians involved in the care of these patients.

On the other hand, given the known antiangiogenic properties of sorafenib, the combination of TACE with sorafenib holds promise and clinical trials investigating this therapeutic approach are ongoing (Sorafenib or Placebo in Combination with Transarterial Chemoembolization for Intermediate-stage HCC [SPACE] trial. Indeed, given that DEB (Drug-Eluting Bead) -TACE has shown better tolerability than TACE, the combination of sorafenib with DEB-TACE is also promising.

3.4 Antiangiogenic agents

HCC is a hypervascular tumor with overexpression of several proangiogenic factors such as vascular endothelial growth factor (VEGF). On the other hand, high microvessel density have been observed in HCC tissue samples. Because of VEGF expression levels are directly associated with low survival rates, the inhibition of angiogenesis can represent a potential target in HCC and several antiangiogenic agents have entered clinical studies.

3.4.1 Sunitinib

Is an oral multikinase inhibitor, approved for the treatment of GIST after progression or intolerance to imatinib mesylate and also for the treatment of advanced or metastatic kidney cancer, that targets receptors of tirosine kinases including VEGFR-1 and -2, PDGFRalpha/beta, c-KIT, FLT3, and RET kinases.

Sunitinib has been shown to possess antitumoral activity and an acceptable safety profile in several Phase II trials in patients with advanced HCC. But, a higher toxicity and a greater number of side effects were observed in HCC patients than in patients with other neoplasias. For this reason, the drug usually was administered in a lower dose in HCC trials (37.5mg vs 50 mg).

In a phase II European/Asian study on 37 patients, the original starting dose was 50 mg/d for 4 consecutive weeks followed by two rest periods. The primary end point was the evaluation of the overall response rate according to Response Evaluation Criteria in Solid Tumours criteria. The main grade grade 3 and 4 toxicities observed were thrombocytopenia (43%), neutropenia (24%), neurological symptoms (24%), fatigue (22%) and hemorrhages (14%). Forty-three percent of patients required a dose reduction and 4 patients died due to the treatment. Median TTP was 5.3 months and OS was 9.3 months. (Faivre et al., 2009).

Another phase II study evaluated the efficacy and tolerability of sunitinib at the initial dose of 37.5 mg/d for 4 consecutive weeks followed by two rest periods in 34 patients with advanced HCC. Grade 3 and 4 toxicities observed were neutropenia (12%), thrombocytopenia (12%), fatigue (12%), rash (6%), hand-foot syndrome (6%), hyperbilirubinemia (6%) and hypertension (6%). One patient died of liver failure due to a rapid disease progression. Stable disease was highlighted in 47% of patients for at least 12 weeks. Progression free survival was 4 months and the median overall survival of 9.9 months. (Zhu et al., 2009).

Thus, the efficacy and tolerability of the drug were tested recently in a phase III trial, but the study was stopped prematurely because of lack of efficacy and significant adverse events (Table 3).

Dose schedule and sample size	37.5 mg 4 weeks on/2 weeks off (n = 34)	50 mg 4 weeks on/2 weeks off (n = 37)	37.5 mg 4 weeks on/2 weeks off (n = 17)	37.5 mg continuous (n = 45)
Objective response rate, n (%)	1 (2.9)	1 (2.7)	1 (5.9)	1 (2.2)
Disease control rate*	52%	38%	53%	42%
Overall survival (months)	9.8	8.0	-	9.3
Time to progression (months)	4.1	-	-	2.8
Progression-free survival (months)	3.9	3.7	-	2.8

Table 3. Phase II trials of SUNITINIB in advanced HCC

3.4.2 Brivanib

Is an oral dual inhibitor of VEGF and fibroblast growth factor (FGF) receptors signaling pathways, effective in mouse HCC xenograft models. A phace II study with Brivanid at the dose of 800 mg daily, as first and second line treatment in 96 patients with advanced HCC (unresectable locally advanced or metastatic disease) who did or did not receive pre-treatment, demonstrated a median TTP of 2.7 months (95% CI, 1.5-3.9), when the drug was administered as first line treatment and a median TTP of 1.4 months (95% CI, 1.4-2.6) when the drug was administered as second line treatment. Interestingly, a 50% decrease in serum AFP from baseline was seen in 40% of all patients. Additionally, reduction in collagen IV (a new serum angiogenesis biomarker) levels was observed to be associated with long term outcome. Most frequently observed grade 3-4 adverse events included fatigue (16%), high levels of AST (19%), hyponatremia (41%), hypertension (7.3%), diarrhoea (4.9%), and headache (4.9%). (Park et al., 2011).

Thus, Brivanib is now under evaluation in phase III studies in both the first-line setting in comparison with Sorafenib and in the Sorafenib-refractory setting in comparison with best supportive care in advanced HCC.

3.4.3 ABT-869

Is an orally active, potent and selective inhibitor of VEGF and platelet derived growth factor (PDGF) receptor families. ABT-869 showed potent antiproliferative and apoptotic properties in vitro and in animal cancer xenograft models using tumor cell lines that were "addicted" to signaling of kinases targeted by ABT-869. When given together with chemotherapy or mTOR inhibitors, ABT-869 showed at least additive therapeutic effects.

A Phase II study, when the drug was administered at 0.25 mg/kg daily in patients with Child-Pugh A cirrhosis reported response rate of 8.7% (95% CI, 1.1 - 28). For all patients (Child-Pugh A and B cirrhosis) median TTP was 112 days, median PFS was 112 days (95% CI, 61 - 168) and median OS was 295 days (95% CI, 182 - 333). The most common adverse events (AEs) were hypertension (41%), fatigue (47%), diarrhea (38%), rash (35%), proteinuria (24%), vomiting (24%), cough (24%) and oedema peripheral (24%). The most common grade 3/4 AEs were hypertension (20.6%) and fatigue (11.8%). Most adverse events were mild/moderate and reversible with interruption/dose reductions/or discontinuation of ABT-869. However, additional studies are required to determine the optimal dosing strategy especially in HCC patient population as frequent dose interruption or reduction was observed.

On the other hand, a phase III study comparing efficacy and tolerability of ABT-869 versus Sorafenib is ongoing.

3.4.4 Bevacizumab

Is a recombinant, humanized, monoclonal antibody against VEGF present direct anti-angiogenic activity and may enhance the efficacy of chemotherapy by normalizing the tumor vasculature and decreasing the elevated interstitial pressure in tumors. The drug has been studied both as monotherapy and in combination with cytotoxic and molecular targeted agents in patients with advanced HCC.

In a phase II study bevacuzimab was evaluated as monotherapy at two different dosages (5 mg/kg and 10 mg/kg) intravenously, once every 2 weeks, in patients with HCC with no overt extrahepatic metastases or invasion of major blood vessels. The median PFS was 6.9 months and the median OS was 12.4 months with 65% of patients progression-free at 6 months. (Siegel et al., 2008)

The drug was evaluated also in combination with chemotherapy (gemcitabine, oxaliplatine, capecitabine) in several phase II studies with response rates ranging between 11%-20% and median overall survival ranging between 9.6-10.7 months. (Zhu et al., 2006)

The combination of Bevacuzimab (10 mg/kg intravenously once every 14 days) with Erlotinib (150 mg orally daily) achieved a response rate of 25%, a median overall survival of 68 weeks and a median PFS of 39 weeks (Table 4).

Although the above studies demonstrated early evidence of antitumor activity of Bevacizumab in HCC and the reported tolerability profile was in general good, the increased risk of hypertension, thromboembolic events and bleeding requires further evaluation. On the other hand, because of the non-randomized trials and the small number of patients enrolled, the results must be confirmed in large randomized studies. The contribution, also, of chemotherapy and Erlotinib needs further investigation.

Study	Regimen	No. of patients	RR (%)	Median PFS/TTP (months)	Median survival (months)
Siegel et al.	B	46	13	6.9	12.4
Malka et al.	B	24	12.5	NR	NR
Zhu et al.	GEMOX-B	33	20	5.3	9.6
Sun et al.	CAPEOX-B	30	10	5.4	NR
Hsu et al.	Capecitabine-bevacizumab	25	16	4.1	10.7
Thomas et al.	B + Erlotinib	40	25	9.0	15.6

B: Bevacizumab only; CAPEOX-B: Capecitabine--oxaliplatin--bevacizumab; GEMOX-B: Gemcitabine--oxaliplatin--bevacizumab;
PFS: Progression-free survival;RR: Response rate; TTP: Time to progression.

Table 4. Phase II studies of bevacuzimab-based regimens in HCC

3.4.5 TSU-68

This agent is another oral multikinase inhibitor of VEGF receptor-2, PDGF receptor and fibroblast growth factor receptor, that was tested recently at a dose of 200 mg and 400 mg bid in patients with advanced HCC, in a phase I/II study. Safety and efficacy were evaluated. The median TTP was 2.1 months, and the median OS was 13.1 months. Common adverse events were hypoalbuminemia, diarrhea, anorexia, abdominal pain, malaise, oedema and AST/ALT elevation. The analysis of angiogenesis-related parameters suggests that serum-soluble vascular cell adhesion molecule-1 is a possible marker to show the response. (Kanai et al., 2011)

In another phase II study TSU-68 showed promising efficacy with a high safety profile, even in heavily pretreated (surgery, radiofrequency ablation, transcatheter arterial embolization, chemotherapy, or radiotherapy) HCC patients with Child-Pugh B liver cirrhosis. This study design with stepwise adjustment of doses based on liver function constitutes an appropriate approach for HCC. Additionally, a randomized phase II study of TSU-68 in patients with HCC treated by TACE showed a marginally but statistically significant efficacy to prolong PFS compared to TACE alone. The results suggests that the of TSU- 68 administration may improve the overall survival of patients treated by TACE.

3.4.6 Cediranib

CEDIRANIB is another potent oral inhibitor of vascular endothelial growth factor signalling with activity against platelet derived growth factor receptor beta (PDGFRb) and c-Kit. Also, is a potent inhibitor of both KDR (IC50\0.002 lM) and Flt-1 (IC50=0.005 lM) with activity against Flt-4 at nanomolar concentrations. The agent was evaluated in a phase II trial, but grade 3 toxicity (anorexia, hypertension and fatigue) was reported in the vast majority of patients. Thus, a new study was conducted at a dose of 45 mg once daily, for 28-day cycles, but with low efficacy rates. (Alberts et al., 2011)

A single-arm phase II study that uses AZD2171 at 30 mg daily to assess the tolerability and safety in advanced HCC is also ongoing.

3.4.7 Vatalanib or PTK787/ZK 222584 (PTK/ZK)

Vatalanib or PTK787/ZK 222584 (PTK/ZK) is an oral, anti-angiogenesis compound that blocks tyrosine kinase signaling from all known VEGF receptors (including VEGFR-1/flt-1, VEGFR-2/KDR, and VEGFR-3/ Flt-4, PDGFR, and the c-kit with a higher selectivity for VEGFR-2).

The compound was tested initially in an open-label, multi-center, phase I study to characterize the safety, tolerability, and pharmacokinetic profile. The agent was administered once daily at a dose of 750 mg to 1250 mg in patients with unresectable HCC. Patients were stratified into three groups with mild, moderate, and severe hepatic dysfunction, respectively, on the basis of total bilirubin and AST (aspartate aminotransferase)/alanine aminotransferase levels. The maximal tolerated dose was defined as 750 mg daily and 50% achieved stable disease.

Based on the results of this study, a phase 1-2 trial of PTK787/ZK222584 combined with intravenous doxorubicin was conducted. The results showed encouraging activity of the combination in treating advanced HCC patients and the commonest grade 3 or 4 nonhematological toxicities were mucositis (11%) and alopecia (7%). Grade 3 or 4 neutropenia was observed in 26% of patients and neutropenic sepsis in 7.2%.

3.4.8 Pazopanib (GW786034)

PAZOPANIB (GW786034) is an oral angiogenesis inhibitor targeting VEGFR, PDGFR, and c-Kit.

A Phase I study was conducted to determine the maximum tolerated dose, safety, pharmacokinetics, pharmacodynamics and efficacy of pazopanib in patients with locally unresectable and/or advanced HCC. Eligibility criteria included unresectable and/or metastatic HCC with at least one target lesion, recovery from prior systemic regimens, Eastern Cooperative Oncology Group performance status of 0 or 1, Child Pugh A, and adequate organ function. Doses of pazopanib were escalated from 200 mg once daily to 800 mg daily in a 3 + 3 design. In the 27 Asian patients enrolled, MTD was determined to be 600 mg once daily. The results showed a manageable safety profile in HCC at the maximum tolerated dose of 600mg QD. PR was observed in 7% of patients and stable disease of 4 months in 41% of patients. Median TTP at the maximum tolerated dose was 137.5 days (range, 4–280 days). Changes in tumour dynamic contrast-enhanced MRI parameters were seen following repeated dose pazopanib administration. (Yau et al., 2010)

3.4.9 NGR-hTNF

NGR-hTNF is a novel agent that selectively binds to aminopeptidase N (CD13), which is overexpressed in tumour blood vessels. In a phase II trial this agent was well-tolerated and the OS was 9.1 months. Of note, one complete response was observes in a Sorafenib-refractory patient and one partial response in a cirrhotic Child-Pugh B patient (Rimassa & Santoro 2010).

3.5 Epidermal Growth Factor Receptor (EGFR) inhibitors

The expression of several EGF family members, specifically EGF, TGF-a, heparinbinding epidermal growth factor, and EGFR, has been described in several HCC cell lines and tissues. Multiple strategies to target EGFR signaling pathways have been developed, and two classes of anti-EGFR agents have established clinical activity in cancer: monoclonal antibodies that competitively inhibit extracellular endogenous ligand binding, and small molecules that inhibit the intracellular tyrosine kinase domain.

3.5.1 EGFR tyrosine kinase inhibitors

ERLOTINIB: Two phase II clinical studies have evaluated the safety and efficacy of Erlotinib (Tarceva) provided at 150 mg daily in patients with advanced HCC. Partial response was observed in 9% and 0% of patients, and the median overall survival was 13 months and 25 weeks respectively, from the date of Erlotinib therapy initiation (Rossi et al., 2010).

GEFITINIB provided at 250 mg daily was examined in a single-arm phase II study (E1203) from the Eastern Cooperative Oncology Group. A two-stage design was used, and 31 patients were accrued to the first stage. The median PFS was 2.8 months (95% CI 1.5–3.9) and median OS was 6.5 months (95% CI, 4.4–8.9). The criterion for second stage accrual was not met, and the authors concluded that gefitinib as a single agent was not active in advanced HCC. 3.22% of patients had PR and 22.5% of patients presented stable disease, but the criterion for second stage accrual was not met and thus the study was stopped prematurely because of lack of efficacy.

LAPATINIB, a selective dual inhibitor of both EGFR and HER-2/NEU tyrosine kinases, also demonstrated modest activity in HCC. Among the 40 patients with advanced HCC, the response rate was 5%, the progression free survival 2.3 months, and OS of 6.2 months (Table 5).

3.5.2 Monoclonal antibodies against EGFR

CETUXIMAB is a chimeric monoclonal antibody against EGFR . In two phase II studies in patients with advanced HCC was administered at 400 mg/ m^2 intravenously, followed by weekly intravenous infusions at 250 mg/m^2. The reported median OS was 9.6 months, the median PFS 1.4 months and the median TTP 2 months.

The combination of cetuximab with gemcitabine and oxaliplatin (GEMOX) was evaluated in a phase II study. All patients received cetuximab at an initial dose of 400 mg/m2 followed by 250 mg/m2 weekly, gemcitabine 1000 mg/m2 on day 1, and oxaliplatin at 100 mg/m2 on day 2, repeated every 14 days until disease progression or limiting toxicity. The confirmed response rate was 20%, the disease stabilization rate 40%, the median PFS 4.7 months and the OS 9.5 months. The 1-year survival rate was 40%.

The combination of cetuximab with capecitabine and oxaliplatin was evaluated in a single-arm phase II study. Capecitabine was administered at 850 mg/m^2 twice daily for 14 days, oxaliplatin on day 1 at 130 mg/m^2 intravenously, and cetuximab at 400 mg/m^2 on day 1 followed by 250 mg/m^2 weekly in a 21-day cycle. Response rate was 10%, and TTP 4.3 months. The most common side effects were electrolyte abnormalities and diarrhoea (Table 5).

	Year	Pts.	RR (%)	Median PFS (months)	Median OS (months)
Erlotinib	2005	38	9	3.2	13
Erlotinib	2007	40	0	3.1	6.3
Lapatinib	2009	40	5	2.3	6.2
Lapatinib	2009	26	0	1.9	12.6
Cetuximab	2007	32	0	2	-
Cetuximab	2007	30	0	1.4	9.6
GEMOX + Cetuximab	2008	45	20	4.7	9.5
CAPEOX + Cetuximab	2008	25	10	4.3	-

CAPEOX: Capecitabine--oxaliplatin; GEMOX: Gemcitabine--oxaliplatin;
OS: Overall survival; PFS: Progression-free survival; RR: Response rate

Table 5. Phase II trials of EGFR inhibitors in HCC

3.6 Additional potential therapeutic targets

During hepatocarcinogenesis, multiple genetic and epigenetic changes occur, and different pathways are involved such as the PI3/Akt/mTOR, hepatocyte growth factor (HGF)/cMET, insuline-like groth factor (IGF) and its receptor (IGFR) pathways and finally the Wnt-β catenin pathway. Several agents targeting these pathways are in clinical development in advanced HCC.

3.6.1 mTOR Inhibitors (mammalian target of rapamycin)

During hepatocarcinogenesis, several genetic and epigenetic changes occur and multiple pathways are involved such as PI3K/Akt/mTOR. The mTOR is a key regulator of Growth Factor signaling pathways. Is an intracellular serine/threonine kinase in the PI3K/Akt signaling pathway.

mTOR activation promotes cell growth and proliferation, angiogenesis and cancer cell metabolism through increased nutrient uptake and utilization. Preclinical data have demonstrated that mTOR inhibitors were effective in inhibiting cell growth and tumour vascularity in HCC cell lines and HCC tumour models. The importance of the mTOR pathway in HCC was examined in a large comprehensive study with HCC and nontumoral tissues. Aberrant mTOR signalling (p-RPS6) was present in 50% of the cases and chromosomal gains in rapamycininsensitive companion of mTOR (RICTOR) in 25%. Positive p-RPS6 staining was found to correlated with HCC recurrence after resection.

SIROLIMUS (Rapamycin): Retrospective studies in patients who underwent liver transplantation for HCC have shown that patients who received sirolimus for immunosuppression had a much lower rate of tumour recurrence than those who received calcineurin inhibitors. In a pilot study Sirolimus was administered in patients advanced hepatocellular carcinoma. Overall, therapy with rapamycin was well tolerated. Most common toxicities were thrombocytopaenia and anaemia. The observed median OS was 5.27 months and the median TTP was 3 months.

TEMSIROLIMUS: Temsirolimus is a soluble ester analogue of sirolimus. Temsirolimus has been approved by the FDA for treatment of advanced renal cell carcinoma and demonstrated a survival benefit as monotherapy by comparison with interferon alpha in a multicenter phase III trial. At the moment several studies with the drug as monotherapy or in combination (with Sorafenib or Bevacuzimab) are ongoing in patients with advanced HCC.

EVEROLIMUS (RAD001): This agent, an orally administered mTOR inhibitor, was evaluated initially in a phase I study. Totally 36 patients were treated at different dose levels on a daily or weekly schedule and data reported that the drug is moderately active in this setting. Dose-limiting toxicities observed included hyperbilirubinemia, high levels of alanine aminotransferase, thrombocytopenia, infection, diarrhea, and cardiac ischemia. On the other hand, reactivation of hepatitis B and C virus was observed in four and one patients, respectively. The disease control rate of 31 evaluable patients was 61% (10 of 16) and 46.7% (7 of 15, including one case of partial response) of patients receiving daily and weekly treatment, respectively.

In a phase I/II study everolimus was administered in 28 patients with advanced HCC and adequate hematologic, hepatic, and renal functions at 5 mg/day or 10 mg/day orally (6 weeks/cycle). The primary end points were determination of a safe dosage of everolimus (phase 1) and progression free survival at 24 weeks (phase 2). Grade 3-4 adverse events included lymphopenia , ALT and AST elevation, hyponatremia, anemia, hyperglycemia, proteinuria, rash, and hypoxia. One patient (4%) had partial response . The median progression free survival and overall survival were 3.8 months 8.4 months, respectively. The estimated progression free survival rate at 24 weeks was 28.6%.

Thus, a randomized phase III, double-blind, placebo-controlled, multicenter study to evaluate the efficacy of everolimus in adult patients with advanced hepatocellular carcinoma after failure of Sorafenib treatment (EVOLVE-1 Study) is ongoing (Tazi et al., 2011).

3.6.2 MEK inhibitors

HCC is characterized by frequent MEK/ERK activation in the absence of RAF or RAS mutation. A multicenter, single arm phase II study with a two-stage design was conducted with AZD6244, a specific inhibitor of MEK, in advanced HCC. The primary end point was response rate. The agent was administered orally at a dose of 100 mg twice a day. Despite the good tolerability, minimal activity was observed (no response, and stable disease in 37.5% of the patients). The median TTP was reported to be 8 weeks.

3.7 Immunomodulatory agents

Immunomodulation is another promising strategy against HCC. Thymostimulin (a standardized low molecular protein fraction containing thymosin-a1 and thymic humoral factor) has been demonstrated to induce a selective, dose-dependent, cytotoxic immune reaction against HCC cell lines in vitro. Based on the experimental data, two single-center phase II trials using thymostimulin in patients with locally advanced and metastasised HCC not amenable to or failing surgical and/or local therapy have been published, with 63% and

79%, respectively, both depicted tumor control rates even in metastatic disease and without side-effects. Both of them, however, lacked control groups.

Recently, a multi-center, randomised, placebo-controlled phase III study in HCC patients according to the same eligibility criteria with the studies reported above. Liver function (Child-Pugh classification) was used for stratification and subgroup analysis. The aim was to evaluate if the tumor control by thymostimulin observed in the phase II trials would translate into improved survival as compared with best supportive care and placebo. Thymostimulin was administered in a dose of 75 mg subcutaneously 5 days a week for one year. Twelve-month survival was 28% for the thymostimulin group and 32% for the control group with no significant differences in median OS (5.0 vs. 5.2 months)or TTP (5.3 vs. 2.9 months). Adjustment for liver function, Karnofsky status or tumor stage did not affect results. While quality of life was similar in both groups, fewer patients on thymostimulin suffered from accumulating ascites and renal failure (Dollinger et al., 2010).

3.8 Radioembolization

Attempts to improve locoregional therapies for patients with unresectable HCC are ongoing; as a result, novel liver directed therapies are emerging. Radioembolization is one such therapy, comprising a catheter-based delivery of yttrium-90 (90 Y)-embedded microspheres into the hepatic artery. Once administered, these microspheres selectively emit high-energy, low-penetration radiation to the tumor, resulting in necrosis. Currently, phase I and phase II studies are under way to evaluate the efficacy of this approach, and a number of cohort studies, retrospective analyses, and case reports have already been published. Indeed, a recent literature review showed that there is a growing body of literature to suggest that radioembolization might be an effective treatment approach for patients with HCC.

A phase II study evaluated radioembolization with 90 Y glass microspheres in patients with unresectable HCC with and without portal vein thrombosis. Treatment was well tolerated, with liver-related adverse events reported more frequently among patients with cirrhosis and main portal vein thrombosis (elevation of bilirubin, 40%; ascites, 18%; hepatic encephalopathy, 4%, compared with 4%, 4%, and 0%, respectively, for patients without main portal vein thrombosis or cirrhosis). Tumor response rates according to the World Health Organization and EASL criteria were 42.2% and 70%, respectively; median survival times for patients with main portal vein thrombosis and thrombosis were 304 days and 813 days for those without cirrhosis. These findings therefore suggest that treatment with 90 Y glass microspheres could be an effective locoregional treatment option, especially for patients with portal vein thrombosis, for whom TAE/TACE is not suitable. However, further evaluation of this novel approach, including direct comparisons with established locoregional therapies (i.e., TAE or TACE), is needed (Lencioni et al., 2010) .

3.9 Radiotherapy

Technological advances and a better understanding of partial liver tolerance of radiation therapy (RT) have improved our ability to deliver tumoricidal doses of RT safely to HCCs, and have led to a resurgence of interest in curative-intent treatment of HCC using RT.

3.9.1 Partial liver irradiation

The development of three-dimensional conformal RT has enabled high dose RT to be directed to the tumour while sparing the nontumour-bearing surrounding liver parenchyma from these high doses.

Using a mathematical model that predicts the risk of radiation-induced liver disease based on dose and fractional volume receiving a given dose, the probability of radiation toxicity can be minimized while still being able to escalate the dose to a small volume.

3.9.2 Image-guidance and targeting

Technological advances in RT now facilitate greater ability to account for respiratory movement of liver tumours during treatment. Tumors can be localized during breathing by using the diaphragm as a surrogate for liver position, via four-dimensional (4D) CT scanning to define the spatial coordinates of the tumour during all phases of respiration, via volumetric cone-beam CT scanning, or using radiopaque fiducials implanted in the vicinity of the tumour. Tumours can be treated during free breathing based on 4D CT derived composite target volumes (coordinates of the tumour during all phases of breathing) or via real-time tracking of tumour motion and gating or robotic control of the treatment beam, during breath holds using active breathing control, or during end-expiratory gating.

These techniques improve the precision of radiation delivery and thereby limit collateral normal tissue toxicity.

3.9.3 External beam radiation therapy

Promising clinical data from multiple studies suggest that HCCs are indeed radiosensitive. Sustained local control rates ranging from 71% to 100% have been reported following 30–90 Gy delivered over 1–8 weeks.

Combination of conformal RT (1.5 Gy twice daily over 6–8 weeks) with concurrent hepatic arterial fluorodeoxyuridine to treat HCCs safely to doses as high as 90 Gy, reported median survival of 15.2 months. Analysis of these data suggested that doses greater than 75 Gy resulted in more durable in-field local control than lower doses. In a prospective phase II trial 66 Gy in 33 fractions were administered to HCC patients ineligible for curative therapies and 92% tumour responses and 78% 1-year local control rates were noted.

With the use of higher doses and fewer fractions (hypofractionated RT), excellent local control rates ranging from 70% to 90% have been reported when the radiation beam can be directed from multiple planes (stereotactic RT) converging on the tumour, the majority of the liver can be spared from irradiation, and treatment is image-guided. Across all partial liver radiation paradigms, the most common site of first recurrence is intrahepatic, however outside the high dose-irradiated volume; toxicity is greater in Child-Pugh B compared to Child-Pugh A patients.

3.9.4 Proton irradiation

In contrast to photon irradiation, where the dose delivered to the tumour is limited by the entrance and exit doses that can potentially harm normal tissues, accelerated proton beams deposit dose within the tumour without exiting through normal tissues beyond the tumour. With the administration of 72 Gy in 16 fractions of proton beam therapy in Japanese patients with unresectable HCC a 5-year local control rate of 87% and an overall survival rate of 23.5% in the absence of significant toxicity were noted. Furthermore, a 5-year survival rate of 53.5% was achieved in almost 25% of 50 patients with solitary tumours and Child-Pugh A cirrhosis suggesting that proton beam therapy is safe and efficacious in the treatment of HCC, and that the results may compare favorably to other curative treatments. Other groups have reported similar results with proton beam therapy of HCCs as well.

3.9.5 Combination of RT with other therapies

Tumours treated with TACE, an established treatment for unresectable HCC, often do not achieve durable local responses. RT has been combined with TACE to overcome treatment resistance. A greater than 60% response rates and a significant drop in tumour markers levels using this combination treatment strategy were noted . TACE followed by RT was reported to improve overall survival over TACE alone in a retrospective analysis of this experience. Similar results have been reported by other groups.

To address the persisting challenge of out-of-field intraheptic failures despite improved in-field local control, concurrent intra-arterial 5-FU and RT followed by monthly 5-FU and cisplatin has shown some promise (Schwarz et al., 2010)

4. Conclusion

Today, Sorafenib is the only approved systemic drug for the treatment of advanced HCC and is considered the new reference standard in the care of patients with this disease and preserved liver function. Several other molecular targeted agents are in different stages of clinical and preclinical development, or as single agents or in combinations.

The efficacy and safety of these agents is under investigation.

5. References

Abou-Alfa GK, Johnson P, Knox JJ, Capanu M, Davidenko I, Lacava J, Leung T, Gansukh B, Saltz LB (2010) Doxorubicin plus sorafenib vs doxorubicin alone in patients with advanced hepatocellular carcinoma: a randomized trial. *JAMA*, Vol. 304, No 19, (Nov 2010), pp 2154-2160, ISSN 0098-7484

Alberts SR, Fitch TR, Kim GP, Morlan BW, Dakhil SR, Gross HM, Nair S (2011) Cediranib (AZD2171) in Patients With Advanced Hepatocellular Carcinoma: A Phase II North Central Cancer Treatment Group Clinical Trial. *Am J Clin Oncol* (Mar 2011) [Epub ahead of print] ISSN 0277-3732

Bruix J, Sherman M (2011) Management of hepatocellular carcinoma: An update. *Hepatology*, Vol . 53, No 3, (Mar 2011), pp 1020-1022, ISSN 0270-9139

Cheng AL, Kang YK, Chen Z, Tsao CJ, Qin S, Kim JS, Luo R, Feng J, Ye S, Yang TS, Xu J, Sun Y, Liang H, Liu J, Wang J, Tak WY, Pan H, Burock K, Zou J, Voliotis D, Guan Z (2009) Efficacy and safety of sorafenib in patients in the Asia-Pacific region with advanced hepatocellular carcinoma: a phase III randomised, double-blind, placebo-controlled trial. *Lancet Oncol.*, Vol. 10, No 1, (Jan 2009), pp 25-34 ISSN 1470-2045

Dollinger MM, Lautenschlaeger C, Lesske J, Tannapfel A, Wagner AD, Schoppmeyer K, Nehls O, Welker MW, Wiest R, Fleig WE; AIO Hepatobiliary Study Group (2010) Thymostimulin versus placebo for palliative treatment of locally advanced or metastasised hepatocellular carcinoma: a phase III clinical trial. *BMC Cancer*, Vol. 24, No 10, (Aug 2010), pp 457-468

El-Serag HB, Marrero JA, Rudolph L, Reddy KR (2008) Diagnosis and treatment of hepatocellular carcinoma. *Gastroenterology* Vol 134, No 6, (May 2008), pp 1752-1763, ISSN 0016-5085

Faivre S, Raymond E, Boucher E, Douillard J, Lim HY, Kim JS, Zappa M, Lanzalone S, Lin X, Deprimo S, Harmon C, Ruiz-Garcia A, Lechuga MJ, Cheng AL (2009) Safety and efficacy of sunitinib in patients with advanced hepatocellular carcinoma: an open-label, multicentre, phase II study. *Lancet Oncol.* Vol. 10, No 8, (Aug 2009), pp 794-800, ISSN 1470-2045

Forner A, Reig M.E, Rodriguez de Lope C, Bruix J (2010) Current strategy for staging and treatment: The BCLC update and future prospects. *Semin Liv Dis.*, Vol. 30, No 1, (Feb 2010), pp 61-74, ISSN 0272-8087

Lencioni R, Chen XP, Dagher L, Venook AP (2010) Treatment of intermediate/advanced hepatocellular carcinoma in the clinic: how can outcomes be improved? *Oncologist*, Vol. 15, Suppl 4, (Nov 2010), pp 42-52, ISSN 1549490X

Kanai F, Yoshida H, Tateishi R, Sato S, Kawabe T, Obi S, Kondo Y, Taniguchi M, Tagawa K, Ikeda M, Morizane C, Okusaka T, Arioka H, Shiina S, Omata M (2011) A phase I/II trial of the oral antiangiogenic agent TSU-68 in patients with advanced hepatocellular carcinoma. *Cancer Chemother Pharmacol*, Vol. 67, No 2, (Feb 2011), pp 315-324, ISSN 0344-5704

Llovet JM, Brú C, Bruix J (1999) Prognosis of hepatocellular carcinoma: the BCLC staging classification. *Semin Liver Dis.*, Vol. 19, No 3, (1999), pp 329-338, ISSN 0272-8087

Llovet JM, Ricci S, Mazzaferro V, Hilgard P, Gane E, Blanc JF, de Oliveira AC, Santoro A, Raoul JL, Forner A, Schwartz M, Porta C, Zeuzem S, Bolondi L, Greten TF, Galle PR, Seitz JF, Borbath I, Häussinger D, Giannaris T, Shan M, Moscovici M, Voliotis D, Bruix J; SHARP Investigators Study Group (2008) Sorafenib in advanced hepatocellular carcinoma *N Engl J Med.*, Vol 359, No 4, (Jul 2008), pp 378-390, ISSN 15334406

Liu JH, Chen PW, Asch SM, Busuttil RW, Ko CY (2004) Surgery for hepatocellular carcinoma: does it improve survival? *Ann Surg Oncol.*, Vol 11, No 3, (Mar 2004), pp 298-303, ISSN 1068-9265

Mazzaferro V, Llovet JM, Miceli R, Bhoori S, Schiavo M, Mariani L, Camerini T, Roayaie S, Schwartz ME, Grazi GL, Adam R, Neuhaus P, Salizzoni M, Bruix J, Forner A, De Carlis L, Cillo U, Burroughs AK, Troisi R, Rossi M, Gerunda GE, Lerut J, Belghiti J, Boin I, Gugenheim J, Rochling F, Van Hoek B, Majno P; Metroticket Investigator Study Group (2009) Predicting survival after liver transplantation in patients with hepatocellular carcinoma beyond the Milan criteria: a retrospective, exploratory analysis. *Lancet Oncol.* , Vol 10, No 1, (Jan 2009), pp 35-43, ISSN 1470-2045

Park JW, Finn RS, Kim JS, Karwal M, Li RK, Ismail F, Thomas M, Harris R, Baudelet C, Walters I, Raoul JL (2011) Phase II, open-label study of brivanib as first-line therapy in patients with advanced hepatocellular carcinoma *Clin Cancer Res* , Vol. 17, No 7, (Apr 2011), pp 1973-1983, ISSN 1078-0432

Parkin DM, Bray F, Ferlay J, Pisani P (2005) Global cancer statistics, 2002. *CA Cancer J Clin*, Vol. 55, No 2, (Mar-Apr 2005), pp 74-108, ISSN 1542-486

Raoul J-L, Sangro B, Forner A, Mazzaferro V, Piscaglia F, Bolondi L, Lencioni R (2011) Evolving strategies for the management of intermediate-stage hepatocellular carcinoma: Available evidence and expert opinion on the use of transarterial chemoembolization. *Cancer Treat Rev*, Vol . 37, No 3, (May 2011), pp 212-220, ISSN 0305-7372

Rimassa L, Santoro A (2010) The present and future landscape of treatment of advanced hepatocellular carcinoma. *Dig Liver Dis*, Vol .42, Suppl 3, (Jul 2010), S273-S280, ISSN 1590-8658

Rossi L, Zoratto F, Papa A, Iodice F, Minozzi M, Frati L, Tomao S (2010) Current approach in the treatment of hepatocellular carcinoma. *World J Gastrointest Oncol*, Vol. 2, No 9, (Sep 2010), pp 348-359, ISSN 1948-5204

Schwarz RE, Abou-Alfa GK, Geschwind JF, Krishnan S, Salem R, Venook AP; American Hepato-Pancreato-Biliary Association; Society of Surgical Oncology; Society for Surgery of the Alimentary Tract (2010) Nonoperative therapies for combined modality treatment of hepatocellular cancer: expert consensus statement. *HPB (Oxford)*, Vol. 12, No 5, (Jun 2010), pp 313-320, ISSN 1365-182X

Siegel AB, Cohen EI, Ocean A, Lehrer D, Goldenberg A, Knox JJ, Chen H, Clark-Garvey S, Weinberg A, Mandeli J, Christos P, Mazumdar M, Popa E, Brown RS Jr, Rafii S, Schwartz JD (2008) Phase II trial evaluating the clinical and biologic effects of bevacizumab in unresectable hepatocellular carcinoma *J Clin Oncol*, Vol 26, No 18, (Jun 2008), pp 2992-2998 , ISSN 0732-183X

Tazi EM, Essadi I, M'rabti H, Touyar A, Errihani H (2011) Systemic treatment and targeted therapy in patients with advanced hepatocellular carcinoma. *North Am J Med Sci* , Vol. 3, No 4, (Apr 2011), pp 167-175, ISSN 1947– 2714

Villanueva A, Llovet JM (2011) Targeted therapies for hepatocellular carcinoma. *Gastroenterology*, Vol. 140, No 5, (May 2011), pp 1410-1426, ISSN 0016-5085

Yau T, Pang R, Chan P, Poon RT Molecular targeted therapy of advanced hepatocellular carcinoma beyond sorafenib (2010) *Expert Opin Pharmacother*, Vol. 11, No 13, (Sep 2010), pp 2187-2198, ISSN 1465-6566

Zhu AX, Blaszkowsky LS, Ryan DP, Clark JW, Muzikansky A, Horgan K, Sheehan S, Hale KE, Enzinger PC, Bhargava P, Stuart K (2006) Phase II study of gemcitabine and oxaliplatin in combination with bevacizumab in patients with advanced hepatocellular carcinoma. *J Clin Oncol* ,Vol. 24, No 12, (Apr 2006), pp 1898-1903, ISSN 0732-183X

Zhu AX, Sahani DV, Duda DG, di Tomaso E, Ancukiewicz M, Catalano OA, Sindhwani V, Blaszkowsky LS, Yoon SS,Lahdenranta J, Bhargava P, Meyerhardt J, Clark JW, Kwak EL, Hezel AF, Miksad R, Abrams TA, Enzinger PC, Fuchs CS, Ryan DP, Jain RK (2009) Efficacy, safety, and potential biomarkers of sunitinib monotherapy in advanced hepatocellular carcinoma: a phase II study *J Clin Oncol.* , Vol. 27, No 18, (Jun 2009), pp 3027-3035, ISSN 0732-183X

18

Systemic Management of Advanced Hepatocellular Carcinoma Patients: The Role of Multi-Targeted Anti-Angiogenic Inhibitors

Joanne Chiu, Roberta Pang, Ronnie Poon and Thomas Yau

University of Hong Kong
Hong Kong

1. Introduction

Hepatocellular carcinoma (HCC) is the third leading cause of cancer-related death worldwide resulting in between 250,000 to one million deaths per annum. It carries dismal prognosis and the number death is close to the incidence of disease owing to the aggressive nature of this tumor. The incidence of HCC is highest in China, eastern Asia, and Saharan African. The main etiology of HCC in these regions is chronic hepatitis B viral infection. In most Western countries, HCC is mainly related to hepatitis C infection and alcoholic liver disease. Nonalcoholic steato-hepatitis and exposure to aflatoxins are also known risk factors for development of HCC.

Advanced non-resectable HCC has a median survival of only 6 months [1]. Traditional cytotoxic chemotherapy has not been found to be effective in prolonging overall survival and is associated with significant hematological toxicities. The use of systemic chemotherapy is also limited by liver cirrhosis which often coexists in these patients.

2. Molecular biology and mechanism of HCC

Pathogenesis of HCC is a complex process. HCC is believed to be related to genetic alterations caused by chronic liver injury and inflammation. Cytokines release induced by death of hepatocytes, fibrogenesis, and liver cirrhosis are the early events marking hepatocarcinogenesis. Occasionally, however, HCC can arise in liver without evidence of chronic cirrhosis. Chronic infections with hepatitis B or C viruses are 2 important etiologies in development of this tumor. Integration of viral DNA in the human genome can potentially induce chromosomal instability, activate oncogenes or deactivate tumor-suppressor genes, promoting cancer formation. Known examples of mutations in the tumor suppressor genes or proto-oncogenes in HCC include p53, p73, APC, Rb, c-myc and cycline D1 [2]. Various viral proteins, such as HBs or preS in hepatitis B and core protein in HCV, have been linked to activation of transcription and cellular proliferation, although the exact mechanism is not known.

Cytogenic studies have shown chromosomal amplification or deletions are common in HCC. HCC is associated with high prevalent amplifications in 1q, 6p, 9q, 11q (contains areas encoding cyclin D1), 17q, and 20q [2, 3], and high prevalent deletions in 4q, 6p (contains areas encoding VEGFA), 8p, 13q, 16q, and 17p [3]. Increase in tolemerase activity leading to telomere shortening and genomic instability, was also observed in nearly 90% of HCC [4]. The significance of these chromosomal alteration remains to be elucidated.

The advance of microarray in the last 2 decades have revolutionized oncological studies and shed light on the molecular mechanisms behind development of cancer. In many tumors, molecular studies successfully identified specific genes that drive the growth of malignancies, leading to development of targeted therapies for each tumor subtypes. For instance, imatinib was designed to block the tyrosine kinase activity associated with the kinase fusion protein BCR-ABL in chronic myeloid leukemia and became the standard of care for this tumor. Gefitinib and erlotinib targeting the tyrosine kinase activation caused by mutated EGFR in adenocarcinoma of lung, and significantly prolonged the life expectancy of patients carrying this genetic abnormality. However such pattern of oncogene addiction has not been identified in HCC. Today, a large body of knowledge have been accumulated to stratify specific gene expressions involved in various stages of HCC tumorgenesis [5]. For instance, early HCC development is marked by down-regulation of Toll-like receptor pathway, Jak/STAT pathway, TGF pathway, and the insulin-signaling pathway, with up-regulation of Wnt signaling pathway. Poorly differentiated HCC is characterized by decreased level of apoptosis-related proteins compared with well differentiated counterpart [6]. Furthermore, many scientists have demonstrated that HCC can be divided into prognostic significant subgroups based on gene signatures [7-11]. Although there is yet consensus on genetic classification of HCC, these data suggested HCC is a group of heterogeneous tumors each with distinct characteristics. This knowledge can path the future development of personalized medicine in treatment of HCC.

While our knowledge on genetic features of HCC continue to expand, much research focus on factors that govern more universal processes such as tumor cells proliferation, neovascularization, tumor invasion, and metastasis. Today, growth of HCC is considered as a result of dysregulation of pleiotropic growth factor signaling [12]. Implicated pathways include insulin-like growth factor/IGF-1 receptor (IGF/IGF-1R), hepatocyte growth factor (HGF/c-MET), stem cell growth factor receptor (c-kit), Wingless (Wnt/β-catenin/FZD), transforming growth factor β (TGFβ/TβR), epidermal growth factor/EGF receptor (EGF/EGFR), and many growth factor regulated angiogenic signaling such as fibroblast growth factor/FGF receptor (FGF/FGFR), platelet growth factor/PDGF receptor (PDGF/PDGFR), and vascular endothelial growth factor/VEGF receptor (VEGF/VEGFR). Activation by ligand binding on the extracellular portion of these transmembrane receptors results in phosphorylation of cytoplastic components, triggering downstream signaling cascades. These pathways are multifunctional and crosstalk to each other. The RAF/MEK/ERK pathway and phosphatidylinositol-3 kinase (P13K)/AKT/mammalian target of rapamycin (mTOR) pathway are some of the major intracellular cascades implicated in HCC.

3. Anti-angiogenic therapy

HCC is a characterized by its high vascularity and anti-angiogenesis becomes an intense area of study in the quest of new therapy for HCC. Angiogenesis plays a pivotal role in the growth to solid tumor. It is a complex multi-step process mediated by various proangiogenic growth factors such as BEFG, FGFs, TGFβ, interleukin-8 (IL8),

Systemic Management of Advanced Hepatocellular Carcinoma Patients: The Role of Multi-Targeted
Anti-Angiogenic Inhibitors

311

metalloproteinase-2 (MMP-2), angiopoietin (Ang), and PDGF. Genetic changes in tumor cells and hypoxia induced by rapid tumor growth could lead to increased secretion of these mediators, which promote migration, proliferation and survival of endothelial cells, as well as growth of stromal cells and extracellular matrix favoring these processes.

3.1 Sorafenib

Sorafenib (Bayer 43-9006; Nexavar) is a multikinase inhibitor of the VEGR-2, VEGFR-3, and PDGF receptor β, and blocks cellular proliferation mediated by the Raf/MAPK/ERK signaling pathway [13]. Two Phase III randomized placebo-controlled trails, the SHARP trial and the Asian-Pacific trial, have shown overall survival benefit using single agent sorafenib as first line treatment in advanced HCC [14, 15]. The SHARP trial contains mainly Westerners, whose etiology factors were predominantly HCV infection and alcoholic liver cirrhosis. It demonstrated sorafenib led to an improvement of median time to progression (TTP) from 2.8 to 5.5 months and overall survival (OS) from 7.9 to 10.7 months, when compared with the placebo group. The Asian-Pacific trial, where most subjects were Orientals, also found sorafenib improved median TTP from 1.4 to 2.8 months and OS from 4.2 to 6.5 months when compared with the placebo group. Based on these 2 independent studies, sorafenib become the first systemic treatment approved by the U.S. Food and Drug Administration (FDA) and many regulatory authorities worldwide for first line management of advanced HCC. It should be noted that, however, the absolute benefit of sorafenib in HCC remains modest. In both studies the OS improvement was between 2.3 to 2.8 months. The overall response rate was 24% in the Western study and 57% in the Asia-Pacific study, but most patients had stable disease and only 3% had partial response. Furthermore, over 95% of subjects in these 2 studies had Child-Pugh class A liver function, rendering the effect in those with poorer liver function controversial. Child-Pugh B or C liver cirrhosis commonly coexist in patients with HCC. A number of small retrospective series showed patients with Child-Pugh B liver function were more likely to have hyperbilirubinemia, encephalopathy, worsening of ascites, and shorter survival when given sorafenib [16-18]. Since patients with poor liver function would naturally have more of these complications and shorter survival, the safety and survival benefit of sorafenib in these patients is not known. A recently published abstract of the GIDEON study probably provides more insight on this issue. It is so far the largest prospective non-interventional study of sorafenib involving over 3000 patients with unresectable HCC. Patients were stratified according to different Child-Pugh status, with the safety and outcome of sorafenib treatment evaluated [19]. Interim analysis showed Child-Pugh B patients, compared with Child-Pugh A patients, did not have a higher incidence of drug-related adverse events (AEs), but had a higher incidence of liver-associated AEs. Kaplan Meier estimate showed similar TTP between 2 groups, and an obviously worse OS in patients with Child-Pugh B or C liver cirrhosis. Most deaths were due to HCC or underlying liver disorders and the differences in patient outcomes across Child-Pugh groups appeared to be attributed by differences in prognosis.

Combination therapy has been a common approach in cancer treatment. By acting on multiple sites of the cell proliferation pathways, there are potential for enhanced efficacy by synergistic effect, reducing the emergence of resistance clones, or minimizing the accumulated toxicities of high dose therapy.

In an attempt to enhance the effect of sorafenib, many clinical trials are undergoing to evaluate the addition of other biological agents to this drug. For example, SEARCH is a Phase III randomized placebo controlled, double blind trial of sorafenib plus erlotinib versus sorafenib plus placebo as first line systemic treatment for hepatocellular carcinoma.

Sorafenib has been combined with a number of chemotherapy. Abou-Alfa's team has published a double-blinded randomized phase II trial comparing doxorubicin with or without sorafenib. Doxorubicin was extensively studied in treatment of advanced HCC in the pre-sorafenib era. It showed minimal efficacy with significant toxicities. In this phase II study, combination sorafenib and doxorubicin showed some activity but only gave a 4% response rate, and the additional effect of chemotherapy was questionable since this study used doxorubicin as the control arm [20].

3.2 Bevacizumab

HCC is a highly vascularized tumor and it correlates with high level of VEGF expression [21], which is thought to be the most important proangiogenic growth factors. Bevacizumab is a humanized recombinant monoclonal antibiody against VEGF with high affinity [22] and has been shown to have efficacy in many solid tumors. Bevacizumab as a single agent has been shown to have activity in advanced HCC. In Siegel's Phase II study which enrolled 46 patients with HCC, bevacizumab (5 mg/kg or 10 mg/kg every 2 weeks) had a response rate of 13%, gave a PFS of 6.9 months and median OS of 12.4 months [23]. However, the use of this drug is complicated by significant hemorrhage in 11% and thrombosis in 6% of subjects. Interestingly, when bevacizumab (10 mg/kg every 2 weeks) was combined with chemotherapy gencitabine and oxaliplatin, the combination achieved an apparently higher RR of 20%, but yielded a median PFS and medial OS of only 5.3 months and 9.6 months respectively with major complications being leucopenia, transaminitis, hypertension and fatigue [24]. As chemotherapy appears to have limited role in the development of systemic treatment of HCC, the M.D. Anderson group brought forward the concept of combining bevacizumab with another biological agent. In their Phase II trial using bevacizumab with erlotinib which involved 57 patients [25], the combination gave a median PFS of 7.9 months and medial OS of 12.8 months. It is worth noting that 6 patients in this trial terminated treatment due to toxicities, but there were an impressive stable disease (SD) rate of 62% and partial response (PR) rate of 28%. This study also included both Child-Pugh A and Child-Pugh B patients although the proportion was not mentioned in the abstract. Meanwhile the same research group is exploring the effect of this drug combination compared with sorafenib as first line treatment in advanced HCC in a Phase II trial. In summary, early clinical trials showed that bevacizumab has some activity in HCC, but efficacy and safety of this drug needs to be clarified as it can potentially be associated with major complication such as thrombosis, hemorrhage and even death.

3.3 Sunitinib

The VEGF family is the most important proangiogenic mechanism known today. VEGF binds to cell surface receptors VEGFR-1, 2, and 3 on endothelial cells. Among these 3 receptors, VEGFR-2 is the primary tyrosine kinase receptor mediating the VEGF signaling. Sunitinib is another anti-angiogenic agent with potent anti-VEGF-2 activity. The concentration required to produce 50% inhibition (IC_{50}) of human VEGFR-2 kinase activity is 0.009 μM compared with 0.09 μM for sorafenib [13, 26]. It is also an oral multi-targeted tyrosine kinase inhibitor with overlapping TKI activities with those of sorafenib, including VEGF receptors, RET kinases, PDGFR-α and β, c-Kit, Flt-3 and colony-stimulating factor receptor type 1 [26]. It was first approved for treatment of advanced renal cell carcinoma (RCC) [27], which is a highly vascularized tumor also resistant to traditional chemotherapy. In RCC, sunitinib and sorafenib demonstrated similar efficacy, thus it was suggested that they might also have comparable effect in advanced HCC. The use of single agent sunitinib as first line treatment in advanced HCC has been tested in a number of Phase II trials (see Table 1 for details) [28-30]. In these trials, sunitinib was given at 37.5 mg daily or 50 mg daily for 4 weeks out of a 6-week cycle, or continuously at 37.5 mg daily. The RR was relative low, with medial PFS between 2.8-5.3 months, and medial OS between 8 to 9.8 months. These data showed preliminarily encouraging survival time approximate those of sorafenib. Nevertheless, use of sunitnib in HCC requires vigorous testing in randomized controlled trial. Cheng et al. released their early Phase III data comparing sunitinib and sorafenib as first line treatment in an abstract form recently [31]. In their open-label trial involving over 1000 Child-Pugh A patients with advanced HCC, patients were randomized 1:1 to receive sunitinib 37.5 mg daily or sorafenib 400 mg BID. The primary end point was OS and secondary endpoint was PFS, time to progression (TTP) and safety. The trial was terminated prematurely, as interim analysis showed sunitinib had significantly shorter OS of 8.1 months compared with 10.0 months of sorafenib (p=0.019). There was no difference in PFS and TTP between 2 groups. Serious adverse events (AEs) in sunitnib and sorafenib groups were found in 44% and 36% of patients, and grade 5 AEs in 18% and 16% of patients respectively. Thus sunitinib failed its primary OS endpoint and was associated with more significant toxicities. Worth noting is that in this study, there was no OS difference between 2 groups among hepatitis B carriers. Formal report of toxicity profile is pending. These results did not support using sunitib as first line treatment in advanced HCC and sorafenib remains the standard choice. Use of sunitnib as second line treatment after sorafenib failure has also been reported by Yau et al. In this Phase II study which enrolled 35 patients, the RR was 6%, TTP was 2.9 months and OS was 5.2 months [32]. More clinical data is needed to elucidate the role of this TKI in treatment of advanced HCC.

3.4 Brivanib

Besides VEGF, the fibroblast growth factor (FGF) pathway is another key driver of angiogenesis. FGF is a potent angiogenic growth factor which stimulates induction and migration of endothelial cell precursors during vascular development [33]. It is also secreted by HCC and contributes to tumor growth [34]. Experiences from other cancers showed the expression of FGF and other angiogenic factors were upregulated upon anti-VEGF treatment, suggesting FGF pathway is one of the alternate escape mechanisms that contributes to resistance or failure of anti-VEGF treatment [35]. Brivanib (BMS-582664) is a novel TKI of both VEGF and Basic FGF (bFGF). In a Phase II open-label study of brivanib as first line treatment of unresectable HCC involving 55 patients, brivanib achieved a median PFS of 2.7 months and median OS of 10 months. Stable disease, partial response, and complete response were found in 22, 3, and 1 patients respectively [36]. Common adverse events included fatigue, hypertension and diarrhea. In view of shown activity and manageable toxicity profile, brivanib has been carried on to a Phase III multi-center double-blinded randomized controlled trial (BRISK FL study) which compares this drug with sorafenib as first line treatment of HCC. This trial has completed recruitment in July 2011 and data collection is underway. The same group of researchers who performed the Phase II brivanib trial also tested the efficacy of this drug in patients who failed prior antiangiogenic therapy. They recruited 22 such patients; of the 19 patients who were assessed for efficacy, 58% had stable disease. Alpha fetoprotein reduction of more than half was also found in 43% of patients [37]. This VEGF / FGF dual targeting agent can potentially become a new anti-angiogenic therapy in advanced HCC.

3.5 Pazopanib

Pazopanib (GW786034) is multi-targeted TKI of VEGFR1-3, PDGFR-α and β, and c-kit [38]. It shares with sunitinib and sorafenib similar preclinical activity in various xenograft tumors models including RCC, thyroid cancer, pancreatic cancer, and HCC [39]. Since it has no significant in vitro effect in proliferation of most tumor cell lines, it is believed its anti-tumor property owes to its anti-angiogenic activity. Clinically pazopanib has been approved by the U.S. FDA for treatment of advanced RCC [40] and has been shown to have promising activity in thyroid cancer [41] and urothelial cancer. Its use in HCC is still under preliminary research. Our group has recently published a Phase I tudy evaluating the early efficacy and pharmacological properties of pazopanib in HCC patients [42]. In this study of 28 patients, the maximum tolerated dose was 600 mg daily. The most common adverse events were diarrhea, skin hypopigmentation, and AST elevation. Grade 3 dose-limiting toxicities were observed in only 2 patients at the 800 mg dose level. Furthermore, 73% of patients responded with either partial response or stable disease. These results suggested pazopanib has acceptable toxicity and can potentially be a candidate for treatment of advanced HCC.

3.6 Other anti-angiogenic agents

Linifanib (ABT-869) is a novel and potent selective inhibitor of the EGF and PDGF families of RTKs. In a Phase II open-label trial, 44 Child-Pugh A or B patients with unresectable HCC were given linifanib at 0.25 mg/kg daily and 0.25 mg/kg alternate day respectively [43]. The overall response rate was 6.8%. For Child-Pugh A patients, median TTP was 5.4 months and median OS was 9.7 months. The most common grade 3 or 4 adverse events were hypertension and fatigue. A Phase III trial comparing linifanib with sorafenib is undergoing.

TSU-68 is another multi-targeted TKI with activity against VEGFR, PDGFR, and FGFR. In a Phase I/II trial, Kanai et al. reported an overall response rate of 51% with 2.9% complete response, 5.7% partial response and 42.8% stable disease. The median TTP was 2.1 months and median OS was 13.1 months [44]. Adverse events include diarrhea, malaise, and ALT / AST elevation, and were similar to other TKIs. This drug showed preliminary efficacy with acceptable safety profile.

Cediranib (AZD2171) is another investigational TKI activity against pan-VEGFR, PDGFR, c-kit an FLT-4 pathways. Recently published Phase II data suggested cediranib at 45 mg daily bared significant toxicity and did not show clinical response [45].

Axitinib (AG013736) is a multi-targated TKI with activity against VEGFR1-3, PDGFR and c-kit. This drug has encouraging survival data as both first and second line treatment in advanced RCC, and has shown promising activity in thyroid cancer [46, 47]. Phase II/III trials testing this drug in HCC is under planning.

The hepatocyte growth factor (HGF) and its receptor called mesenchymal epithelial transition factor (c-MET) is another potential target for treatment of HCC. The HGF/c-MET is involved in growth of hepatocytes [48]. The c-MET mediates cell growth, survival, motility and morphogeneis during early development of liver, as well as repair and regeneration in liver injury [49]. Foretinib (GSK1363089) is a novel receptor TKI targeting c-MET and VEGFR2/KDR in a Phase 1-2 clinical trial for systemic treatment of HCC.

4. Resistance to antiangogenic therapy

The mechanism underlying resistance to antiangiogenic treatment in HCC is still poorly understood. The proposed mechanisms include:

4.1 Redundancy of angiogenic signaling pathways

Tumour dependence on pro-angiogenic factors may be altered after the treatment with sorafenib [50]. The vascular remodeling that due to pericytic over-coverage renders the neovasculature less responsive to VEGF for growth dependence effectively circumventing a blocked signaling pathway with greater dependence on other alternate mechanisms [51].

4.2 Resistance occur at the tumour endothelial cell level

Published evidence has shown that tumour endothelial cells may harbor unstable genome [52]. These aberrant genomes may lead to an increase in genetic alterations and result in mutations in the endothelial cells. Thus, the mutated endothelial cells may acquire resistance to molecularly targeted therapy.

4.3 Increase the biological aggressiveness of the tumour following antiangioneic use

It has been shown that the inhibition of VEGF receptors may result in an increased propensity for metastatic dissemination as the hypoxic microenvironment associated with the sorafenib use selects for highly aggressive, invasive tumour cells [53, 54]

4.4 Splitting of pre-existing vasculature

Antiangiogenic agents inhibit sprouting angiogensis which heavily relies on the need for endothelial cell proliferation and migration. Tumour cells can potentially evade these pruning effects by the splitting of pre-existing vasculature into new blood vessels without a need for VEGF expression and endothelial cell proliferation[55] or form blood vessels without the need for endothelial cell proliferation [56].

4.5 Increase in the expression of the resistance efflux proteins

Resistance efflux proteins are members of the ATP binding cassette transporters, especially multidrug resistance protein 2(MRP2) may partly account for the development of sorafenib resistance. In vitro experiment performed by Shibayama et al. demonstrated that sorafenib is a substrate for MRP2 and thus MRP2 may implicate in the development of drug resistance to Sorafenib [57].

4.6 Presence of cancer stem cell

Cancer stem cells are typified by a capacity for self-renewal, relative quiescence and the ability to differentiate. Evidence has suggested that CSCs are involved in carcinogenesis, tumour invasion and metastases, and resistance to various forms of therapies, including chemotherapy[58].

5. Conclusion

The development of sorafenib marked an important milestone in the systemic treatment of advanced HCC. This drug remains the only approved targeted therapy shown to have survival advance in randomized controlled studies. Hepatocarcinogenesis is a complex process involving multiple growth factor systems which interact with each other. Early clinial trials suggested that agents with single-target activity probably cannot block HCC growth and multi-targeted therapies might be the trend for future drug development. As HCC in different stages demonstrated different molecular characteristics, and knowledge on molecular subgroups of HCC is expanding, we see the vast varieties of potential for development of HCC treatment.

Agents	Study	n	Response rate (%)	Median PFS (months)	Median OS (months)
Sorafenib					
Sorafenib vs. placebo	SHARP	602	24.4	5.5	10.7
Sorafenib vs. placebo	Asia-Pacific	226	57.3	5.5	6.5
Sorafenib + erlotinib Vs Sorafenib + placebo	SEARCH		Ongoing		
Bevacizumab					
Bevacizumab	Siegel 2008	46	13	6.9	12.4
Bevacizumab+gemcitabine & oxaliplatin	Zhu 2006	33	20 (SD 27%)	5.3	9.6
Bevacizumab+erlotinib	Kaseb	57	(SD 62%, PR 28%)	7.9	12.8
Sunitinib					
Sunitinib (37.5mg daily 4/6 weeks)	Zhu [28]	34	2.9	3.9	9.8
Sunitinib (50mg daily 4/6 weeks)	Faivre [29]	37	2.7%	5.3	8
Sunitinib (37.5mg daily continuous)	Koeberle [30]	45		2.8	9.3
Sunitinib vs. sorafenib	Cheng 2011	1073	Not a/v	3.6 vs. 2.9	8.1 vs. 10.0 (p < 0.01)
Brivanib					
Brivanib (800 mg daily)	Park 2011	55	47%	2.7	10
Brivanib vs. sorafenib	BRISK FL		Ongoing		

Table 1. First line trials for major antiangiogenic agents (shaded trials indicate Phase III studies)

Systemic Management of Advanced Hepatocellular Carcinoma Patients: The Role of Multi-Targeted
Anti-Angiogenic Inhibitors

317

6. References

[1] Lopez, P.M., A. Villanueva, and J.M. Llovet, *Systematic review: evidence-based management of hepatocellular carcinoma--an updated analysis of randomized controlled trials*. Aliment Pharmacol Ther, 2006. 23(11): p. 1535-47.

[2] Thorgeirsson, S.S. and J.W. Grisham, *Molecular pathogenesis of human hepatocellular carcinoma.* Nat Genet, 2002. 31(4): p. 339-46.

[3] Chiang, D.Y., et al., *Focal gains of VEGFA and molecular classification of hepatocellular carcinoma.* Cancer Res, 2008. 68(16): p. 6779-88.

[4] Farazi, P.A., et al., *Differential impact of telomere dysfunction on initiation and progression of hepatocellular carcinoma.* Cancer Res, 2003. 63(16): p. 5021-7.

[5] Maass, T., et al., *Microarray-based gene expression analysis of hepatocellular carcinoma.* Curr Genomics, 2010. 11(4): p. 261-8.

[6] Okabe, H., et al., *Genome-wide analysis of gene expression in human hepatocellular carcinomas using cDNA microarray: identification of genes involved in viral carcinogenesis and tumor progression.* Cancer Res, 2001. 61(5): p. 2129-37.

[7] Lee, J.S., et al., *A novel prognostic subtype of human hepatocellular carcinoma derived from hepatic progenitor cells.* Nat Med, 2006. 12(4): p. 410-6.

[8] Yamashita, T., et al., *EpCAM and alpha-fetoprotein expression defines novel prognostic subtypes of hepatocellular carcinoma.* Cancer Res, 2008. 68(5): p. 1451-61.

[9] Kim, J.W., et al., *Cancer-associated molecular signature in the tissue samples of patients with cirrhosis.* Hepatology, 2004. 39(2): p. 518-27.

[10] Hoshida, Y., et al., *Molecular classification and novel targets in hepatocellular carcinoma: recent advancements.* Semin Liver Dis, 2010. 30(1): p. 35-51.

[11] Villanueva, A., et al., *New strategies in hepatocellular carcinoma: genomic prognostic markers.* Clin Cancer Res, 2010. 16(19): p. 4688-94.

[12] Breuhahn, K., T. Longerich, and P. Schirmacher, *Dysregulation of growth factor signaling in human hepatocellular carcinoma.* Oncogene, 2006. 25(27): p. 3787-800.

[13] Wilhelm, S.M., et al., *BAY 43-9006 exhibits broad spectrum oral antitumor activity and targets the RAF/MEK/ERK pathway and receptor tyrosine kinases involved in tumor progression and angiogenesis.* Cancer Res, 2004. 64(19): p. 7099-109.

[14] Cheng, A.L., et al., *Efficacy and safety of sorafenib in patients in the Asia-Pacific region with advanced hepatocellular carcinoma: a phase III randomised, double-blind, placebo-controlled trial.* Lancet Oncol, 2009. 10(1): p. 25-34.

[15] Llovet, J.M., et al., *Sorafenib in advanced hepatocellular carcinoma.* N Engl J Med, 2008. 359(4): p. 378-90.

[16] Abou-Alfa, G.K., Amadori, D., Santoro, A., Figer, A., De Greve, J., Lathia, C., Voliotis, D., Anderson, S., Moscovici, M. and Ricci, S., *Is sorafenib safe and effective in patients with hepatocellular carcinoma and Child-Pugh B cirrhosis.* Journal of Clinical Oncology, 2008 ASCO Annual Meeting Proceedings, 2008. 26(15S (May 20 Supp)): p. 4518.

[17] Worns, M.A., et al., *Safety and efficacy of sorafenib in patients with advanced hepatocellular carcinoma in consideration of concomitant stage of liver cirrhosis.* J Clin Gastroenterol, 2009. 43(5): p. 489-95.

[18] Pinter, M., et al., *Sorafenib in unresectable hepatocellular carcinoma from mild to advanced stage liver cirrhosis.* Oncologist, 2009. 14(1): p. 70-6.

[19] Marrero, J.A., et al., *Global Investigation of Therapeutic Decisions in Hepatocellular Carcinoma and of its Treatment with Sorafenib (GIDEON) second interim analysis in more*

than 1,500 patients: Clinical findings in patients with liver dysfunction. J Clin Oncol 2011. 20 (suppl; abstr 4001)

[20] Abou-Alfa, G.K., et al., *Doxorubicin plus sorafenib vs doxorubicin alone in patients with advanced hepatocellular carcinoma: a randomized trial.* JAMA, 2010. 304(19): p. 2154-60.

[21] Torimura, T., et al., *Increased expression of vascular endothelial growth factor is associated with tumor progression in hepatocellular carcinoma.* Hum Pathol, 1998. 29(9): p. 986-91.

[22] Ferrara, N., K.J. Hillan, and W. Novotny, *Bevacizumab (Avastin), a humanized anti-VEGF monoclonal antibody for cancer therapy.* Biochem Biophys Res Commun, 2005. 333(2): p. 328-35.

[23] Siegel, A.B., et al., *Phase II trial evaluating the clinical and biologic effects of bevacizumab in unresectable hepatocellular carcinoma.* J Clin Oncol, 2008. 26(18): p. 2992-8.

[24] Zhu, A.X., et al., *Phase II study of gemcitabine and oxaliplatin in combination with bevacizumab in patients with advanced hepatocellular carcinoma.* J Clin Oncol, 2006. 24(12): p. 1898-903.

[25] Kaseb, A.O., et al., *Biological activity of bevacizumab and erlotinib in patients with advanced hepatocellular carcinoma (HCC)* J Clin Oncol 2009. 27:15s (suppl; abstr 4522)

[26] Mendel, D.B., et al., *In vivo antitumor activity of SU11248, a novel tyrosine kinase inhibitor targeting vascular endothelial growth factor and platelet-derived growth factor receptors: determination of a pharmacokinetic/pharmacodynamic relationship.* Clin Cancer Res, 2003. 9(1): p. 327-37.

[27] Motzer, R.J., et al., *Sunitinib versus interferon alfa in metastatic renal-cell carcinoma.* N Engl J Med, 2007. 356(2): p. 115-24.

[28] Zhu, A.X., et al., *Efficacy, safety, and potential biomarkers of sunitinib monotherapy in advanced hepatocellular carcinoma: a phase II study.* J Clin Oncol, 2009. 27(18): p. 3027-35.

[29] Faivre, S., et al., *Safety and efficacy of sunitinib in patients with advanced hepatocellular carcinoma: an open-label, multicentre, phase II study.* Lancet Oncol, 2009. 10(8): p. 794-800.

[30] Koeberle, D., et al., *Continuous Sunitinib treatment in patients with advanced hepatocellular carcinoma: a Swiss Group for Clinical Cancer Research (SAKK) and Swiss Association for the Study of the Liver (SASL) multicenter phase II trial (SAKK 77/06).* Oncologist, 2010. 15(3): p. 285-92.

[31] Cheng, A., et al., *Phase III trial of sunitinib (Su) versus sorafenib (So) in advanced hepatocellular carcinoma (HCC).* J Clin Oncol, 2011. 29((suppl; abstr 4000)).

[32] Yau, T., et al., *Efficacy and safety of single-agent sunitinib in treating patients with advanced hepatocelluar carcinoma after sorafenib failure: A prospective, open-label, phase II study. Print this page* J Clin Oncol 2011. 29 (suppl; abstr 4082)

[33] Poole, T.J., E.B. Finkelstein, and C.M. Cox, *The role of FGF and VEGF in angioblast induction and migration during vascular development.* Dev Dyn, 2001. 220(1): p. 1-17.

[34] Uematsu, S., et al., *Altered expression of vascular endothelial growth factor, fibroblast growth factor-2 and endostatin in patients with hepatocellular carcinoma.* J Gastroenterol Hepatol, 2005. 20(4): p. 583-8.

[35] Loges, S., T. Schmidt, and P. Carmeliet, *Mechanisms of resistance to anti-angiogenic therapy and development of third-generation anti-angiogenic drug candidates.* Genes Cancer, 2010. 1(1): p. 12-25.

[36] Park, J.W., et al., *Phase II, open-label study of brivanib as first-line therapy in patients with advanced hepatocellular carcinoma.* Clin Cancer Res, 2011. 17(7): p. 1973-83.

[37] Finn, R.S., et al., *Phase II, open label study of brivanib alaninate in patients (pts) with hepatocellular carcinoma (HCC) who failed prior antiangiogenic therapy.* Gastrointestinal Cancers Symposium (abstract #200), 2009.

[38] Kumar, R., et al., *Pharmacokinetic-pharmacodynamic correlation from mouse to human with pazopanib, a multikinase angiogenesis inhibitor with potent antitumor and antiangiogenic activity.* Mol Cancer Ther, 2007. 6(7): p. 2012-21.

[39] Zhu, X.D., et al., *Antiangiogenic effects of pazopanib in xenograft hepatocellular carcinoma models: evaluation by quantitative contrast-enhanced ultrasonography.* BMC Cancer, 2011. 11: p. 28.

[40] Sternberg, C.N., et al., *Pazopanib in locally advanced or metastatic renal cell carcinoma: results of a randomized phase III trial.* J Clin Oncol, 2010. 28(6): p. 1061-8.

[41] Bible, K.C., et al., *Efficacy of pazopanib in progressive, radioiodine-refractory, metastatic differentiated thyroid cancers: results of a phase 2 consortium study.* Lancet Oncol, 2010. 11(10): p. 962-72.

[42] Yau, T.C., et al., *Phase I Dose-Finding Study of Pazopanib in Hepatocellular Carcinoma: Evaluation of Early Efficacy, Pharmacokinetics, and Pharmacodynamics.* Clin Cancer Res, 2011.

[43] Toh, H., et al., *Linifanib phase II trial in patients with advanced hepatocellular carcinoma (HCC).* J Clin Oncol 2010. 28(15s): p. (suppl; abstr 4038.

[44] Kanai, F., et al., *A phase I/II trial of the oral antiangiogenic agent TSU-68 in patients with advanced hepatocellular carcinoma.* Cancer Chemother Pharmacol, 2011. 67(2): p. 315-24.

[45] Alberts, S.R., et al., *Cediranib (AZD2171) in Patients With Advanced Hepatocellular Carcinoma: A Phase II North Central Cancer Treatment Group Clinical Trial.* Am J Clin Oncol, 2011.

[46] Escudier, B. and M. Gore, *Axitinib for the management of metastatic renal cell carcinoma.* Drugs R D, 2011. 11(2): p. 113-26.

[47] Deshpande, H.A., S. Gettinger, and J.A. Sosa, *Axitinib: The evidence of its potential in the treatment of advanced thyroid cancer.* Core Evid, 2010. 4: p. 43-8.

[48] Michalopoulos, G.K. and M. DeFrances, *Liver regeneration.* Adv Biochem Eng Biotechnol, 2005. 93: p. 101-34.

[49] Birchmeier, C., et al., *Met, metastasis, motility and more.* Nat Rev Mol Cell Biol, 2003. 4(12): p. 915-25.

[50] Raza, A., M.J. Franklin, and A.Z. Dudek, *Pericytes and vessel maturation during tumor angiogenesis and metastasis.* Am J Hematol. 85(8): p. 593-8.

[51] Wenger, J.B., et al., *Can we develop effective combination antiangiogenic therapy for patients with hepatocellular carcinoma?* Oncol Rev. 5(3): p. 177-184.

[52] Streubel, B., et al., *Lymphoma-specific genetic aberrations in microvascular endothelial cells in B-cell lymphomas.* N Engl J Med, 2004. 351(3): p. 250-9.

[53] Blagosklonny, M.V., *Antiangiogenic therapy and tumor progression.* Cancer Cell, 2004. 5(1): p. 13-7.

[54] Paez-Ribes, M., et al., *Antiangiogenic therapy elicits malignant progression of tumors to increased local invasion and distant metastasis.* Cancer Cell, 2009. 15(3): p. 220-31.

[55] Rubenstein, J.L., et al., *Anti-VEGF antibody treatment of glioblastoma prolongs survival but results in increased vascular cooption.* Neoplasia, 2000. 2(4): p. 306-14.

[56] Hendrix, M.J., et al., *Vasculogenic mimicry and tumour-cell plasticity: lessons from melanoma.* Nat Rev Cancer, 2003. 3(6): p. 411-21.

[57] Shibayama, Y., et al., *Multidrug resistance protein 2 implicates anticancer drug-resistance to sorafenib.* Biol Pharm Bull. 34(3): p. 433-5.

[58] Trumpp, A. and O.D. Wiestler, *Mechanisms of Disease: cancer stem cells--targeting the evil twin.* Nat Clin Pract Oncol, 2008. 5(6): p. 337-47.

19

Molecular Targeted Therapy for Growth Factors in Hepatocellular Carcinoma

Junji Furuse
Department of Internal Medicine, Medical Oncology,
Kyorin University School of Medicine
Japan

1. Introduction

Treatments for HCC are classified into local and systemic therapies. Various local treatment modalities, such as resection, local ablation, transcatheter arterial chemoembolization (TACE), and liver transplantation, are available at present. The most suitable treatment modality for HCC is selected according to the tumor stage, grade of liver dysfunction, and performance status of the patient [1,2]. Although the local approaches have been demonstrated to yield good outcomes in patients with earlier-stage disease, the usefulness is limited to patients with early-stage HCC [3]. TACE is the most widely used for patients with HCC who are not suitable candidates for curative surgical resection or local ablation therapy, and have preserved liver function (Child-Pugh class A or B). Randomized clinical trials (RCTs) and meta-analysis of RCTs on TACE have shown that this treatment modality yields a statistically significant improvement of survival in properly selected candidates, e.g., patients with multinodular asymptomatic tumors [4,5].

Despite the local therapies mentioned above yielding successful outcomes at first, the patients often develop recurrences or disease progression subsequently. Locoregional treatments for intra- and/or extrahepatic tumors in HCC patients with extrahepatic metastases may yield some survival benefit; the reported 3- and 5-year survival rates are 31.0, 9.2 and 4.5%, respectively, in patients administered locoregional treatments [6]. However, the survival rate is often dismal in patients with extrahepatic metastases, with the median survival time in HCC patients with metastases being 4.6 months. Despite the poor survival of patients with major vascular invasion, no effective treatment(s) has been established for these patients [3]. Thus, systemic therapy is needed to improve the survival of patients with advanced HCC, including those with major vascular invasion and/or extrahepatic metastases.

Chemotherapy is applied for patients with advanced HCC patients who are TACE-refractory or show major vascular invasion and/or extrahepatic metastases. Various studies have investigated the usefulness of combined therapy with anthracycline antitumor antibiotic agents, cisplatin and/or fluorouracil, with the reported response rates ranging from 14% to 26% and median overall survival (OS) ranging from 8.9 to 11.6 months [7-9]. However, despite the better response in phase III trials to combination chemotherapy as compared to doxorubicin monotherapy, no standard chemotherapy was identified that could clearly prolong the survival [10]. On the other hand, in Japan, various hepatic arterial infusion chemotherapy regimens have been applied for patients with very advanced HCCs, such as those with extensive portal vein tumor thrombosis, and for some of these regimens, responses rates of more than 40% have been reported [11,12]. However, so far, no standard regimen has been identified based on large prospective clinical trials that can clearly prolong the survival in patients with advanced HCC.

Some growth factors and various signal transduction pathways have been identified in HCCs, and various targeted agents have been investigated for the treatment of patients with HCC. These therapies may target not only tumor cell proliferation, but also angiogenesis. Sorafenib is a small-molecule multikinase inhibitor that inhibits kinases such as Raf kinase, vascular endothelial growth factor receptor (VEGFR), and platelet-derived growth factor receptor (PDGFR)-β tyrosine kinases. It is the first agent that was demonstrated to yield survival benefit in patients with unresectable advanced HCC [13,14]. Subsequently, various targeted agents have been investigated for the treatment of HCC in various stages of progression. On the other hand, various characteristic toxicities of molecular targeted agents, such as hand-foot syndrome or hypertension, have been reported [13,14,15]. It is important to understand the efficacy and safety of molecular targeted therapy to gauge their true benefit.

2. Systemic therapy using targeted agents for advanced HCC

2.1 Summary of pivotal trilas of sorafenib

Sorafenib is a small-molecule multikinase inhibitor that inhibits kinases such as Raf kinase, vascular endothelial growth factor receptor (VEGFR), and platelet-derived growth factor receptor (PDGFR)-β tyrosine kinases [16]. In a phase I study of sorafenib conducted in 69 patients with solid malignant tumors, diarrhea was the most commonly encountered treatment-related adverse event, and the dose-limiting toxicities were diarrhea, fatigue, and skin toxicities, namely, hand-foot syndrome and rash [17]. The maximum tolerated dose was found to be 400 mg bid continuous and the recommended dose of sorafenib for future studies was also 400 mg bid as a continuous dosing schedule. In regard to the efficacy, even a partial response (PR) was observed in only one of the 45 patients treated continuously with sorafenib at doses of $\geq$ 100 mg bid, who was a patient of HCC treated with the drug at 400 mg bid. In this phase I study, six HCC patients were assessable for efficacy, of which one showed PR, 4 showed stable disease (SD), and one showed progressive disease (PD). Based on these preclinical results and the results of the phase I study of sorafenib, a phase II study was performed in 137 patients with advanced HCC [18]. Although the response rate was low (2.2%), the time-to progression (TTP) and overall survival (OS) were more promising (Table 1).

Based on these results, a large randomized controlled trial (RCT) of sorafenib versus placebo (the SHARP trial) was conducted in patients with advanced HCC and good liver function (Child-Pugh A)[13]. Six hundred two patients were randomized into two arms, namely, the sorafenib arm and the placebo arm (Table 1). The TTP was 5.5 months for sorafenib and 2.8

months for placebo, and the hazard ratio in the sorafenib arm was 0.58 (95% CI: 0.45-0.74; p<0.001). The median OS was 10.7 months in the sorafenib arm and 7.9 months in the placebo arm, and the hazard ratio for OS in the sorafenib arm was 0.69 (95% CI: 0.55-0.87; p<0.001). Thus, sorafenib was the first systemic chemotherapeutic agent demonstrated to prolong survival in patients with advanced HCC.

Agent	Study setting	n	Response rate	Median TTP	Median OS	p-value (HR, 95%CI)	Author (year)
Sorafenib	Phase II	137	2%	4.2 mo	9.2 mo	-	Abou-Alfa (2006) [18]
Sorafenib	Phase I	27	4%	4.9 mo	15.6 mo	-	Furuse (2008) [19]
Sorafenib	Phase III	299	2.3%	5.5 mo	10.7 mo	P < 0.001 (0.69, 0.55-0.87)	Llovet (2008) [13]
Placebo		303	0.7%	2.8 mo	7.9 mo		
Sorafenib	Phase III	150	3.3%	2.8 mo	6.5 mob	P = 0.0155 (0.67, 0.49-0.93)	Cheng (2009) [14]
Placebo		76	1.3%	1.4 mo	4.2 mo		

TTP, time-to progression; OS, overall survival; HR, hazard ratio; CI, confidence interval

Table 1. Clinical trials of sorafenib for hepatocellular carcinoma.

In the SHARP trial, approximately 90% of the patients enrolled were from Europe or Australia. The differences in the efficacy and safety was a concern in relation to the application of sorafenib as a global standard therapeutic agent for advanced HCC, as the etiology and treatment strategies for HCC vary among regions in the world. Therefore, to confirm the efficacy and safety of the drug in Asian populations, a RCT of sorafenib was conducted in the Asia-Pacific region (the Asia-Pacific trial)[14]. The dosing schedule of sorafenib was the same as that used in the SHARP trial, namely, continuous administration of 400 mg bid, and the patients were randomized 2:1 to sorafenib or placebo. The median OS, which was the primary endpoint, was 6.5 months for sorafenib and 4.2 months for placebo, and the hazard ratio for OS in the sorafenib arm was 0.67 (95% CI: 0.49-0.93; p=0.0155) [14].

Despite the equivalent hazard ratio for OS and TTP in the two RCTs, the median OS and TTP were very poor in the Asia-Pacific trial as compared with that in the SHARP trial. This was considered to be attributable to the differences in the patient characteristics, such as the poorer performance status (69% of ECOG PS) and more advanced stage of the cancer in the latter trial (96% with BCLC stage C, 52% with lung metastases).

Since patients enrolled in the SHARP trial and Asia-Pacific trial were limited to those with good liver function (Child-Pugh A), the usefulness of sorafenib needed to be examined in patients with Child-Pugh class B, or moderate liver dysfunction. In a phase II study of sorafenib, 38 out of the 137 patients enrolled were classified into Child-Pugh class B [18]. This study revealed some variability in the AUC and Cmax values, which were slightly greater in the Child-Pugh class B patients than in the Child-Pugh class A patients, however, the differences were not significant [18]. In Japan, a phase I study of sorafenib was conducted to investigate the pharmacokinetics, safety and efficacy of the drug in Japanese patients with advanced HCC; the study included an equal number of Child-Pugh class A and B patients [19]. In regard to the differences in the pharmacokinetics between the Child-Pugh class A and B patients, although both the area under the concentration-time curve for 0-12 h and the maximal concentration in the steady state were slightly lower in the Child-Pugh class B patients than in the Child-Pugh class A patients, there were no major differences in the incidence or grade of drug-related adverse events between the Child-Pugh class A and B groups; however, hypertension, hand-foot skin reactions, and rash were reported more frequently in the Child-Pugh class B group [18]. Especially, grade 3-4 adverse events of elevated bilirubin, ascites, and encephalopathy occurred at a greater frequency in Child-Pugh class B patients than in the Child-Pugh class A patients [20]. Thus, the efficacy or safety of sorafenib in HCC patients categorized as Child-Pugh class B are not clear yet.

The most commonly reported toxicities of sorafenib are transient elevation of lipase and/or amylase, rash/desquamation, hand-foot skin reaction, diarrhea, anorexia, weight loss, alopecia, and voice changes. The reported drug-related adverse events of grade 3 or greater severity are diarrhea, hand-foot skin reaction, hypertension and rash.

2.2 Indications of sorafenib in the treatment of HCC

The Barcelona Clinic Liver Cancer (BCLC) staging classification has been employed as a guide for treatment selection in HCC patients [21]. Based on the results of RCTs of sorafenib, BCLS Stage C (advanced stage), which includes portal invasion, lymph node metastasis, and/or distant metastasis, has been reported as a suitable criterion for the selection of sorafenib. The Japanese consensus-based treatment algorithm also recommends treatment for HCC according to the tumor stage and degree of impairment of liver function [2]. In this algorithm, sorafenib is recommended as the first-line therapy for advanced HCC patients classified as Child-Pugh class A, who show extrahepatic spread or major vascular invasion and/or are TACE-refractory.

2.3 Recent trials using new targeted agents

Phase I, phase II studies have been conducted to investigate the usefulness of various new targeted agents for the treatment of advanced HCC (Table 2). Some large phase III studies of new targeted agents alone or such agents in combination with sorafenib vs. sorafenib alone have also been conducted. Some multikinase inhibitors, such as sunitinib, brivanib and linifanib, that have shown promising antitumor activity against HCC in phase II studies [22-25] have been investigated in head-to-head study comparisons with sorafenib (Table 3). Some phase III studies comparing sorafenib in combination with another molecular targeted agent or cytotoxic agent vs. sorafenib alone are also under way.

Agent	Study setting	n	Response rate	Median TTP/PFS	Median OS	Author (Year)
Sunitinib	Phase II	37	2.7%	5.3 mo	8.0 mo	Faivre (2009) [22]
	Phase II	45	2.9%	3.9 mo	9.3 mo	Zhu (2009) [23]
Brivanib	Phase II	55	7.3%	2.7 mo	10.0 mo	Park (2011) [24]
Linifanib	Phase II	44	6.8%	3.7 mo	9.3 mo	Toh (2009) [25]
Everolimus	Phase I/II	28	4%	3.8 mo	8.4 mo	Zhu (2010) [26]
TSU-68	Phase I/II	35	2.9%	2.1 mo	13.1 mo	Kanai (2010) [27]
Sunitinib	Phase III	529	6%	4.1 mo	8.1 mo*	Cheng (2011) [28]
Sorafenib		554	6%	4.0 mo	10.0 mo	

TTP, time-to progression; PFS, progression-free survival; OS, overall survival
*hazard ratio 1.31 (95% confidence interval: 1.13-1.52), P = 0.0019

Table 2. Clinical trials of new molecular targeted agents for hepatocellular carcinoma.

Study setting	Agent
1. First-line chemotherapy	sunitinib, brivanib, linifanib
2. Second-line chemotherapy	brivanib, everolimus, ramcirumab, axitinib*
3. Combination with TACE	sorafenib, brivanib, TSU-68
4. Adjuvant therapy after resection or ablation	sorafenib

TACE, transarterial chemoembolization
* randomized phase II study

Table 3. Molecular targeted agents developing in randomized clinical trials

The estimated time-to progression in patinets treated with sorafenib ranges from 2.8 to 5.5 months and some patients may accrue benefits of second-line chemotherapy after being labeled as sorafenib-refractory. Some large phase III studies of new targeted agents, such as brivanib, everolimus and ramcirumab, as second-line treatment have also been conducted (Table 3).

Among these phase III studies, the results of a phase III study comparing sunitinib with sorafenib was reported in 2011. The trial did not show any survival advantage of sunitinib in pateints with advanced HCC; in fact, the survival in the sunitinib group was inferior to that in the sorafenib group (Table 3) [28].

3. Combined molecular targeted therapy with local therapy

3.1 Combination with TACE

Transcatheter arterial chemoembolization is widely applied for the treatment of HCC as one of the standard treatments along with resection and local ablation. One-third of all patients with primary HCC are treated by TAE/TACE as the first-line treatment [2]. However, the Nationwide Follow-up Survey by the Liver Cancer Study Group of Japan (LCSGJ) revealed that the 5-year survival rates for resection, ablation and TACE were 59.2%, 48.4% and 29.7%, respectively, for single tumors, and 46.4%, 37.3% and 23.0%, respectively, for two tumors; thus, the efficacy in terms of survival prolongation of TACE was limited as compared with that of resection and ablation [2]. It is difficult to obtain complete necrosis of tumors by TACE, and the reported objective response rate to TACE ranges from 15%-55% [29]. Thus, to improve the efficacy of TACE, combined use of TACE with molecular targeted therapy has been investigated.

Regarding the increment of the serum VEGF level associated with TACE, it was reported that the serum VEGF increased within 1 to 2 days after TACE and recovered by one month later; also, an association between the serum VEGF level and the prognosis after TACE in HCC patients has been reported. Therefore, it may be reasonable to suppress the effects of VEGF by VEGFR inhibitors to improve the survival benefit yielded by TACE in patients with HCC [30].

The first trial of combined TACE with molecular targeted agents was a placebo-controlled phase III study of sorafenib (post TACE study) conducted in Japan and Korea [31]. The primary endpoint was the TTP, and to prove the assumption that the median TTP would be 50% higher in the sorafenib than in the placebo group. The median TTP in the sorafenib and placebo groups was 5.4 and 3.7 months, respectively (hazard ratio (HR), 0.87; 95% confidence interval, 0.70-1.09; P = 0.252). Although the TTP in the sorafenib group was better than that in the placebo group, the drug yielded no statistically significant prolongation of the TTP after TACE. This study was designed before the results of the SHARP and Asia-Pacific trials of sorafenib were reported, and only patients who responded to TACE were included as the subjects of this study. As a result, it took a median of 9.3 weeks from TACE to randomization, because the efficacy of TACE could only be evaluated by CT one month after the procedure, and a central review of CT findings was required.

Currently, many comparative studies between TACE plus a targeted agent and TACE alone are under way (Table 3). In these studies, administration of targeted agents is initiated before TACE or as soon as possible after TACE.

3.2 Adjuvant therapy with targeted agents after curative treatments

One of characteristics of HCC is the very high recurrence rate after regional therapies. Even for early-stage HCCs (smaller than 3 cm and 3 or less in number), the reported cumulative 1- and 5-year recurrence rates after resection are 24.5% and 74.3%, respectively [32]. There are two mechanisms of recurrence after curative treatments, that is, metastasis from the primary

HCC lesion and new multicentric development. Patients with HCC have microscopic lesions, and intrahepatic metastases often develop rather early after curative treatments. On the other hand, patients with HCC are also at a greater risk of multicentric hepatocarcinogenesis and de novo development of HCC tumors [33].

Thus, various adjuvant therapies have been investigated to suppress the risk of recurrence after curative treatments, including resection and ablation therapy. An acyclic retinoid, polyprenoic acid, was reported to prevent the development of second primary hepatomas after surgical resection or percutaneous injection of ethanol in a small randomized comparison trial [34]. Peretinoin, an acyclic retinoid, administered at the dose of 600 mg statistically significantly decreased the 2-year recurrence rate as compared with placebo in a large RCT, however, no improvement of the primary endpoint, that is, of the recurrence-free survival, was observed, therefore, the efficacy is still unclear [35]. It was reported that adoptive immunotherapy may also improve the recurrence-free outcomes after surgery for HCC [36], but it has not yet been applied for adjuvant therapy in the clinical setting because of the complicated method of its use. While interferon or vitamin K have been suggested as having potential activity for suppressing recurrence, so far, no standard adjuvant therapy regimen including these agents has been established [37-39].

In a prospective study consisting 57 patients with HCC who underwent resection, high expression levels of PDGFR-α and PDGFR-β were independently associated with decreased survival [40]. Molecular targeted agents are expected to suppress the recurrence rate of HCC after curative treatments. Sorafenib is also currently under investigation as an adjuvant therapy after curative treatment(s).

4. References

[1] Bruix J, Llovet JM. Prognostic prediction and treatment strategy in Hepatocellular carcinoma. Hepatology 2002;35:519-524

[2] Arii S, Sata M, Sakamoto M, et al. Management of hepatocellular carcinoma: Report of Consensus Meeting in the 45th Annual Meeting of the Japan Society of Hepatology (2009). Hepatol Res 2010;40:667-685

[3] Ikai I, Arii S, Okazaki M, et al. Report of the 17th Nationwide Follow-up Survey of Primary Liver Cancer in Japan. Hepatol Res 2007;37:676-691.

[4] Llovet JM, Real MI, Montaña X, et al. Arterial embolisation or chemoembolisation versus symptomatic treatment in patients with unresectable hepatocellular carcinoma: a randomised controlled trial. Lancet 2002;359:1734-1739

[5] Llovet JM, Bruix J. Systematic review of randomized trials for unresectable hepatocellular carcinoma: Chemoembolization improves survival. Hepatology 2003;37:429-442

[6] Ishii H, Furuse J, Kinoshita T, et al. Extrahepatic spread from hepatocellular carcinoma: who are candidates for aggressive anti-cancer treatment? Jpn J Clin Oncol 2004;34:733-739

[7] Leung TW, Patt YZ, Lau WY, et al. Complete pathological remission is possible with systemic combination chemotherapy for inoperable hepatocellular carcinoma. Clin Cancer Res 1999;5:1676-1681

[8] Boucher E, Corbinais S, Brissot P, et al. Treatment of hepatocellular carcinoma (HCC) with systemic chemotherapy combining epirubicin, cisplatinum and infusional 5-fluorouracil (ECF regimen). Cancer Chemother Pharmacol 2002;50:305-308.

[9] Ikeda M, Okusaka T, Ueno H, et al. A phase II trial of continuous infusion of 5-fluorouracil, mitoxantrone, and cisplatin for metastatic hepatocellular carcinoma. Cancer 2005;103:756-762

[10] Yeo W, Mok TS, Zee B, et al. A randomized phase III study of doxorubicin versus cisplatin/interferon alpha-2b/doxorubicin/fluorouracil (PIAF) combination chemotherapy for unresectable hepatocellular carcinoma. J Natl Cancer Inst 2005;97:1532-1538

[11] Ando E, Tanaka M, Yamashita F, et al. Hepatic arterial infusion chemotherapy for advanced hepatocellular carcinoma with portal vein tumor thrombosis: analysis of 48 cases. Cancer 2002;95:588-595

[12] Ota H, Nagano H, Sakon M, et al. Treatment of hepatocellular carcinoma with major portal vein thrombosis by combined therapy with subcutaneous interferon-alpha and intra-arterial 5-fluorouracil; role of type 1 interferon receptor expression. Br J Cancer 2005;93:557-564

[13] Llovet JM, Ricci S, Mazzaferro V, et al. Sorafenib in advanced hepatocellular carcinoma. N Engl J Med 2008;359:378-390

[14] Cheng AL, Kang YK, Chen Z, et al. Efficacy and safety of sorafenib in patients in the Asia-Pacific region with advanced hepatocellular carcinoma: a phase III randomised, double-blind, placebo-controlled trial. Lancet Oncol 2009;10:25-34

[15] Iijima M, Fukino K, Adachi M, et al. Sorafenib-associated hand-foot syndrome in Japanese patients. J Dermatol 2011;38:261-266

[16] Wilhelm SM, Carter C, Tang L, et al. BAY 43-9006 exhibits broad spectrum oral antitumor activity and targets the RAF/MEK/ERK pathway and receptor tyrosine kinases involved in tumor progression and angiogenesis. Cancer Res 2004;64:7099-7109.

[17] Strumberg D, Richly H, Hilger RA, et al. Phase I clinical and pharmacokinetic study of the Novel Raf kinase and vascular endothelial growth factor receptor inhibitor BAY 43-9006 in patients with advanced refractory solid tumors. J Clin Oncol 2005;23:965-972

[18] Abou-Alfa GK, Schwartz L, Ricci S, et al. Phase II study of sorafenib in patients with advanced hepatocellular carcinoma. J Clin Oncol 2006;24:4293-300

[19] Furuse J, Ishii H, Nakachi K, et al. Phase I study of sorafenib in Japanese patients with hepatocellular carcinoma. Cancer Sci 2008;99:159-165.

[20] Abou-Alfa GK, Amadori D, Santoro A, et al. Safety and Efficacy of Sorafenib in Patients with Hepatocellular Carcinoma (HCC) and Child-Pugh A versus B Cirrhosis. Gastrointest Cancer Res 2011;4:40-44

[21] Bruix J, Sherman M. Management of hepatocellular carcinoma: an update. Hepatology 2011;53:1020-1022

[22] Faivre S, Raymond E, Boucher E, et al. Safety and efficacy of sunitinib in patients with advanced hepatocellular carcinoma: an open-label, multicentre, phase II study. Lancet Oncol 2009;10:794-800

[23] Zhu AX, Sahani DV, Duda DG, et al. Efficacy, safety, and potential biomarkers of sunitinib monotherapy in advanced hepatocellular carcinoma: a phase II study. J Clin Oncol 2009;27:3027-3035

[24] Park JW, Finn RS, Kim JS, et al. Phase II, open-label study of brivanib as first-line therapy in patients with advanced hepatocellular carcinoma. Clin Cancer Res 2011;17:1973-1983

[25] Toh HC, Chen P, Knox JJ, et al: International phase 2 trial of ABT-869 in patients with advanced hepatocellular carcinoma (HCC). Eur J Cancer Supple 7; 366 (abstr PD-6517)

[26] Zhu AX, Abrams TA, Miksad R, et al. Phase 1/2 study of everolimus in advanced hepatocellular carcinoma. Cancer 2011 Apr 27. [Epub ahead of print]

[27] Kanai F, Yoshida H, Tateishi R, et al. A phase I/II trial of the oral antiangiogenic agent TSU-68 in patients with advanced hepatocellular carcinoma. Cancer Chemother Pharmacol 2010 Apr 14. [Epub ahead of print]

[28] Cheng A, Kang Y, Lin D, et al. Phase III trial of sunitinib (Su) versus sorafenib (So) in advanced hepatocellular carcinoma (HCC). J Clin Oncol 29: 2011 (suppl; abstr 4000)

[29] Bruix J, Sala M, Llovet JM. Chemoembolization for hepatocellular carcinoma. Gastroenterology. 2004 Nov;127(5 Suppl 1):S179-188

[30] Shim JH, Park JW, Kim JH, et al. Association between increment of serum VEGF level and prognosis after transcatheter arterial chemoembolization in hepatocellular carcinoma patients. Cancer Sci 2008;99:2037-2044

[31] Kudo M, Imanaka K, Chida N, et al. Phase III study of sorafenib after transarterial chemoembolisation in Japanese and Korean patients with unresectable hepatocellular carcinoma. Eur J Cancer. 2011 Jun 9. [Epub ahead of print]

[32] Yamamoto J, Okada S, Shimada K, et al. Treatment strategy for small hepatocellular carcinoma: comparison of long-term results after percutaneous ethanol injection therapy and surgical resection. Hepatology 2001;34:707-713

[33] Takayama T, Makuuchi M, Hirohashi S, et al. Early hepatocellular carcinoma as an entity with a high rate of surgical cure. Hepatology 1998;28:1241-1246

[34] Muto Y, Moriwaki H, Ninomiya M, et al. Prevention of second primary tumors by an acyclic retinoid, polyprenoic acid, in patients with hepatocellular carcinoma. Hepatoma Prevention Study Group. N Engl J Med 1996;334:1561-1567

[35] Okita K, Matsui O, Kumada H, et al. Effect of peretinoin on recurrence of hepatocellular carcinoma (HCC): Results of a phase II/III randomized placebo-controlled trial. Oncol 28:15s, 2010 (suppl; abstr 4024)

[36] Takayama T, Sekine T, Makuuchi M, et al. Adoptive immunotherapy to lower postsurgical recurrence rates of hepatocellular carcinoma: a randomised trial. Lancet 2000;356:802-807

[37] Kubo S, Nishiguchi S, Hirohashi K, et al. Effects of long-term postoperative interferon-alpha therapy on intrahepatic recurrence after resection of hepatitis C virus-related hepatocellular carcinoma. A randomized, controlled trial. Ann Intern Med 2001;134:963-967

[38] Mazzaferro V, Romito R, Schiavo M, et al. Prevention of hepatocellular carcinoma recurrence with alpha-interferon after liver resection in HCV cirrhosis. Hepatology 2006;44:1543-1554

[39] Mizuta T, Ozaki I, Eguchi Y, et al. The effect of menatetrenone, a vitamin K2 analog, on disease recurrence and survival in patients with hepatocellular carcinoma after curative treatment: a pilot study. Cancer 2006;106:867-872

[40] Patel SH, Kneuertz PJ, Delgado M, et al. Clinically Relevant Biomarkers to Select Patients for Targeted Inhibitor Therapy after Resection of Hepatocellular Carcinoma. Ann Surg Oncol 2011 May 18. [Epub ahead of print]

Permissions

The contributors of this book come from diverse backgrounds, making this book a truly international effort. This book will bring forth new frontiers with its revolutionizing research information and detailed analysis of the nascent developments around the world.

We would like to thank Dr. Wan-Yee Lau, for lending his expertise to make the book truly unique. He has played a crucial role in the development of this book. Without his invaluable contribution this book wouldn't have been possible. He has made vital efforts to compile up to date information on the varied aspects of this subject to make this book a valuable addition to the collection of many professionals and students.

This book was conceptualized with the vision of imparting up-to-date information and advanced data in this field. To ensure the same, a matchless editorial board was set up. Every individual on the board went through rigorous rounds of assessment to prove their worth. After which they invested a large part of their time researching and compiling the most relevant data for our readers. Conferences and sessions were held from time to time between the editorial board and the contributing authors to present the data in the most comprehensible form. The editorial team has worked tirelessly to provide valuable and valid information to help people across the globe.

Every chapter published in this book has been scrutinized by our experts. Their significance has been extensively debated. The topics covered herein carry significant findings which will fuel the growth of the discipline. They may even be implemented as practical applications or may be referred to as a beginning point for another development. Chapters in this book were first published by InTech; hereby published with permission under the Creative Commons Attribution License or equivalent.

The editorial board has been involved in producing this book since its inception. They have spent rigorous hours researching and exploring the diverse topics which have resulted in the successful publishing of this book. They have passed on their knowledge of decades through this book. To expedite this challenging task, the publisher supported the team at every step. A small team of assistant editors was also appointed to further simplify the editing procedure and attain best results for the readers.

Our editorial team has been hand-picked from every corner of the world. Their multi-ethnicity adds dynamic inputs to the discussions which result in innovative outcomes. These outcomes are then further discussed with the researchers and contributors who give their valuable feedback and opinion regarding the same. The feedback is then collaborated with the researches and they are edited in a comprehensive manner to aid the understanding of the subject.

Apart from the editorial board, the designing team has also invested a significant amount of their time in understanding the subject and creating the most relevant covers. They scrutinized every image to scout for the most suitable representation of the subject and create an appropriate cover for the book.

The publishing team has been involved in this book since its early stages. They were actively engaged in every process, be it collecting the data, connecting with the contributors or procuring relevant information. The team has been an ardent support to the editorial, designing and production team. Their endless efforts to recruit the best for this project, has resulted in the accomplishment of this book. They are a veteran in the field of academics and their pool of knowledge is as vast as their experience in printing. Their expertise and guidance has proved useful at every step. Their uncompromising quality standards have made this book an exceptional effort. Their encouragement from time to time has been an inspiration for everyone.

The publisher and the editorial board hope that this book will prove to be a valuable piece of knowledge for researchers, students, practitioners and scholars across the globe.

List of Contributors

Davide Degli Esposti and Antoinette Lemoine
AP-HP, Hôpital Paul Brousse, Service de Biochimie et Biologie, Moléculaire, Inserm; Université Paris-Sud 11; PRES Universud-Paris; Paul Vaillant Couturier, France
Laboratoire de Biochimie et Biologie Cellulaire, Faculté de Pharmacie, Université Paris-Sud 11, Jean Baptiste Clément, France

Morando Soffritti, Eva Tibaldi and Marco Manservigi
Cesare Maltoni Cancer Research Center, Ramazzini Institute, Castello di Bentivoglio, Via Saliceto, Bentivoglio, Bologna, Italy

Misael Uribe, Jesús Román-Sandoval, Norberto C. Chávez-Tapia and Nahum Méndez-Sánchez
Medica Sur Clinic and Foundation, Biomedical Research, Department and Liver Research Unit, Mexico City, Mexico

Daniela Fanni, Clara Gerosa and Gavino Faa
University of Cagliari, Italy

Péter Tátrai, Ilona Kovalszky and András Kiss
Semmelweis University, Hungary

Kristina Zviniene
Lithuanian University of Health Sciences, Lithuania

Keiko Sakamoto, Yoshinobu Shinagawa, Ritsuko Fujimitsu, Mikiko Ida, Hideyuki Hiashihara, Kouichi Takano and Kengo Yoshimitsu
Department of Radiology, Faculty of Medicine, Fukuoka University, Nanakuma, Johnan-ku, Fukuoka, Japan

Helena Y. Lin, Surbhi Jain and Ying-Hsiu Su
Department of Microbiology and Immunology, Drexel University College of Medicine, Doylestown, PA, USA

Wei Song
BS Science Inc, Doylestown, PA, USA

Chi-Tan Hu
Department of Gastroenterology and Hepatology, Buddhist Tzu Chi General Hospital and Tzu Chi University, Hualien, Taiwan

Atsushi Miyoshi, Kenji Kitahara, Kohji Miyazaki and Hirokazu Noshiro
Department of Surgery, Saga University Faculty of Medicine, Japan

Keita Kai and Osamu Tokunaga
Department of Pathology & Microbiology, Japan

Jing An Rui
Peking Union Medical College Hospital, Chinese Academy of Medical Sciences, China

Zenichi Morise
Department of Surgery, Fujita Health University School of Medicine, Banbuntane Houto-kukai Hospital, Otobashi Nakagawa-ku, Nagoya Aichi, Japan

Mehmet Sitki Copur
Medical Director, Saint Francis Cancer Center, Grand Island, Nebraska, USA
University of Nebraska Medical Center, Omaha, Nebraska, USA

Angela Mae Obermiller
Pharmacy Supervisor, Saint Francis Medical Center, Grand Island, Nebraska, USA
University of Nebraska Medical Center, Omaha, Nebraska, USA

Federico Cattin, Alessandro Uzzau and Dino De Anna
Department of General Surgery, University of Udine School of Medicine, Italy

Kazuhiro Kasai and Kazuyuki Suzuki
Division of Gastroenterology and Hepatology, Department of Internal Medicine, Iwate Medical University, Japan

Maurizio Grosso, Fulvio Pedrazzini, Alberto Balderi, Alberto Antonietti, Enrico Peano, Luigi Ferro and Davide Sortino
A. O. S. Croce e Carle, Cuneo, Italy

Kiyoshi Mochizuki
Department of Gastroenterology and Hepatology, Kansai Rousai Hospital, Hyogo, Japan

Hojjat Ahmadzadehfar, Amir Sabet and Hans Jürgen Biersack
Department of Nuclear Medicine, University Hospital Bonn, Germany

Jörn Risse
Radiology and Nuclear Medicine Institute, Bad Honnef, Germany

Dimitrios Dimitroulopoulos and Aikaterini Fotopoulou
Gastroenterology Dpt., "Agios Savvas" Cancer Hospital, Greece
Radiation-Oncology Dpt.,"Hygia" Hospital, Athens, Greece

Joanne Chiu, Roberta Pang, Ronnie Poon and Thomas Yau
University of Hong Kong, Hong Kong

Junji Furuse
Department of Internal Medicine, Medical Oncology, Kyorin University School of Medicine, Japan

www.ingramcontent.com/pod-product-compliance
Lightning Source LLC
Chambersburg PA
CBHW070726190326
41458CB00004B/1050